Service Quality Improvement

The Customer Satisfaction Strategy for Health Care

Wendy Leebov, Ed.D., and Gail Scott, M.A.

AHA books are published by
American Hospital Publishing, Inc.,
an American Hospital Association company

The views expressed in this publication are strictly those of the authors and do not necessarily represent official positions of the American Hospital Association.

Library of Congress Cataloging-in-Publication Data

Leebov, Wendy
    Service quality improvement : the customer satisfaction strategy
for health care / Wendy Leebov and Gail Scott.
      p.   cm.
    Includes bibliographical references.
    ISBN 1-55648-110-1 (pbk.)
    1. Health services administration.   2. Patient satisfaction.
I. Scott, Gail, 1946–   . II. Title.
    RA971.L373 1993
    362.T068′5 – dc20
    DNLM/DLC
    for Library of Congress   93-32889
                                              CIP

Catalog no. 136107

©1994 by American Hospital Publishing, Inc.,
an American Hospital Association company

Printed in the USA

AHA is a service mark of the American Hospital Association used under license by American Hospital Publishing, Inc.

Text set in Palatino
5M – 12/93 – 0359

Audrey Kaufman, Acquisitions and Development Editor
Nancy Charpentier, Production Editor
Peggy DuMais, Production Coordinator
Cheryl Kusek, Cover Designer
Marcia Bottoms, Books Division Assistant Director
Brian Schenk, Books Division Director

Contents

List of Figures

About the Authors

Wendy Leebov, Ed.D., is associate vice-president of human resources in charge of organization and staff development for the Albert Einstein Healthcare Network in Philadelphia. The founder of The Einstein Consulting Group, Dr. Leebov is a nationally recognized expert on service and quality improvement in health care. She has appeared in three teleconferences on customer-oriented management and quality improvement sponsored by the American Hospital Association and has coauthored a number of books: with C. J. Ersoz, *The Health Care Manager's Guide to Continuous Quality Improvement* (American Hospital Publishing, 1991); with Gail Scott, *Health Care Managers in Transition: Shifting Roles and Changing Organizations* (Jossey-Bass, 1990); and with Michael Vergare and Gail Scott, *Patient Satisfaction: A Guide to Practice Enhancement* (Medical Economics Books, 1989). In addition, her booklet series on customer relations (American Hospital Publishing, 1990–1991) has achieved great popularity as workbooks for staff training and development on such topics as customer relations, complaint management, telephone tactics, practical assertiveness, and coworker relationships. Dr. Leebov is also editor of *The Service/Quality Connection*, a national subscription newsletter published by the National Society for Patient Representation and Consumer Affairs. She has a doctorate in human development from Harvard University.

Gail Scott, M.A., is currently president of The Einstein Consulting Group, a subsidiary of the Albert Einstein Healthcare Foundation in Philadelphia. She has more than 20 years' experience in training and organizational change and currently provides a variety of consulting and training services to health care organizations and businesses nationwide. An organization development expert, Ms. Scott has helped more than 300 hospitals, ambulatory care centers, and nursing homes nationwide to institute service and quality improvement strategies and management development systems that extend beyond the classroom to improve on-the-job performance. With Wendy Leebov, she has authored two books (*Health Care Managers in Transition*, 1990, and *Patient Satisfaction: A Guide to Practice Enhancement*, 1989). Ms. Scott earned her M.A. degree in communications from Beaver College (Glenside, Pennsylvania).

Acknowledgments

We want to thank all the wonderful people who've educated us about the world of service quality improvement and supported us during the writing of this book. Many inspirational, incisive, and demanding hospital clients and service improvement leaders who made this book possible by teaching us the realities and the possibilities.

Martin Goldsmith, Janine Kilty, and Robert Stutz, who provided institutional support and encouragement during our process of learning, experimentation, and application.

Lori Anderson, Kelly Yeager, Sheila Wallace, Marcia Melincoff, and the talented consultants who comprise The Einstein Consulting Group, whose help and experiences in the field have added insights to our understanding of how to improve service quality.

Mary Ellen Kelly, who typed, boosted, researched, and kept us laughing so we could churn out the words.

Audrey Kaufman from American Hospital Publishing, Inc., who once again provided superb editorial direction and encouraged us throughout the process.

Florence and Mike Leebov, Liz Dunn, Nikki Gollub, Pepper, and Tom Quinlan for their blind confidence and unwavering support.

Thanks to you all.

Preface

In its few years of existence in hospitals, service improvement in health care has evolved into more of a science than an art. Starting as a focus on customer relations, or guest relations, it evolved into an expanded approach to service quality—the key to health care customer satisfaction. Today, the burgeoning activity in the service and quality improvement field attests to the importance and strength of the service premise in health care. Over the past few years, *most* hospitals, ambulatory care centers, and other health care organizations have included service excellence in their missions. Many have instituted formally designed, explicit service strategies to advance that goal.

☐ A Smorgasbord of Approaches

Many hospitals have looked to the hospitality industries for their approach to service excellence. This is because they see that hospitals and hotels share many characteristics: overnight guests, food and housekeeping services, amenities that add to comfort and well-being, and a complex, interlocking system of procedures that have to run smoothly and work for the customer's convenience and satisfaction.

In promoting excellence, some hospitals have focused on skill building by reinforcing key interpersonal skills (such as techniques for meeting and greeting, anticipating needs, and listening to and coping with complaints). Other facilities have focused on motivation, not training, on the premise that people have the skills but have to be motivated to use them. This premise leads to approaches aimed at inspiring employee commitment by informing employees about the organization's challenges and encouraging them to do all they can to ensure their hospital's future.

A number of hospitals have focused primarily on top management to spearhead the service strategy and integrate it into the organization's culture and everyday management practices. Others say that service excellence is for frontline people. Still others insist it must include every person in the organization, whether or not the person interacts directly with patients.

In certain facilities, entire departments are devoted to service improvement. In others, advancing service quality is only a small part of a particular worker's overall responsibilities.

Some health care organizations use all of the tools of quality improvement to improve service processes so that they reach ever-higher levels of customer satisfaction. In short, there are almost as many approaches to service improvement as there are organizations engaged in it. That situation is both a blessing and a curse.

In the past 10 years, we have coached more than 300 hospitals nationwide in their organizational change efforts and, as a result, have learned a great deal about the vision, planning, ongoing assessment, and change in the internal culture that is needed to drive enduring improvement. We have learned a great deal from clients about specific practical tactics that health care leaders can use to expedite service improvement. We've also learned from false starts and failed efforts.

One thing is perfectly clear: Raising awareness without follow-through is worthless and doomed for failure. Successful efforts create a culture of continuous improvement with an infrastructure of vision, expectations, and systems to support it. Strategies fizzled in hospitals that limited their efforts to workshops that were excellently run and positively perceived. They left in their wake the questions, "Is this all there is? Now what?"

☐ A Successful Approach

A successful service improvement strategy starts with raising awareness about what constitutes service excellence and why it matters to the customer, the organization, the employee, and the physician. Beyond that, the successful strategy also follows these guidelines:

- Set clear expectations and standards. People need to know what constitutes service excellence in systems, routines, and individual performance. Specifically, they need to know what is expected of them in their everyday interactions.
- Establish efficient and effective service processes. Service processes need to meet customer expectations in ways that don't make staff uneasy. Endless training of staff on interpersonal skills is a Band-Aid approach when staff are victimized by systems and work processes that make no sense and that create barriers to customer satisfaction. Health care staff can't be expected to apologize over and over to customers for faulty systems. Service strategies must include tactics that address these process problems and make them ever better.
- Build skills. Training at all levels is a crucial part of service excellence strategies. However, it must be practical and job-specific, and training emphasis must be on implementation, not on learning. Staff at all levels can develop their skills and upgrade the service they provide if the organization invests in their development and supports it until new skills become habits.
- Institute mechanisms for continuous problem solving and process improvement. Service quality slips unless it is continuously improved, and improvement doesn't just happen. Organizations with distinctive service provision work at it ruthlessly.
- Engage middle managers centrally. Many strategies of the past worked *around* middle managers, but the successful strategies worked *through* them. This book focuses attention on training, mind-set shifts, and support systems to help managers be drivers of service improvement, not barriers to it.
- Measure and use data to drive improvement. People need to know how they're doing. Feedback systems need to be installed and used to celebrate achievements, track trends, and pinpoint opportunities for improvement. Some organizations don't regularly consult customers for feedback, or if they do, they bury it or refute the data. Service strategies can't work in systems that resist change and support maintaining the status quo.
- Build internal, not just external, customer relationships. Many strategies in the past focused on extending excellent service to patients and physicians to the exclusion

of internal customers. Because of the degree of specialization of functions in health care organizations, bridges must be built between departments so that service is "seamless." "Turfdoms" must be eliminated; communication must be strengthened; and collaborative process improvement and problem solving must be taught, expected, and supported in order to achieve excellent service.

- Reinforce, reinforce, reinforce. Given the weight of their work loads and the many issues that compete for attention, people need to be acknowledged and appreciated for their efforts in the direction of service excellence. This way, the employees who make service legendary not only feel intrinsic satisfaction but also receive positive attention for their contributions.

☐ Follow-Up and Follow-Through

Some organizations stopped their efforts toward quality improvement as soon as they experienced the sweet smell of success. Many organizations with well-crafted service strategies that focused on behavioral improvement achieved measurable and noticeable results but stopped short once they did. Administrators besieged with other priorities seemed to conclude that the "service problem" was now taken care of, so they could move on to the next priority. This short-term and finite orientation was doomed to failure because customer expectations are a moving target, and service improvement strategies must strive for continuous improvement in order to keep up. Thus, our emphasis in this book is on "continuous service improvement" as the *process* by which people approach service excellence. This process is driven by several factors:

- Service improvement needs to be the responsibility of everyone at all levels. In many organizations we observed, service strategies were something the top told the middle to do for the bottom! Effective service strategies demand that everyone participate and that everyone be both teacher and learner in the quest for service improvement.
- The corporate culture needs to support service quality improvement. Everyday practices and policies need to align with the facility's service mission. In the past six years, we've seen the difference between a "learning organization" and one that is ambitious but stagnant. Only a "learning" organization makes service improvement a continual reality.
- Mechanistic approaches don't work. Successful strategies are grounded in a powerful and far-reaching service vision, an openness at all levels to ongoing learning, belief in the potential and responsibility of staff at all levels to make service excellence a reality, and a commitment to teamwork for the sake of patients. These "soft" factors that focus on people and their motivations and capabilities need to be addressed in organizational change strategies, or meticulous work on the "hard" factors breaks down. Strategies need to include the kind of careful planning, vision development, and team building up front that help everyone feel, "We're all in this together and we're all going in the same direction."

Given all of these factors, it's no wonder that *effective* service quality improvement strategies are uncommon. Building on knowledge gained about these and other factors, this book is designed to help health care leaders strengthen their strategies by learning from other people's often costly experiences. Tailored to the needs of service improvement strategy coaches, executives, middle managers, consultants, and team and task force members, this book presents the nuts and bolts of a systems approach to service quality improvement. The processes described should help you align your organization's cultural practices and every program, department, and individual's behavior with your service mission.

Part one, "Introduction to Service Quality Improvement," introduces compelling reasons for focusing organizational attention and resources on continuous service improvement and articulates the mental models that are the foundation of a comprehensive service excellence strategy.

Part two, "The 10 Pillars of Continuous Improvement," provides a comprehensive array of concrete tactics that have been used by health care organizations to strengthen these pillars in pursuit of service excellence. Included are examples of practices related to developing and communicating management vision and commitment, accountability, measurement and feedback, problem solving and process improvement, communication, staff development and training, physician involvement, reward and recognition, employee involvement and empowerment, and reminders and refreshers.

Part three, "Operational Strategies," addresses a variety of topics that are key to executing a strategy tailored to your organization's needs. Included are how to plan your strategy, how to build an effective infrastructure, how middle managers can align their departments and programs with your service mission (using a service quality culture check provided as a chapter appendix), how to strengthen internal customer relationships, how to handle employee resistance, and innovative breakthroughs in service improvement. The final chapter addresses the follow-through challenge by describing strategies to fit various scenarios and safeguards you can install to make sure your strategy has eternal life.

This book, the new edition of *Service Excellence: The Customer Relations Strategy for Health Care*, has been designed to provide readers with state-of-the-art service improvement tactics. We describe what we believe to be the best practices in service quality improvement, with enough detail to allow you to use them to augment or refine your current practices. There's still so much that health care organizations can and need to learn about service excellence and the process of service quality improvement that it makes little sense to devote time to reinventing wheels that are already rolling.

Part One

Introduction to Service Quality Improvement

Chapter 1

The Quest for Customer Satisfaction

Forward-moving corporations and health care organizations are shifting their attention away from outdoing their competitors toward satisfying their customers. This trend is talked about by today's business thinkers:

> The winners are companies that have learned that the best way to become externally focused and internally aligned is to focus their organization on the customer. . . . The externally focused, internally aligned organization will dominate the future. Put even stronger, this is the only kind of organization that may survive the future.[1]

> The purpose of a business is to create and keep customers; all else is derivative.[2]

> Getting the organization to be externally focused and internally aligned is critical for advancing any business strategy. It's only once you have laid that foundation that the organization will be able to respond to change as rapidly as it needs to.[3]

> Everyone has to be linked to our customer in one way or another. . . . A customer-driven point of view ensures the survival of the corporation. Those who do will prosper and grow. Those who don't will die.[4]

Successful corporations recognize the importance of a customer focus and the direct relationship between a customer focus and business success. The 3M Company cites five business essentials, the first three of which (listed below) reinforce the importance of customer satisfaction and respect for customer perceptions of quality:[5]

- Quality is consistent conformance to customer expectations.
- Measurements of quality are indicators of customer satisfaction, rather than indicators of self-gratification.
- The objective is consistent conformance to customer expectations 100 percent of the time.

The relationship between quality and profitability has been firmly demonstrated by the Strategic Planning Institute in its ground-breaking Profit Impact of Marketing Strategies

(PIMS) data base. According to the PIMS study, "relative perceived quality" is the factor most highly related to market share and profitability. Relative perceived quality is quality *from the customer's perspective.*[6]

☐ The Customers' Definition of Quality

If customers select health care institutions based on quality, the most influential factor in their choice is *service.* That's what they know best. Health care consumers know how to evaluate the service they receive even though they may not always know how to evaluate the quality of health care provided.

Just look at the range of options available for consumers planning to take a trip or purchase a computer. The single factor by which consumers make their choices, assuming price and availability are similar, is *service.* The same is true for health care. When all technical variables are equal, consumers select health care organizations that provide services they can see and experience rather than organizations that emphasize medical and technical services they can't see or judge adequately.

According to Tom Peters and Nancy Austin, customers tend to use service dimensions to judge overall quality.[7] In other words, they evaluate the technical aspects of a product or service (even when they lack the expertise to do so directly) by judging service features as indirect proxy measures of quality. In health care such features include promptness of service, level of confidence projected by personnel, and the completeness of explanations offered by technicians and clinicians. Patients' perceptions must be taken seriously and considered important though indirect indicators of the quality of care provided by the health care organization. Although most patients still follow their physicians' advice in choosing health care facilities, there is a growing trend toward customer independence. Health care consumers are becoming more likely to shop around for physicians with admitting privileges at facilities with reputations for service excellence as well as medical and technical excellence.

For example, research at Thomas Jefferson University Hospital in Philadelphia indicates that at Jefferson, clinical factors do not correlate highly with reported patient loyalty.[8] When Jerald Young of the University of Florida called 2,500 households and asked the question, "Why would you change health care providers?" The results were:[9]

- Sixty percent said that they would change if they had concerns about the quality of the medical care offered by the provider.
- Forty percent said that they would change if they were dissatisfied with the quality of personal treatment they received.
- Twenty percent said that they would change if they had concerns about time issues.

When he asked people who actually had changed health care providers why they did so, however, their responses broke down as follows:

- Fifty-four percent said that they changed as a result of the personal treatment they received.
- Twenty-three percent said that they changed as a result of time issues.
- Twenty percent said that they changed as a result of the quality of medical care offered by the provider.

Typically, patients cite service problems among their reasons for not returning to a particular hospital—problems such as unsupportive staff behavior (coldness, impatience, and annoyance, for example); service delays; impersonal behavior; and confusing and incorrect bills combined with insensitive handling of financial questions. Karl Albrecht describes the "Seven Sins of Service"—the key criteria customers use to explain their loss of loyalty to a particular service provider:[10]

1. Apathy
2. Brush-off
3. Coldness
4. Condescension
5. Robotism
6. Rule book
7. Runaround

Many service experts would add to this list time problems. For a lot of people, like the author of the novel *Postcards from the Edge,* "instant gratification isn't fast enough."[11] Although it may seem counterintuitive, speed and quality do go hand in hand, because process snags are the major impediments to fast and efficient service delivery. An advertisement from United Technologies put it well: "We no longer live in an era of caveat emptor; this is the era of caveat vendor. The lesson is clear: the vendor who fails to provide excellent service loses to a competitor who does—a competitor who has listened better, heard better, and had the courage to act even when such action necessitated change."[12]

The health care consumer is more sophisticated, demanding, and educated than ever before. Consumers are free to choose from a veritable smorgasbord of hospitals, outpatient services, health maintenance organizations, and holistic health centers. If your organization is to be among those health care providers that survive the decade, payers and consumers must consider it an acceptable choice. Therefore, success for today's health care providers depends on the following factors:

- How well the organization manages to instill a commitment to customer service in every employee
- How well executives and managers at all levels enlist every manager, physician, and employee in patient retention strategies that have personal meaning for everyone involved
- How well the organization listens to its customers and makes continuous improvements with the goal of ever-improving levels of customer satisfaction
- How well customer service commitment can be translated into actions, processes, and performance tracking that everyone understands, shares responsibility for, and embraces wholeheartedly
- How seriously the organization's leadership is invested in developing employees who excel in fulfilling customer needs and meeting the complex challenges of today's changing health care environment

Despite recent advances, the emphasis on customer service has not yet been fully accepted in health care. Only since the 1980s have health care providers begun to consider patient satisfaction as an important indicator of quality and a factor in successful competition. As Donabedian has stated, "Patient satisfaction may be considered to be one of the desired outcomes of care, even an element in health status itself. It is futile to argue about the validity of patient satisfaction as a measure of quality. Whatever its strengths and limitations as an indicator of quality, information about patient satisfaction should be as indispensable to assessments of quality as to the design and management of health care systems."[13] Two measures of service excellence, competition and compassion, are explored below.

Service Excellence as a Competitive Edge

Organizations that consistently provide excellent service are winners for several reasons. For example:

- They earn customer loyalty, and customer loyalty translates into repeat customers.
- They are less vulnerable to price wars. There is even evidence that they have historically been able to command higher prices without losing market share.
- They don't have to spend as much on marketing because customers spread the good word about them.
- They are profitable. *The PIMS Principles*[14] reported that relative service quality is positively correlated with profitability and drives business performance. It further points out that there are substantial differences in relative quality between market leaders and followers. "Attaining a superior quality position does not seem to involve many of the strategic tradeoffs, such as higher relative direct costs or marketing expenditures, that business analysts often attribute to quality strategies."[15] (Figure 1-1 illustrates these relationships graphically.)

Confirming the PIMS findings in health care specifically, the *National Consumer Trends Report* concluded that perceived quality is the main reason consumers prefer one hospital over another.[16]

Service Excellence as a Reflection of Compassion

People who need hospitals are sick, vulnerable, and worried. For an endless variety of understandable reasons, hospitals run the risk of forgetting about their patients. If hospital professionals were patients, they wouldn't settle for less than the most humanistic treatment. If their loved ones were in those beds, they would fight to the death for the best the hospital could offer. All hospital providers, no matter what their jobs are, should be guided by what most believe to be the physician's duty: to cure sometimes, relieve often, but comfort always. That philosophy has been at the heart of the healing arts since the beginning of recorded history.

For all the recent turmoil in health care and the medical professions, one fact remains unmistakably clear and irrefutable: medicine and health care are humanistic activities. No matter how much high technology or how many machines and microchips are involved in the diagnostic process, the backbone of health care is its "laying on of hands." Experiences at the hands of a physician, nurse, or other member of the health care profession are intensely personal, intensely human. A patient—whether inpatient or outpatient—needs that human touch, that caring, compassion, and love that in itself can work miracles even when technical and professional skills can do nothing.

Today, people live in a highly technical, often impersonal world. Machines have taken over to an extent that even H. G. Wells did not foresee. Hospitals are caught in a crunch.

Figure 1-1. Winning with Superior Perceived Quality

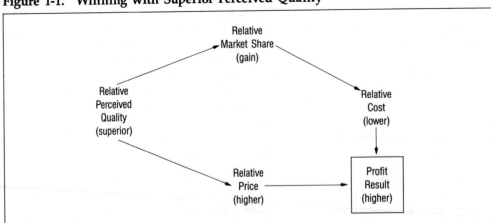

On the one hand, a health care institution must provide its users with state-of-the-art diagnostic and procedural services. That's what the public expects. On the other hand, however, people still expect the tender loving care that has been part of the care-giving culture since the days of Florence Nightingale.

The more high-tech equipment and technology in a facility, the harder it is for health care providers to remain close to their patients. Technicians stand behind computer screens; printouts offer diagnostic information; and a complex series of buzzers, beepers, and other "newfangled" devices stand between the patient and the provider. Because hospitals must provide the best possible medical care that contemporary technology makes available, high tech has become king.

The advent of high tech at first seemed to make high touch less important in the preservation of human health and human life. But in the mid-1980s this picture began to change. Because of massive fiscal and market pressures, hospitals were forced to start scrambling for patients. Because most hospitals offered the same services—high-tech miracles, digital diagnostics, and all the other trappings of modern medicine—providers had to look for a way to distinguish themselves. Each hospital needed to identify a factor that would attract and secure a loyal following of patients and physicians and solidify its wavering census. The time was right for the appearance of innovative service options. Only the fittest and feistiest facilities would survive. In all likelihood, everything legal, ethical, and profitable had probably been tried in the past decade. One of the most promising ideas to appear was customer relations.

How ironic that the care and love that had traditionally epitomized medicine needed a strong, external, market-driven motive to regain their rightful places in modern health care. Because both patients and caregivers experienced severe frustration during this period, the climate became ripe for increased attention to service quality in the hope of reducing tensions. Hospital leaders wanted to build a new image of hospitals as service-oriented organizations intent on achieving excellence. Their strategy was built on the premise that the quality of caring and warmth and the comforts and personal attention offered by service-oriented caregivers could go a long way in making both patients and staff feel human in a high-tech setting.

☐ The Hospital's Tarnished Image

According to the Washington-based Technical Assistance Research Programs (TARP), if you satisfy one customer, he or she tells four others. If you alienate one customer, he or she tells ten, or even more if the problem is serious. Thus, when you annoy one customer, you have to satisfy three just to stay even. The TARP findings also indicate that 30 percent of customers who experience service problems don't complain because complaining is "too much trouble," or they can't find an easy channel, or they think no one cares. Of that 30 percent, only 9 percent will return to the organization in question. Both of these dynamics explain the loss of market share experienced by organizations that disappoint their customers by offering questionable customer service.[17]

In a competitive environment, health care organizations have a stake in making sure that the grapevine draws people to them instead of turning them away to their competitors. Consider the 10-10-10 principle used in business: It takes **$10,000** to get a customer; it takes **10 seconds** to lose one; it takes **10 years** for the problem to go away.

In the June 30, 1986, *Newsweek*, Meg Greenfield wrote that the hospital experience is "a maddening combination of individual excellence and systematic incompetence, the one tirelessly and heroically saving life and limb, the other forever putting both at mindless risk." She went on to say that hospitals "are presided over and manned by human beings and that they are at a minimum fallible because the good guys and good instincts don't always prevail. . . . They and their technological equipment operate against a background of remorseless human shortcoming, bureaucratic inefficiency and indifference.

That, not some need to understand the exotic equipment or science, is the problem. What is required is a fundamental, painstaking re-education process on the part of the whole institution—a relearning of attentiveness, individual accountability, care."[18]

The public no longer idealizes the health care organization or the caregiver. Media coverage and people's own experiences have pushed health care off its former pedestal of uncritical respect and destined it to endless scrutiny. One reason for this change is the disappointing quality of health care service; the other is the public's unrealistically high expectations of health care providers.

In a Conference Board study reported by K. Pallarito and in an article by C. Bell— both in 1990 issues of *Modern Healthcare*—it is suggested that consumers expect miracles. They expect a positive outcome from hospital services no matter what the severity, intensity, or complexity of their health problems. Hospitals find themselves with far fewer grateful patients and many more angry ones because of such impossible expectations.[19,20]

If customers say they find little value in a service, conventional wisdom suggests either lowering the price or offering greater value for the money. In hospitals, because price reduction is becoming increasingly difficult, the only remaining remedy is to close the gap between price and satisfaction—through improved service. Arthur Sturm of the Sturm Communications Group reports on a Conference Board study that showed that hospitals have lost their "halo of goodness." According to Sturm, "Pressure on hospitals to moderate prices reflects the marketplace's frustration with value. Initially, much of the price pressure comes from pent-up hostility caused by successive years of tremendous increases in price for little or no perceived increase in outcomes, service, and responsiveness—issues that often drive the perception of value."[21]

While the media emphasize the skyrocketing cost of health care, the public increasingly sees hospitals as money-hungry businesses that have lost their charitable roots and concern for human welfare. Members of the public bring this mind-set with them when they seek care or visit hospitalized friends or relatives.

Hospital employees have to recognize these negative stereotypes, not be infuriated by them, and recognize the many ways in which poor service can be costly. For example, it costs five times as much to get a customer than to keep one.[22] According to Philip Crosby, 25 to 50 percent of a company's operating expense can be attributed to poor service quality—to the cost of not delivering service right the first time.[23] Hospitals spend megabucks on cumbersome systems, redundant tests and treatments, lost results and charts, complaint handling, billing problems, and marketing expense targeted at acquiring new patients and referral sources. An all-out focus on service improvement can prove expensive initially, but this expense represents a powerful and savvy long-term investment with the potential to reduce the cost-of-service problems dramatically in the long run. Hospitals and their employees must create a new reality, one that shows their continued concern for helping people as well as needing to remain financially viable institutions.

☐ The Only Constant Is Change

Hospitals sprinted through a period of rapid growth that has been followed recently by a period of traumatic cutbacks, downsizing, and change, change, change. Things aren't as they were. People who entered health care because it was "secure" are now overwhelmed with anxiety and the disappointment of broken promises at the same time that they are being pushed to work even harder.

Change has brought uncertainty about the future of the health care industry, and uncertainty generates fear. Mergers and acquisitions, hospital closings, and intense competition have created a tense atmosphere, and the prospect of facing a radically changed, national health system of managed care sometime in the next 10 years looms in the background. Add to these elements the challenge of working with increasingly demanding consumers and the result is clear: Most health care organizations acknowledge that they must become increasingly customer driven and must consciously and conscientiously strive for service excellence.

The challenge is to provide high-quality care and caring in the face of extreme pressure. The reputation of your organization and the self-esteem of your employees rest on making your patients' needs the hospital's paramount responsibility and not letting the hospital become either self-absorbed with anxiety and disillusionment or obsessed with the bottom line. Your hospital must back up clinically excellent health care with a concerted effort to satisfy your customers and bolster the caring attitude, job satisfaction, and self-esteem of all your employees. That's what service improvement strategies are all about.

□ Final Thoughts

Few people would question the fact that service quality is critical to an organization's success. Yet people complain vehemently about the lack of service quality, and health care organizations are hard pressed to deliver consistent service quality to their numerous customers. The reason may be that *high-quality service is much harder to achieve than high-quality products.*

Service expert Ron Zemke argues that service problems stem from a misconception on the part of organizational leaders that services are like products and can be managed similarly.[24] Figure 1-2 summarizes Zemke's discussion of seven important differences between products and services—differences that have far-reaching implications for management action. Frederick Reichheld and W. Earl Sasser contrast a zero-defects approach to product quality with the need for a "zero-defections" approach to service quality.[25] These approaches are summarized by Zemke and illustrated in figure 1-3.

When we are cognizant of these differences, it becomes possible to engineer dramatic improvements in service quality through systematic intervention. Private-sector businesses have achieved it and so have hospitals. What it takes is a long-term, systematic approach that puts customers first and realigns the organization's people and systems to heighten customer satisfaction.

Figure 1-2. Services versus Products

Services	Products
1. The customer owns a memory. The experience cannot be sold or passed on to a third party.	1. The customer owns an object.
2. The goal of service is uniqueness; each customer and each contact is "special."	2. The goal of product production is uniformity.
3. A service happens in the moment; it cannot be stockpiled.	3. A product can be put into inventory; a sample can be sent in advance for review.
4. The customer is a coproducer who acts as a partner in creating the service.	4. The customer is an end-user, who is not involved in the production process.
5. Customers conduct quality control by comparing expectations to experience.	5. Quality control is conducted by comparing output to specifications.
6. If services are improperly performed, apologies and reparations are the only means of recall.	6. If improperly made, a product can be pulled off of the line.
7. The morale of service employees is critical.	7. The morale of production employees is important.

Figure 1-3. Zero Defects versus Zero Defections

Zero Defects Is About:	Zero Defections Is About:
Technical quality	Customer's judgment of quality
Precise standards and performance	Transactions that delight the customer
Treating errors as mortal sins	Treating errors as opportunities to excel
Minimizing the human element	Capitalizing on the human element
Creating standards and protocols for every aspect of a transaction	Creating standards for technical quality and empowerment and recovery strategies for customer quality
No surprises, standard operating procedures, rote and drill	Speed, flexibility, and ability to respond reliably to unique demands
Production quality	Performance quality
Developing satisfactory and mutually beneficial relationships	Building lasting, creative customer partnerships
Customer satisfaction	Customer retention
Reworking every policy and procedure to perfection; creating absolutely seamless performance	Experimenting; leapfrogging the competition; taking measured risks and then learning from them

Reprinted, with permission, from the Jan. 1992 issue of *TRAINING* magazine. Lakewood Publications, Minneapolis, MN. All rights reserved.

Notes and References

1. Forum Corporation. *Leading the Customer-Focused Company: Lessons Learned from Listening to the Voices of Leaders.* Boston, MA: Forum Corporation, 1992.

2. Levitt, T. *The Marketing Imagination.* New York City: Free Press, 1983, p. 105.

3. Buzzell, R., and Gale, B. GE Medical Systems ASIA. In: *The PIMS Principles.* New York City: Free Press, 1987.

4. Reported in the Forum Corporation (One Exchange Place, Boston, MA 02109) company brochure, 1992, p. 5.

5. 3M Company.

6. Buzzell, R., and Gale, B. *The PIMS Principles.* New York City: Free Press, 1987, p. 103.

7. Peters, T., and Austin, N. *Passion for Excellence.* New York City: Random House, 1985.

8. Fisk, T., Brown, C., Cannizzaro, K., and Naftal, B. Creating patient satisfaction and loyalty. *JHCM* 10(2):5–15, June 1990.

9. As reported by Ron Zemke, Closing the Service Gap III Conference, Memphis, TN, Oct. 31, 1990.

10. Albrecht, K. *At America's Service.* Homewood, IL: Dow Jones-Irwin, 1989.

11. Fisher, C. *Postcards from the Edge.* New York City: Pocket Books, Simon and Schuster, 1990.

12. United Technologies ad, 1987.

13. Donabedian, A. The quality of care: how it can be assessed. *JAMA* 260:1,743–48, 1988.

14. Buzzell and Gale, p. 81.

15. Buzzell and Gale, p. 82.

16. 1984–1987 National Consumer Trends Report. Professional Research Consultants, Dec. 1987.

17. Goodman, J. Customer-driven quality: quantifying the payoff of quality actions. Speech given at Closing the Service Gap III Conference, Memphis, TN, Oct. 29–30, 1990.

18. Greenfield, M. The land of hospital. *Newsweek* 107(26):74, June 30, 1986.

19. Pallarito, K. Hospital charges rate low in value. *Modern Healthcare* 20(23):3, June 11, 1990.

20. Bell, C. Hospitals need image makeover. *Modern Healthcare* 20(24):17, June 18, 1990.

21. Sturm, A. Hospitals must close the gap between high price, low regard. *Modern Healthcare* 20(36):89, Sept. 10, 1990.

22. Liswood, L. *Service Them Right: Innovative and Powerful Ways to Keep Your Customers.* New York City: Harper and Row, 1989.

23. Crosby, P. *Quality without Tears.* New York City: McGraw-Hill, 1984.

24. Zemke, R. The emerging art of service management. *Training* (Lakewood Publications, Minneapolis, MN) 29(1):37–42, Jan. 1992.

25. Reichheld, F. F., and Sasser, W. E., Jr. Zero defections: quality comes to services. *Harvard Business Review* 60(5):105–11, Sept.–Oct. 1990.

Chapter 2

The Process of Service Quality Improvement

The theoretical framework used to drive service quality improvement is based on how the key elements of service quality are integrated into a comprehensive "systems approach." From the start of the improvement process, it is important to make the distinction between *service quality, service excellence,* and *service quality improvement*—terms that are used repeatedly throughout this book, but are not used interchangeably. Each has a distinct meaning.

Service quality is the extent to which an organization meets customer expectations. It is one dimension of organizational performance that ranges from "poor" service quality to "excellent" service quality. *Service excellence,* on the other hand, marks the upper end of the service quality continuum. It is service that is flawless from the customer's point of view, given the customer's criteria for judging service quality. Service excellence is the result of making continuous service improvements successfully. *Service quality improvement* is the *process* that moves an organization up the service quality continuum to achieve service excellence.

Inevitably, service quality remains a moving target because the health care industry itself is in perpetual motion. Our services and techniques are complex and changing. The rules of reimbursement are unpredictable and beyond the health care organization's control. There is a great deal of turnover and evolution in the work force. Patients and families want change. And the strain or harmony in relationships between administrators and physicians, between physicians and employees, and among employees themselves continues to shift. Because service quality is not static, the organization that gets complacent about service quality can expect not only slippage, but also a rapid decline in competitive position as the organization down the street seizes the service quality challenge and strides forward.

This chapter will discuss the key elements of service quality, the four facets of service quality improvement strategies, and the mind-set required to implement change. The chapter will close with clarifying the distinction between service improvement versus quality improvement.

☐ The Key Elements of Service Quality

In health care, service quality means focusing on two activities. Those actions are *doing the right things right* and *making continuous improvements.*

The Right Things Done Right

As the matrix in figure 2-1 suggests, your organization and everyone in it can do the right or wrong things, and these things can be done in either the right or the wrong way. *Processes* that meet customer expectations in a streamlined, cost-effective manner are the right things. *Performance* by people and departments that conforms to these processes is doing things right. Fortunately, process and performance interact. When you clarify and improve processes, performance improves as a result. The following examples demonstrate the four possibilities:

1. *Doing the right things wrong:* You have a piece of equipment that can produce very accurate test results, but when you use the equipment incorrectly, you're doing the right thing wrong. Or, your organization has designed a very efficient discharge planning process, but the people using it don't follow the procedures specified.
2. *Doing the wrong things wrong:* Your organization has a very inefficient system for scheduling patients for preadmission tests, and the people using this inefficient system make numerous mistakes entering patients' names and appointment times.
3. *Doing the wrong things right:* Your organization has a very inefficient system for scheduling patients for preadmission tests, but the people do a perfect job of entering patients' names and appointment times as well as other information.
4. *Doing the right things right:* You have a great piece of equipment that is capable of producing very accurate and valuable test results; employees know when to use it, and they use it correctly 100 percent of the time. Your organization is doing the right things right.

When it comes to service quality, both processes and performance matter. Processes, policies, and jobs must be designed to reflect the best, most effective methods for serving customers and eliminating inefficiencies, and the system's design must ensure that the desired quality of service is built into the way things are done. In addition, you must be sure that people and departments have the competence to reliably and consistently carry out processes and procedures so that the way things are actually done is consistent with well-conceived designs.

Figure 2-1. Process–Performance Matrix

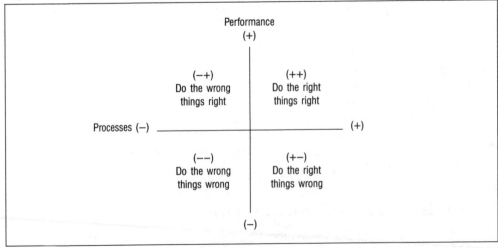

Continuous Improvement

Continuous improvement lies at the heart of the service quality challenge. Perfection may not be possible, but making service better by tackling problem after problem and experimenting with improvement after improvement is possible. Continuous improvement is the responsibility of every person in the organization. There's so much to do for the sake of customers that the energy and ingenuity of every employee at every level are needed to meet the service quality challenge. Excellent service is never an accident; it is always a matter of deliberate effort. That deliberate effort can be labeled "continuous improvement." Doing the right things right and undertaking continuous improvement will result in the following:

- Optimal clinical outcomes for patients
- Satisfaction for all customers
- Retention of talented staff
- Financial viability

Optimal Clinical Outcomes

Optimal clinical outcome is expected by all patients and their families. Even though patients want optimal clinical outcomes, they often cannot evaluate clinical outcomes because they have limited clinical knowledge. But the professionals in your organization can (and do) apply their standards of clinical quality on the patients' behalf. In the clinical arena, doing the right things right is analogous to doing the "appropriate things effectively." The question is, "is this action necessary [required], and if it is, "how can we be sure it will be done right [effectively]?" The matrix in figure 2-1 can be revised to reflect the clinical arena. (See figure 2-2.)

Satisfaction for All Customers

Using the word *customer* to refer to patients and their families offends many health care professionals. But the customer concept is key to understanding the importance of focusing on customer expectations. Patients are customers of health care services in that they choose among health care services, and they have certain expectations for these services. When their expectations are not met, they do not consider the service to be of quality.

Figure 2-2.   Appropriateness–Effectiveness Matrix

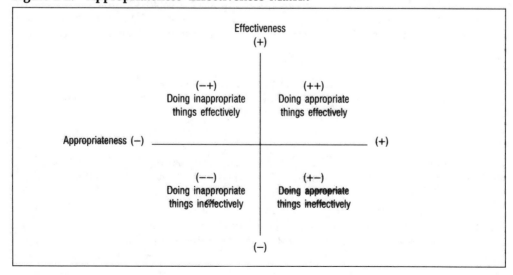

The use of the broad and inclusive term *customer* also helps to focus improvement on the numerous customers important to a complex health care organization. Many different groups of customers judge the quality of health care services—patients, families and friends, physicians, internal customers, payers, and members of the community. Each of these customer groups has expectations of the organization's services. They judge service quality by assessing the extent to which their needs and expectations, or their "requirements," are met.

Strategically speaking, customers need to be understood as distinct groups with different needs and expectations in relation to health care. For the purposes of this book, five key customer segments are considered the targets of service excellence strategies:

1. Patients
2. Visitors
3. Physicians
4. Employees
5. Payers

Referral sources and community groups, vendors, volunteers, trustees, and others may also be considered key customer groups. Each organization must identify which customer groups to target in their service improvement strategies.

Patients

Patients make up the first and foremost customer group key to the success of your organization. Of all the customer groups, patients experience the most direct and intense contact with your staff and services. For four main reasons, you need to concern yourself with patients' perceptions and satisfaction with your services:

- *The humanistic reason:* Patients deserve excellent quality of care and service because, more often than not, they are quite vulnerable. They come to the hospital sick, worried, pained, concerned, and anxious about their physical, emotional, and economic well-being: "Am I well? Can I get through this emotionally? Can I afford this?" Excellent service is therapeutic.
- *The economic reason:* Patients are customers. They think like customers, they have options that they consider more carefully than ever, and they expect value for their money.
- *The marketing reason:* Patients serve as your organization's informal public relations and sales force. They control the grapevine that influences future business.
- *The efficiency reason:* Satisfied patients are easier to serve. Dissatisfied patients consume valuable staff time, time that could be better spent serving more people more thoroughly.

Most patients want the best state of health they can achieve, as well as convenient, timely service; courteous, compassionate staff; and ample as well as accurate information about their condition.

Visitors

Visiting family and friends are the second key customer group. When they accompany patients to your organization or visit hospitalized patients, they are frequently overlooked by staff members whose primary concern is with the patients.

These visitors also have firsthand experiences with your facility and staff, and they want their presence and importance to be acknowledged. They want information, and they appreciate comforts, amenities, and updates that help what can be agonizing hours of waiting pass more quickly. They may be edgy because they feel powerless to help their loved one. Concerned and anxious, they look for information and reassurance.

They also act on their own protective instincts by scrutinizing employee behavior toward the patients and by zealously advocating patients' rights.

If family and friends are impressed with their own and their loved one's experience with your organization, they may consider using your facility themselves if they need similar services. However, whether they are impressed or not, their word of mouth spreads opinion about your organization to the rest of the community. This kind of free advertising can help or hurt your hospital.

Physicians

Physicians are customers, too. They are direct customers when they serve their patients within the organization, interacting with staff and systems in the process. They are indirect customers when they refer patients to the organization for tests, procedures, or consultations with other physicians. Also, as more physicians become salaried members of care teams, cooperation and a mutual service orientation create the spirit of partnership and teamwork that result in excellent service.

When asked about what matters most to them in their relationships with hospitals, physicians consistently mention *ease-of-practice* issues. That is, the physician who finds it easy to practice in your organization feels positive about your organization. An astute strategy for service excellence can help keep physicians satisfied by facilitating the ease with which they practice in the hospital. Physicians want your organization to be user-friendly and supportive in serving their patients.

Employees

Employees comprise your organization's internal customers insofar as they use the organization to meet their own and their families' health care needs. They spread the word about your organization to community members, families, and friends; they also field questions about the organization from community members who look to them for the inside scoop. To that end, you need to sell your employees on your organization, and one way to do so is to help them achieve job satisfaction.

What do your employees say about your organization on the bus ride home, at family gatherings, at community meetings? As a trusted information source about your organization, employees deserve to be on the receiving end of services, benefits, information, respect, and care that will inspire productive work on your organization's behalf as well as loyalty and support.

These internal customers/employees are also service givers who provide services not only to patients but to other employees as well. In that sense, employees are one another's internal customers, relying on each other to get their jobs done. People who don't serve external customers directly are serving employees who do. If every employee had his or her expectations met by every employee "supplier" of services and products, the work environment would be free of error and aggravation.

Payers

Employers in the United States acknowledge that health care is an expensive item in their annual budgets. A significant portion of the price consumers pay for automobiles, airline tickets, and food from fast-food chains, for example, goes to pay for employee health care benefits.

To stay in business, your organization must satisfy powerful new forces in the health care industry. Third-party payers—including businesses, insurance companies, health maintenance organizations, preferred provider organizations, government programs, unions, and other health care funders—are shopping for the best health care deals they can find for their constituencies. They look for optimal health outcomes for their constituents at the lowest possible cost, and they want satisfied constituents who don't complain. Above all, they expect service: cost information, accurate answers to their questions, and positive reports about the quality of care and caring offered.

Numerous Satisfaction Criteria

The *service quality matrix*, developed by the Albert Einstein Healthcare Foundation, demonstrates how comprehensive this service concept needs to be (see figure 2-3). On the basis of an analysis of research identifying the criteria consumers use to evaluate their health care experiences, the service matrix defines six key components (vertical axis) integral to service excellence as perceived by each of an organization's key customer groups (horizontal axis). An effective service improvement strategy reflects a lasting commitment to excellent performance on all six components of the service matrix:

- *People skills:* In the past, most efforts to improve customer relations focused primarily on people skills, specifically the courtesy, care, and concern that personnel in the organization extend to patients, visitors, physicians, and one another. No doubt, people skills have a dramatic impact on consumer satisfaction, the reputation of the organization that spreads through the grapevine, and the consumer's future choices about where to go for care. A rude receptionist can turn away a patient faster than parking problems or even a questionable diagnosis.

- *Amenities:* Amenities (such as coffee in the waiting room, toys and a play area for the kids, a Walkman® in the dental chair, free toothbrush and shampoo in an attractive container, valet parking, videocassette recorders, and colorful linens) can make customers feel more comfortable and special. However, although such amenities may be appreciated by customers, they do not compensate for other service deficiencies. Patients complain bitterly that although the pile of magazines in the waiting room may make the time go faster, they should still not have to suffer long waits (caused by a systems problem) or rude employees (caused by poor people skills). Attention to amenities to the exclusion of a hard-nosed attack on systems problems, such as long waits or misplaced charts and laboratory tests, is misguided and limits the long-term success of your organization's service improvement strategy.

- *Systems and processes:* Even people skills are not enough if the organization's underlying systems do not support them. Many customer relations programs have failed

Figure 2-3. Service Quality Matrix

| Key Components | Customers | | | | |
	Patients	Family and Friends	Physicians	Internal Customers	Payers
People skills					
Amenities					
Systems and processes					
Environment					
Technical and clinical competence					
Cost					

because of inattention to the underlying work processes that make it anywhere from difficult to impossible to serve a customer. Employees get frustrated apologizing to patients for long waits day after day and year after year. Especially in an atmosphere of increased concern for the customer, employees resent underlying systems problems and inconveniences that interfere with their ability to extend appropriate care and attention to customers. Long waits, cumbersome and interminable decision-making processes, equipment that doesn't work, poor scheduling practices, circuitous routes from one location to another, and supply shortages exemplify lapses in support systems.

Without attention to underlying systems and process problems, good employees gradually become demoralized and their people skills become less effective. Also, the organization's relationships with employees are perceived as poor by the customer, who has been oppressed by the organization's senseless procedures and practices and drained of time, energy, and patience.

- *Environment:* The physical environment also merits attention. Many organizations instituting customer relations programs have unearthed parking, transportation, and physical access problems. In facilities with such problems, employees feel frustrated because more courteous behavior on their part cannot adequately compensate for environmental deficiencies, and they do not feel inspired to bend over backward to compensate for management's neglect of environmental factors. Obviously, dilapidated, dirty, or overtly unsafe buildings dissuade patients from returning. How comfortable can a patient and visitor feel and how energetic do physicians and employees feel in uncomfortable surroundings? The physical environment, its accessibility and aesthetics, deserves consideration as part of a comprehensive strategy for service excellence.

- *Technical and clinical competence:* More often than not, technical and clinical competence has been the primary focus of health care organizations, which have always been concerned about whether a diagnosis is right, whether laboratory tests are accurate, whether the maintenance worker can fix the air conditioner, and so forth. Increasingly, however, the marketing-oriented health care manager knows that technical and clinical competence is not enough, especially given that consumers are not able to evaluate this component as well as they can evaluate other, more familiar aspects of service such as friendliness, respectful treatment, easy access, attentiveness, and convenience.

- *Cost:* Cost is also a factor in some customers' decision making about health care. When service or quality are questionable, cost is especially influential. When service and quality are perceived as high, cost becomes less important than "value." People will pay more for high-quality service.

Health care leaders need to identify their customers' key expectations and then determine how they can meet or exceed them.

Retention of Talented Staff

Another outcome of doing the right things right and making continuous service improvements is greater success in attracting and retaining talented employees and physicians. Competent, caring health care professionals want to be associated with an organization that strives for service excellence in practice, not only in its rhetoric. By streamlining systems, making the organization and its processes more customer-friendly, relieving turf tensions, and taking better and better care of patients, providers feel better about their work and are much more likely to extend their loyalty to the department and/or organization.

Financial Viability

Finally, optimal clinical outcomes, satisfied customers, and committed staff all pay off financially. You can document efficiencies in cost savings. You can increase business volume by achieving greater customer satisfaction. And you reduce the high cost of turnover and recruitment by enabling your staff to achieve greater pride, quality of work life, and job satisfaction. There's no doubt about it: Providing poor service is extremely costly.

□ The Four Facets of Service Quality Improvement Strategies

A comprehensive approach to achieving service excellence through the process of service quality improvement includes four facets. These components, depicted in figure 2-4, are summarized as follows:

- *Customers and their expectations:* At the heart of the strategy are the customers. It is their expectations that will drive improvement efforts.
- *Performance improvement:* The job of employees and physicians is to serve patients and other customers with competence, caring, and professionalism. An effective service quality improvement strategy focuses on raising performance standards and increasing the consistency of conformance.
- *Process improvement:* To support your staff and customers, you need straightforward, streamlined, cost-effective work processes and systems. An effective strategy

Figure 2-4. Four Facets of Service Quality

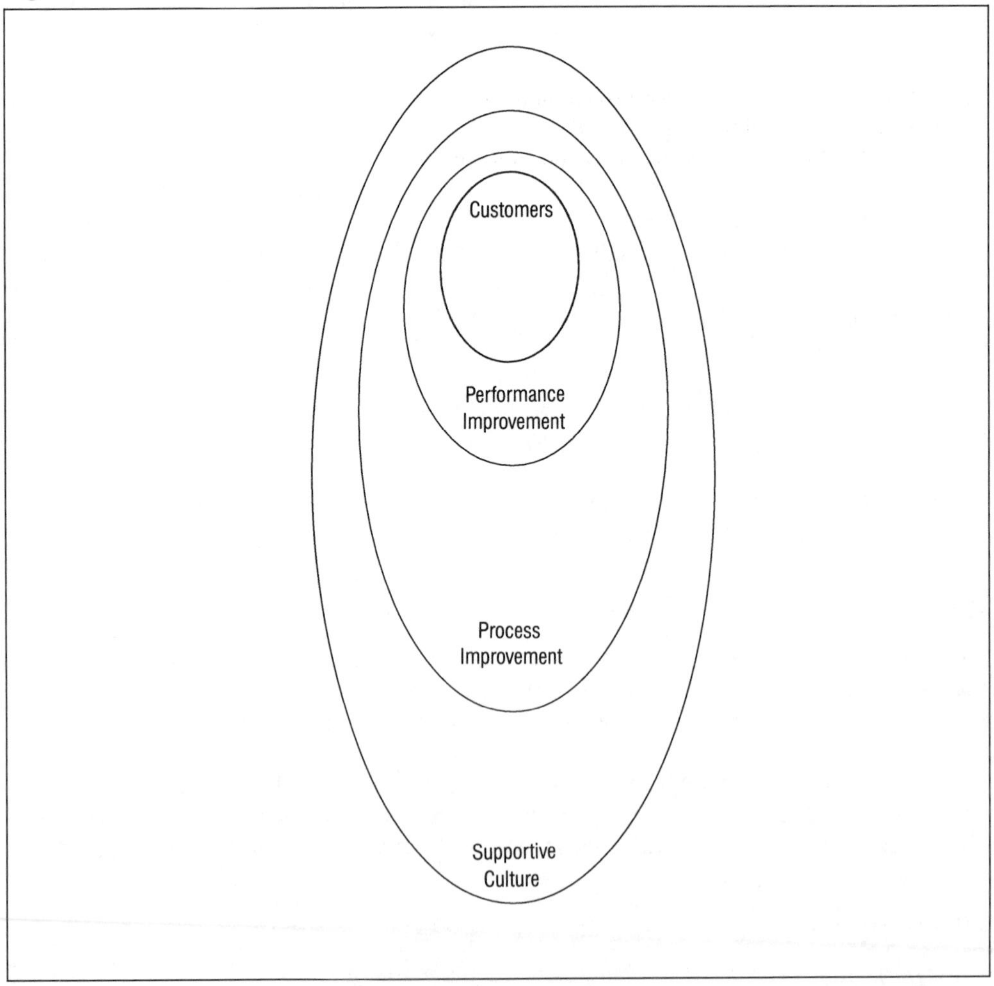

Customers

Performance
Improvement

Process
Improvement

Supportive
Culture

helps people take initiative, experiment, and use state-of-the-art tools to improve processes within and across departments to create a "seamless" organization.
- *A culture that supports continuous improvement:* An optimal strategy achieves change by modifying the organization's cultural practices so that they encourage and support continuous improvement of service quality.

In a comprehensive approach, the preceding facets are further driven by two elements. These are mind-set and process of continuous improvement. The following subsections explain specifically how these two elements interact with expectations, performance, process, and culture. More will be said about mind-set later in the chapter.

Customers and Their Expectations

As already indicated, customer expectations must drive service quality improvement efforts. Health care organizations have numerous customers and potential customers whose expectations must be identified, prioritized, and made the criteria for judging success. The key is to identify key customer targets and their expectations, and then to exceed those expectations.

The organization must build into its mind-set and its everyday operations an ongoing system for ensuring continuous improvement in meeting customer expectations—a regular, reliable process that holds the organization and every department accountable for effective performance related to your customers' expectations.

The most effective service businesses in the United States (Florida Power and Light, Federal Express, 3M Company, Delta Airlines, Xerox Corporation, for example) incorporate a cyclical, systematic, customer-driven improvement process. The management process is central to the success of departments and pivotal to the effectiveness of department managers. One example of such a system is the customer-driven management model illustrated in figure 2-5.

To make customer expectations drive service improvement, to be systematic in your approach, and to ensure *continuous* service improvement, you need to install a cyclical improvement process like the customer-driven management model at both the organization and department levels. You then need to make this process a regularly scheduled approach to quality management and continuous improvement.

Performance Improvement

Once you have identified customer expectations, the next step is to identify and operationalize the level of employee and physician performance that will meet those expectations. This complex process involves setting explicit standards and designing service protocols, role modeling by the manager and supervisor, coaching, training, counseling, recognizing and rewarding excellence, running interference and removing barriers, and much more. Although work processes are certainly important, the role of individual performance should not be neglected as your mind-set begins to attune itself to sorely needed process changes.

Process Improvement

Process improvement is essential. Too often performance is blamed for service problems and dissatisfied customers when the work process itself was never adequately designed to support effective service delivery. The model shown in figure 2-6 is a rational and effective approach to process improvement. With such a model, people involved in key service processes can identify process problems that affect customer satisfaction, diagnose their underlying causes, and identify and test solutions or improvements. With these needs in mind, they can then proceed to institute changes that reap benefits for customers and make service delivery more efficient and less frustrating for staff. (More will be said on process improvement in chapter 7.)

A Culture That Supports Continuous Improvement

It takes an "aligned organization" to achieve excellent service. That's why it is necessary to strengthen your organization's culture so that it supports service quality improvement. To do so, you need to adopt a mind-set that allows you to examine your everyday practices (that is, the current culture) and determine the extent to which these practices support excellent service. These practices then need to be revamped to align with and drive continuous service improvement.

Figure 2-5. Customer-Driven Management Model

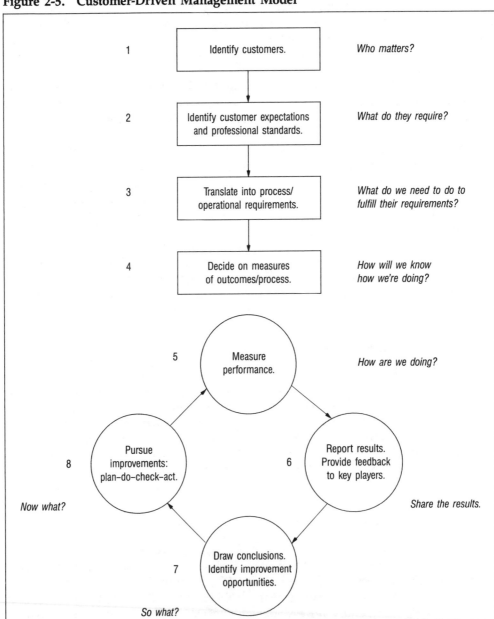

Reprinted, with permission, from The Einstein Consulting Group, Philadelphia, Pennsylvania, 1990.

Figure 2-6. Model for Process Improvement

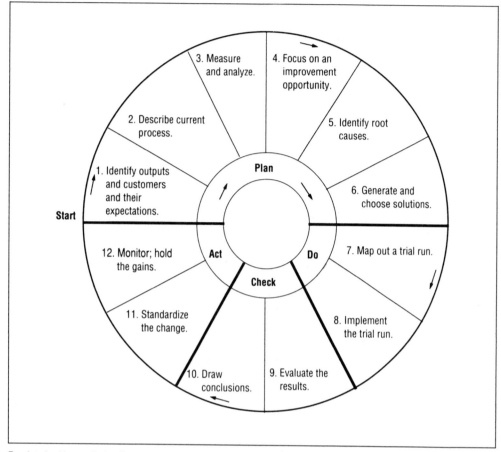

Reprinted, with permission, from Albert Einstein Healthcare Foundation, Philadelphia, Pennsylvania, 1990.

The 10 pillars of continuous improvement are an organizing framework for examining, assessing, and redesigning an organization's everyday cultural practices for continuous service improvement. These pillars, introduced in chapter 3 and examined in depth in part two of this book, include management vision and commitment, accountability, measurement and feedback, problem solving and process improvement, communication, staff development and training, physician involvement, reward and recognition, employee involvement and empowerment, and reminders and refreshers.

To strengthen the institution's culture so that it is service focused, you may need to rethink your practices in the 10 areas reflected by these 10 pillars. In other words, the culture can be rebuilt to become a service culture—by design, laying one new brick after another.

No short-term or quick-fix approach is sufficient to make continuous service improvement happen. Strategies don't work unless they are long-term and enduring. You must do things better and do things differently in an endless cycle of learning and improvement.

□ The Continuous Improvement Mind-Set

Service quality results from deliberate, sustained effort—effort that starts with managers at all levels of the organization. To exert a powerful impact on the organization's service mission and effectiveness and to merit pride in (and recognition for) service excellence throughout the organization, people's energies must be aligned in the direction of continuous service quality improvement. This calls for a special combination of skills and attitudes, many of which require growth and change by health care leaders, managers, physicians, and staff at every level.

The pivotal change required involves the mind-set of every leader and manager in the organization. Leaders might be aware of the skills and models that are important to making continuous improvements, but without the appropriate mind-set—which drives attention and actions—they simply will not take the necessary steps or expend the necessary energy to effect change. In their book *Health Care Managers in Transition*,[1] the authors describe mind-set shifts that are essential to managing for improved service quality and continuous improvement in today's turbulent health care environment. Specifically, executives, managers, physicians, and staff need to make 10 shifts:

1. *From provider to customer orientation:* Customer-oriented people treat customer satisfaction as a much higher priority than what's traditional or convenient for themselves as providers.
2. *From tolerance to higher standards:* People with rising standards believe that "good enough" never is.
3. *From director to empowerer:* Managers who empower rather than direct others increase their own impact by engaging employees in service quality improvement and by allowing employees the latitude to act on behalf of customer satisfaction and fulfillment of other organization objectives.
4. *From employee as expendable resource to employee as customer:* Managers who treat employees as customers recognize that energized, satisfied employees do not jump ship but instead have energy and motivation to contribute to the organization's objectives.
5. *From reactive to proactive:* Proactive managers take initiative and responsibility to make improvements for internal and external customers. In doing so, they anticipate problems before they become fires that must be fought or crises that must be squelched.
6. *From tradition and safety to experimentation and risk:* Managers who experiment and take risks recognize that you move forward only if you stick your neck out and try new ways to make things better.
7. *From "busy-ness" to results:* Results-oriented managers feel accountable for outcomes and measure their own success by answers, solutions, experiments, and initiatives. They do not gauge their worth by how swamped or busy they are.
8. *From turf protection to teamwork across lines:* Teamworking managers cross turf lines to confront and solve problems and improve service to customers. This shift promotes an effort to create the "seamless" organization.
9. *From "we–they" thinking to organizational perspective:* Teamworking managers do not pit their own interests against those of their organizations. Thus, they see resource constraints and improvement priorities from an organizational, not self-interested, perspective and take initiative to build a broader stake in organizational improvement among their staff.
10. *From cynicism to optimism:* Optimistic managers believe in the possibility of new solutions and breakthroughs. By personally devoting energy to pursuing new avenues, these visionary managers make their optimism contagious among staff and peers.

These 10 key shifts are summarized in figure 2-7. These management attitudes are the underpinnings of an effective service improvement strategy. They are so important that many organizations take time early in their strategies to build them throughout their management team. Without a shared mind-set that focuses on customers; embraces risk, experimentation, and change; and strives for continuous improvement, service improvement is empty rhetoric.

To create the possibility of service excellence, leaders must raise their sights and aim for excellence. Otherwise, if you don't strive for excellence your efforts to motivate your work force are doomed to failure. As a guideline, picture a continuum of employee behavior from awful on the left to excellent on the right, with disappointing, inoffensive, and good in between (see figure 2-8).

Many management teams embrace service improvement because they're tired of the small number of people at the left end of the continuum—those whose behavior repels customers. Their rudeness, inattentiveness, indifference, or irritability toward customers cause vehement complaints, guest dissatisfaction, time-consuming troubleshooting, and image problems. Managers who want a service strategy to rehabilitate or eliminate these offenders have one goal—to stop damaging, expensive behavior. In fact, many organizations devote resources to service improvement for just this reason. In a culture that has rarely disciplined employees for mediocre or poor interpersonal skills, such a goal is not unusual. However, it is shortsighted.

Objectives for service excellence need to be ambitious and inspirational. If you move people successfully from awful to inoffensive or even good, you've come some distance along the spectrum, and the temptation is to feel satisfied because offensive behavior and complaints have been eliminated. A facade of positivity exists because of the absence of negativity. However, the absence of negativity does not result automatically in positivity. By reaching for inoffensiveness and not excellence, you limit the potential of your service strategy and your ability to delight customers, because staff are inspired only when they strive toward excellence. In other words, striving for inoffensiveness is not inspirational.

Nor does being "good" help your organization. In a competitive environment, being good is not enough. The competitive edge is *excellence.* Service does not stand out as a competitive strength unless it's so strong in your organization that it captures the attention of the customer. You have to exceed the customers' expectations to the point where they stop short and are impressed by how good you really are. Your message should be to settle for nothing less than excellence:

Good isn't good enough for us. This organization is too good to set our sights on being merely decent to people. We want to *stand out* in our treatment of customers. Only through excellence can we give our customers the treatment they deserve. Only

Figure 2-7.   10 Key Shifts in Management Mind-Set

From	To
Provider orientation	Customer orientation
Tolerance	Higher standards
Directing	Empowering
Employee as expendable resource	Employee as customer
Reactive	Proactive
Tradition and safety	Experimentation and risk
"Busy-ness"	Results
Turf protection	Teamwork across lines
"We–they" thinking	Organizational perspective
Cynicism	Optimism

Reprinted, with permission, from The Einstein Consulting Group, Philadelphia, Pennsylvania, 1990.

Figure 2-8.   Continuum of Employee Behavior toward Customers

Awful	Disappointing	Inoffensive	Good	Excellent

through service excellence will we create a loyal customer following. Only through excellence can we maintain our own integrity as health care givers and hold in high esteem our workplace and ourselves. And only by being open to dramatically different organizational forms and methods of service delivery can we create the possibility of ever better service and ever higher customer satisfaction.

☐ Service Improvement versus Quality Improvement

As mentioned earlier, service quality means doing the right things right and making continuous improvements in order to achieve optimal patient outcomes, satisfaction for all customers, retention of talented staff, and financial viability. If you accept this definition, the state-of-the-art approach to service and quality is one and the same for the future despite historical differences between a service focus and a quality focus. Whether you call it service excellence, total quality management (TQM), continuous quality improvement (CQI), total quality improvement (TQI), service quality improvement, or a homegrown label, customer expectations must be the driving force.

There has been widespread confusion in the health care field about the relationship between service and quality. This confusion most likely stems from perceived differences in motivation and tactics typically associated with hospital service strategies of the past when contrasted to more recent quality improvement strategies. The overarching objectives do not differ, but rather the means used historically to achieve these objectives has changed. A snapshot comparison of past service strategies and current TQI strategies would show marked differences; a moving picture, however, would show that these differences are fading fast.

In the early 1980s, hospitals increased their focus on customers initially through guest relations strategies. They wanted to:

- Compete effectively in the face of diagnosis-related groups (DRGs)
- Meet rising consumer expectations
- Reduce customer complaints and the hassle of dealing with them day after day
- Shift from a "provider" orientation to a "customer" orientation
- Balance the increase in high tech with a counterbalancing emphasis on high touch
- Motivate employees by stretching toward excellence
- Be the provider of choice among patients and physicians and the employer of choice among staff

After focusing their strategies largely on the human behavior dimension, many organizations began to realize that the behavioral focus was not enough because other factors—such as systems, amenities, and demonstrated technical capabilities—affect customer satisfaction. With that realization came the shift in language from "guest relations" to "service excellence." Now, in the 1990s, many providers have turned away from "service" toward *total quality* as the umbrella value that should drive organizational change. Hospitals are focusing on quality because:

- They acknowledge that the Joint Commission on Accreditation of Healthcare Organizations (JCAHO) is focusing on quality issues.
- They want to "keep up with the Joneses" (*quality* is certainly in vogue).
- They want to provide great service at lower cost in the face of severe resource constraints.
- They want to replace operational snags, disruptions, and cumbersome processes with streamlined, efficient, smart systems.
- They want to eliminate costly waste and rework that frustrates customers and employees alike.
- They recognize that quality is a goal that galvanizes everyone, from staff to physicians to patients.

Even though the motivations behind the emphasis on service versus quality have changed, the strategies for the future need not be new or different. Given our current knowledge, it has become clear that *total quality* and *service quality* are interchangeable terms, a matter of semantics. The comprehensive service/quality improvement strategy does the following:

- Makes expectations of the organization's numerous customers its driving force and customer satisfaction its overarching goal
- Addresses customers' nonclinical requirements, as well as clinical performance and outcomes
- Focuses extensive attention on the redesign and improvement of systems and processes
- Pays attention to cost reduction, as waste signifies inefficiencies that interfere not only with customer satisfaction but also with funding of services needed to meet customer needs
- Establishes standards and holds people and systems accountable through measurement, monitoring, feedback, and attentive managers
- Rewards and recognizes individuals and teams who perform well and contribute to improvements
- Engages everyone at every level and empowers them to act in pursuit of quality and customer satisfaction

Although many people claim that quality improvement is a more inclusive term than service quality improvement, many organizations use the term *quality improvement* narrowly to mean only a "process improvement" focus. A focus on processes is essential because, as indicated earlier in this chapter, health care organizations (and other industries as well) have traditionally blamed people and their performance for service problems when systems and work processes were actually at fault. The fact is that work processes, interpersonal behavior, environmental factors, amenities, and technical capabilities are all essential elements of service delivery. For that reason, we use service quality as an all-inclusive term.

☐ Final Thoughts

Only a carefully coordinated, comprehensive strategy can make continuous service quality improvement and satisfied customers the norm. This strategy motivates the entire organization and builds a powerful culture that supports service quality and sustains it over the long run.

In short, to make service quality ever better, you need to not only manage the status quo, but lead the charge of continuous improvement with a mind-set that triggers experimentation, risk taking, and persistence in process improvement. To do this, you need to develop and articulate a vision of service quality, cross turf lines to tackle problems, build effective partnerships with internal customers to expedite needed change, and inspire staff to heightened levels of involvement and action. These are tall orders, yet they are essential to service quality leadership, now a business necessity.

The achievement of service excellence is a process, not a program, for a program has a beginning and an end. An effective service quality improvement strategy is ongoing and enduring. It's a way of doing business that demands not only skillful planning and implementation but also energy, determination, and perseverance so as to bring about substantive change. Service excellence should be a *value* within the organizational culture, one that needs to be firmly instilled and aggressively maintained *forever*.

Reference

1. Leebov, W., and Scott, G. *Health Care Managers in Transition: Shifting Roles and Changing Organizations.* San Francisco: Jossey-Bass, 1990.

Part Two

The 10 Pillars of Continuous Improvement

Chapter 3

The Foundation of Continuous Service Improvement

The Story of Two Carpenters: One of the carpenters was wise. She took a long time to anchor her house on a solid foundation. The other carpenter was foolish. This carpenter was in a hurry. "Foundations are not important," he thought, "except in a storm and a storm may never come." So he built his house on insecure footings. The ensuing storm blew the house down.

Your organizational culture needs a strong infrastructure, or support system, that focuses ongoing attention on service quality and continuous service improvement. As we noted in chapter 1, to foster excellent service and continuous improvement over the long haul, not only do you need a focus on customers, excellent service performance by staff, and well-designed service processes, you also need a supportive organizational culture that does not push for competing or conflicting priorities.

What if you don't have a service-oriented culture now? You can build it by reexamining and revamping your everyday cultural practices so that they align with your quest for service excellence. Because *culture* is simply "the way you do things," the challenge is to analyze your current practices (your current ways of doing things) and revamp them as needed so that they align with your service mission. This rebuilding of everyday practices to support service improvement creates an infrastructure that ensures ongoing service improvement.

☐ The 10 Pillars of Continuous Improvement

To strengthen your culture in this direction, it is helpful to use a blueprint for internal culture change. Figure 3-1 presents a visual model of the components of a service-oriented culture. As the model shows, your service mission is your overall purpose—what you aim to achieve. Your values describe *how* you want to get there (for example, through a focus on customers, with compassion, through teamwork). The "pillars" refer to cultural practices and supports that need to be aligned with your service mission and values. Competing, unaligned, or contradictory practices frustrate personal energy and commitment. You need to align your everyday practices with your quest for continuous service

Figure 3-1. The 10 Pillars of Continuous Service Improvement

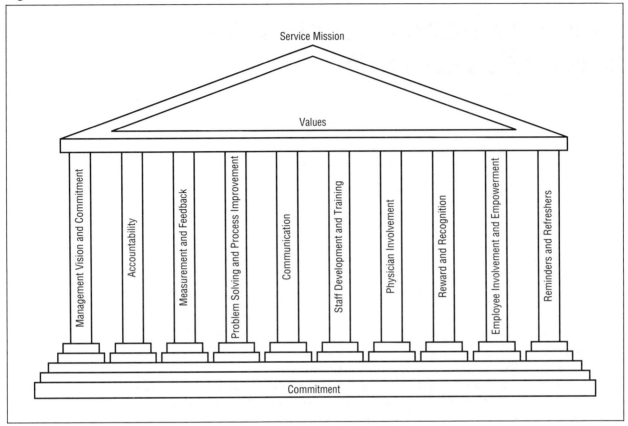

improvement so that everyone's energies move in the same direction, toward your mission. Your everyday practices and policies need to *encourage* excellent individual service performance, attention to service processes, and service improvement initiatives so that these translate into the collective results you want.

The 10 pillars of continuous service improvement break down your cultural practices into manageable clusters so that you can analyze their impact on service quality and rebuild those that work against your service quest. These pillars reflect broad categories of practices and policies that merit rethinking to ensure that they align with and advance your service commitment. The 10 pillars are:

- Management vision and commitment
- Accountability
- Measurement and feedback
- Problem solving and process improvement
- Communication
- Staff development and training
- Physician involvement
- Reward and recognition
- Employee involvement and empowerment
- Reminders and refreshers

The pillars represent 10 powerful forces, all of which need to be working in the same direction. They are the primary forces that determine your degree of success. Each must be solid, long-lasting, and supportive of your quest for service excellence.

Pillar 1. Management Vision and Commitment

The first pillar necessary to support your service strategy is management vision and commitment. Service excellence can't survive if it is conceived as a program with a beginning and end. It needs instead to be an enduring organizational value and a commitment pervasive at every level of the organization. Such a commitment takes leadership, and courageous leadership at that. Top management needs to stick its proverbial neck out to move people toward service excellence.

The power of strong top management commitment is obvious. When departments won't schedule their people into a mandatory workshop, when extra dollars are needed to fund a recognition strategy, when two department heads won't set ambitious service standards with their people because they don't work with patients, when employees have ideas about ways to improve service but no one will listen, that's when your strategy starts to crack and crumble. Management commitment is not an elusive force. Chapter 4 explores the intricacies of knowing when it's there and building it brick by brick.

Pillar 2. Accountability

The second pillar that merits a critical eye is accountability. To hold people accountable to high standards, you first need standards, and your standards need teeth.

Chapter 5 examines key methods for building accountability for service excellence into your human resource management practices:

- Creating a systemwide policy for service excellence
- Hiring service-oriented people in the first place
- Developing and installing service management expectations of all managers and supervisors
- Developing explicit service expectations that apply to all employees and physicians organizationwide
- Developing service standards and protocols
- Developing *job-specific* service expectations
- Building service expectations into job descriptions
- Building service dimensions into the performance appraisal process
- Getting new people off on the right foot through new-employee orientation
- Installing a commendation process that rewards service excellence, not only technical or clinical excellence
- Providing training and support so that managers implement accountability policies

Pillar 3. Measurement and Feedback

Perhaps you support the notion of continuous service improvement as a necessity and priority. But can you track and evaluate progress? Without built-in systems for ongoing evaluation, you can't be sure of how you're doing. You also have inadequate information by which to guide your improvement initiatives. You need to be sure you've installed evaluation methods that tap the perceptions, degree of satisfaction, and suggestions of each of your key customer groups. Also you need to monitor operational processes key to fulfilling your customers' expectations. Otherwise, you're navigating blindly and missing invaluable opportunities to gain constructive feedback that will keep you on course and point the way to important improvements.

Chapter 6 discusses multiple ways to tap into each customer group by using a variety of methods, including focus groups, surveys, interviews, audits, and complaint tracking. Specifically, you'll see options for learning not only from patients, but also from visitors, employees, physicians, and payers. Chapter 6 also identifies a blueprint for other key measurement and feedback systems needed to collect the quantity and quality of data needed to control operational processes and drive improvement initiatives.

Pillar 4. Problem Solving and Process Improvement

The fourth pillar refers to problem solving and process improvement. Timely, organized, and effective systems for handling complaints, systems problems, and sorely needed process improvements increase customer satisfaction.

What happens in your organization when people complain? Is the complaint addressed and tracked so that, if there's a pattern of dissatisfaction, you can take steps to prevent the problem in the future? When people point to service weaknesses or make suggestions about how to make things better, what happens to their input? Systems and procedures that don't work must be weeded out and dealt with promptly before they threaten your strategy and your employees' morale.

Imagine a hospital in which all staff members excel in people skills. However, the hospital is plagued by systems problems. People always have to wait because of understaffing or poor scheduling procedures, the emergency department and front lobby never have enough wheelchairs, charts are lost, computers are down, medications aren't delivered at night, orders are mixed up, the supply of bed linens is never sufficient, people wait endlessly to be assigned a room, and so on.

When a hospital has systems problems, all of its key customer groups are victims: patients aren't happy, visitors aren't happy, physicians aren't happy, and employees are likely to be downright angry. Your organization needs to pay systematic attention to solving systems problems and to refining everyday work processes so that employees are able to provide accessible, convenient, user-friendly, and responsive service to customers—and ensure that they do.

Chapter 7 presents a variety of mechanisms for effective problem solving and process improvement—mechanisms that digest, prioritize, and process the riches of customer complaints, perceptions, and preferences. It also takes a hard look at the difficulties hospitals seem to have in tackling systems problems, the organizational obstacles that make these problems seem insurmountable, and a variety of strategies for making your organization more customer-friendly through process improvement.

Pillar 3 (measurement and feedback) represents ways to generate data from every one of your key customer groups. But what happens with those data? Unless you funnel the information into "improvement" processes—into the hands of people who have the power to listen and act—are you doing anything more than inviting your customers to vent? You need regular methods for making improvements, specifically process improvements, in order to ensure even better customer satisfaction and decreased staff frustration.

Pillar 5. Communication

"Nobody ever tells me anything!" Have you ever heard this said by employees or physicians? Employee attitude surveys show that employee morale is defeated more by no news than by bad news. We want our employees and physicians to be invested in and committed to the organization. But why should they be if managers don't keep them informed about how the organization is doing, what people are doing, and how they can help? People also want to know what is happening as a result of their efforts on the organization's behalf and as a result of their complaints, suggestions, and innovative ideas. In an information vacuum, key people feel ignored, unacknowledged, and unvalued for what they believe are valuable contributions. Finally, without communication about performance using such tools as storyboards and trend charts, staff may find it difficult to stay focused on customer priorities and initiate important improvements.

Chapter 8 identifies regular methods and systems for ensuring communication up, down, and sideways in your organization. Some specific techniques presented are:

- Enabling everyone organizationwide to see the big picture via regular leadership "advances," fireside chats, and employee updates

- Listening and responding to employees and physicians using such vehicles as the employee "sound-off" meeting, the "grapevine," and hotlines
- Reinforcing your service commitment through written devices such as house organs, letters from leaders, and bulletin boards
- Communicating about service performance using results-reporting memos, charts, feedback meetings, storyboards, storytelling, and more

Pillar 6. Staff Development and Training

The sixth pillar, staff development and training, is related to the array of *human* development needs that affect your organization's ability to deliver excellent service and achieve continuous improvement. Typically, managers and supervisors need training in how to install a cyclical customer-driven management system in their departments and programs to ensure continuously improving service. They also need to develop a customer orientation and the drive, spirit, and initiative that will catapult service performance forward. Many staff members need help sharpening their customer relations skills, including the art of meeting and greeting, extending sympathy, handling complaints, easing the stress of long waits, making small talk to ease anxiety, and even in just plain listening.

Chapter 9 identifies typical training needs for administrators, department heads and supervisors, nurses, frontline employees, people with substantial telephone contacts, people who have but a minute with the patient, job-specific groups, and others. It also describes state-of-the-art training delivery systems that go beyond classroom training to build effective habits and reinforce teamwork, mentoring, peer teaching, and support.

Pillar 7. Physician Involvement

Chapter 10 describes options that help physicians commit to active participation in your strategy. Strategies include briefings on service improvement, identification of process improvement priorities key to a physician-friendly institution, team building with nurses and others, feedback devices that shape physician behavior, and more. Chapter 10 also examines the nuances of the different groups (attending physicians, residents, and employed physicians) and identifies planning questions that need to be answered in determining a start-up approach. Then it describes several strategies for involving physicians, including:

- Building up-front commitment
- Helping physicians enhance their own behavior
- Using feedback to improve physician behavior
- Helping physicians build service-oriented practices
- Engaging physicians as partners
- Having physician liaisons who ease the physicians' way
- Helping staff deal with physicians effectively one-on-one

Pillar 8. Reward and Recognition

Excellence in service may be its own reward, but it's better to assume that it isn't. As part of your strategy, you need to align your reward and recognition strategies with your service vision and values so that individuals and teams have incentives to do more for the sake of service excellence.

Do your reward and recognition strategies reinforce the behaviors that reflect outstanding service? Are groups, departments, and individuals all included in the acknowledgment process? Chapter 11 examines a smorgasbord of strategies for recognizing and rewarding employees for excellent performance, contributions to teamwork, and service improvement. Strategies include:

- Auditing your current reward and recognition practices to identify the impact these are having on people's energy to excel on service dimensions, then creating a long-term improvement plan
- Aligning your compensation system with your service mission
- Ensuring that managers provide recognition to staff in their everyday words and deeds
- Recognizing teams for satisfying customers and taking steps to improve service
- Recognizing managers who exemplify your service commitment
- Creating positive feedback loops from external customers (patients and physicians) to staff
- Installing methods that make it easy for coworkers and peers to recognize each other for excellent service
- Using visual and written media to recognize service contributions
- Using recognition campaigns to focus attention and improvement on specific service needs (for example, phone skills)
- Celebrating your service mission and service accomplishments with occasional hoopla

Pillar 9. Employee Involvement and Empowerment

Involved employees are committed employees. Conversely, if your employees are demoralized or feel unappreciated and devalued in your environment, they are unlikely to give their best to their customers. To sustain a satisfied and productive work force, deliberate attention must be devoted to fostering employee involvement and empowerment.

Through participatory staff meetings, improvement teams, suggestion systems, and the like, you can engage employees in service improvement as hired heads, not just hired hands! You also need empowered employees, which means easing your employees into broader levels of authority and latitude to act to serve their customers. Chapter 12 identifies a menu of strategies for involving staff in service innovation and improvement and for helping them to act empowered and exercise excellent judgment as you expand their latitude to act on behalf of customers.

Pillar 10. Reminders and Refreshers

Time passes, and awareness fades. A whole host of other problems and pressures clutter people's busy work lives. This situation is what makes the tenth pillar, reminders and refreshers, so important.

You have to take action to remind people of your service priority and to refresh their minds, mind-set, and approaches. You're in competition for people's attention, and so you need to consciously institute methods that trigger attention to service excellence. Otherwise, well-intentioned people with their hearts in the right place just may not be thinking about it.

Chapter 13 describes a rich variety of ways to pull people's attention back to service excellence periodically so that service excellence does not become a stale or disappearing theme. The chapter describes House Rule of the Month campaigns, posters, pins, and other visual reminders, events and celebrations, refresher staff meetings to improve service, and the service lending library as examples of vehicles to draw attention to service excellence.

☐ Plans for Strengthening the Pillars

The options for strengthening the 10 components of a service-oriented culture can be overwhelming unless you plan carefully, prioritizing your needs and developing plans that suit your schedule and financial resources. Many hospitals have developed pillar-related task forces or subcommittees to develop blueprints for aligning the cultural practices in each area with their service mission. These short-term teams typically consist of a diverse group of executives and managers. The job of each team is to think for the organization about what it needs to do to bring practices related to their assigned pillar into alignment with their service mission. For example:

- The management vision and commitment team identifies the specific management expectations and actions needed to champion, model, and advance the organization's service mission and strategy.
- The accountability think tank figures out what needs to happen to the performance appraisal system, job descriptions, and personnel policies to support alignment with the organization's service mission and to foster continuous service improvement by individuals.
- The measurement and feedback team figures out how to measure progress on service dimensions (so that you can celebrate accomplishments and identify service improvement opportunities) and how to feed back the results so that data drive improvements.
- The problem-solving and process improvement team identifies structures and methods needed to respond effectively to customer problems and complaints, to use multiple data sources to identify service problems and snags, and to make process improvements that affect customer satisfaction.
- The communication team examines your methods of written and face-to-face communication and figures out how to augment them or alter their content to better support service excellence and continuous improvement. They also identify bridges and teams that need to be built among people within your organization.
- The physician involvement team figures out how to incorporate multiple layers of physicians into your service improvement strategy.
- The staff development and training team outlines the content and approach to training that will help people develop the competence and confidence to live your service commitment.
- The reward and recognition team identifies ways to strengthen your reward and recognition practices to align with and advance service by individuals and teams.
- The employee involvement and empowerment team identifies strategies for harnessing employee talent, energy, and ingenuity in making service improvements and in directly intervening with customers to meet their needs.
- The reminders and refreshers team identifies methods for keeping service issues visible so that your service strategy doesn't fade because people are not paying attention to it.

If you form teams to do your organization's thinking and planning related to bolstering these pillars, consider the questions in figure 3-2 as a guide. Throughout the process, ask, "Which other pillar teams do we need to consult because of potential overlap between our plans and theirs?" For example, the training team might want to consult and work with the recognition team when they want some form of recognition to be attached to completion of a training program.

☐ Strong Pillars Make Strong Service Cultures

The next 10 chapters of this book explore the pillars of continuous improvement one by one. You will find a rationale for each pillar as well as alternative approaches, illustrations, and suggestions. Note, please, that these pillars are not sequential or chronological. Read them according to your interests or in any order that appeals to you.

If your service improvement strategy is already in place, read with an eye toward identifying gaps or the telltale signs of crumbling pillars. If you have no strategy in place yet, use these pillars to build the cultural infrastructure you need to achieve an enduring service culture that fosters continuous service improvement.

Figure 3-2. Questions to Guide Planning Teams

1. What are our organization's current practices (both formal and informal) related to the pillar assigned to our team?
   - *Use brainstorming:* The technique of brainstorming gets people to generate as many of their thoughts as possible aloud without stopping to criticize or compliment along the way. By encouraging rapid flow of thoughts without discussion, brainstorming encourages people to speak up and think quickly.
   - *Use interviews or focus groups:* Consult employees/physicians to determine the practices that they perceive.
2. Related to our team's focus, to what extent do our current practices align with and advance our service mission and continuous service improvement?
   - What ARE our current practices?
   - How aligned is each with our service mission?
   - Which need to be strengthened? Maintained as is? Eliminated?

   Conduct interviews or focus groups with staff to find out which practices have positive versus negative effects on service quality. There may be practices that *seem* to advance service, but really don't because they don't have the desired effect on staff.

   Do force-field analysis. The logic that underlies the technique of force-field analysis is the following: To move toward alignment, you have to challenge the status quo. This can be done in two ways. You can:
   —Strengthen the practices that are currently pushing toward excellent service and continuous service improvement (the driving forces), or
   —Weaken or eliminate the practices that are impeding excellent service and continuous service improvement (the restraining forces).

   100% Alignment with Service Mission   0% Alignment

   ←——→

   Practices that *advance* service | Practices that are *consistent* with service mission but don't advance it | Practices that work *against* service mission

3. Related to this team's focus, if we were to start from scratch to build practices that align with and advance our service commitment, which practices would we want to institute?
4. Given everyday realities and the resources at hand in our organization, what do we propose as priorities to strengthen this pillar so that it bolsters our service commitment?
5. Related to each priority, specifically what needs to be done?
6. What human and material resources are needed to accomplish our proposed plan?
7. What would be a reasonable time line for achieving the priorities?

Chapter 4

Management Vision and Commitment

Before reading this chapter, complete the self-test in figure 4-1. Make copies and ask colleagues (including administrators, department heads, nonsupervisory employees, and physicians) to complete one from their perspective. Then count the number of true answers. If the average score is fewer than 10 "true" answers, you need to do some serious work at the management level to bolster your service strategy. Look at the "false" answers to see what you can do to strengthen management vision and commitment in your organization so that managers can effectively drive your service strategy. These results and the information in this chapter can help you engage your management team in a reexamination of the strategic importance they assign to service excellence in your organization and the leadership they demonstrate in the process of mobilizing others.

Progress toward customer satisfaction and continuous improvement is driven by leaders who explicitly communicate their commitment. You as a leader can build commitment to and participation in service quality improvement by modeling appropriate roles, setting standards, being visible and available, using personal clout to "move things," solving problems, holding people accountable, and being willing to take risks for the sake of making things better.

The management team is the most dangerous and most important element, because if you don't have top management support and leadership, you don't have a service strategy with potential to move the organization forward. Management support involves more than signing memos, attending workshops, and allocating money. Ideally, starting with top executives, managers need to *lead* the service strategy and behave as organizational champions for the value of service excellence.

To show long-term effects, service excellence must be made a key organizational value and commitment, pervasive at every level of the organization, but such a long-term commitment requires courageous leadership. Managers at all levels of the organization need to exert energy and direction; they need to be service champions who move people and systems toward service excellence.

This chapter will describe the following leadership functions, which are key building blocks to service improvement strategies:

- Leading with a service vision
- Practicing what you preach

Figure 4-1. Self-Test

Management Vision and Commitment. *Circle the appropriate answer. The more "true" answers, the better. "False" answers indicate areas that need improvement.*

1. Our administrative team communicates often and with feeling about the importance of excellent service and continuous improvement.	True	False
2. Our administrative team makes a deliberate effort to be visible and available to all levels of staff.	True	False
3. Our administrators demonstrate courtesy, concern, and responsiveness in their behavior toward customers and employees—serving as positive role models.	True	False
4. Managers here are obviously committed to meeting customer expectations.	True	False
5. Executives and managers here actively advance our priority of continuous service improvement by allocating significant time to it.	True	False
6. Our administrative team has made a public commitment to becoming more service-oriented and responsive to the needs of key customer groups.	True	False
7. Our administrators have made our service vision and mission very clear to all staff.	True	False
8. Our middle managers communicate that excellent service and continuous service improvement are priorities.	True	False
9. Middle managers actively implement our service strategy reflected by the fact that their departments have organized plans that ensure continuous improvement.	True	False
10. Our administrative team has clearly articulated how service excellence fits within our strategic plan.	True	False
11. Managers here can describe excellent service in concrete terms; they can describe what it looks like.	True	False
Total:	——	——

- Talking service passionately
- Listening and communicating with your employee customers
- Holding people accountable
- Taking risks
- Going for the long haul, not the quick fix

☐ Lead with a Service Vision

One of the most important acts of leaders at the executive level is to create a clear vision for service excellence and to communicate that direction to all staff. Although crucial, this often does not happen. Many organizations have plunged into service strategies without giving adequate attention to such questions as: What's this really for? What are we trying to create and why?

Good Samaritan Hospital in Lexington, Kentucky, is an example of an organization that has thoroughly integrated its service vision into its management and operations. The hospital has a vision of service excellence that celebrates the uniqueness of the contribution of every department in providing service to internal and external customers. To reinforce this vision, a stunning quilt has been placed on display in the hospital's front lobby. Each department crafted a square to express its vision of service excellence, and then hospital auxilians sewed the squares together to form the quilt. Hanging below the quilt, engraved on a bronze plaque, is the hospital's service vision of creating a "seamless" organization for the sake of patients.

Visions can explain strategic directions. A hospital in Texas chose to focus its service strategy on creating great partnerships with physicians. Their vision is: Unity and support in partnerships by which "together, we can deliver wonderful care to patients." This vision helps employees to focus their energies and explains the emphasis placed on relationships with physicians. It also makes managers aware of their responsibility in helping the hospital achieve its vision.

A vivid vision serves as an impetus to change. Duncan Moore, chief executive officer at Tallahassee Memorial Regional Medical Center, expresses his vision as a parable he shares with employees and reinforces with annual "Caring Hands Awards" (figure 4-2). This vision is also referred to when managers are called upon to make difficult decisions, such as supporting a very stringent dress code or participating in the creative redesign of patient care units.

A clearly stated vision provides employees and physicians with an image of an ideal future state that inspires them to work toward making it real. An inspiring vision is sensible and practical on the one hand and emotionally uplifting and compelling on the other hand. A vision creates a sense of security and focus for staff in the midst of change. When inevitable changes happen, leaders can draw everyone's attention toward the vision. It is the energy and commitment of people fueled by their vision that actually *moves* organizations.

Without *shared* focus, people work at cross-purposes and act according to their individual inclinations. Energies in the organization are dispersed in many directions. In contrast, staff in an organization with a shared vision align their energies in one direction, thus reducing conflict and harnessing everyone's energy toward the same ends.

Your organization's leaders need to develop a unique service mission and vision for your organization and then share them with every employee and physician. A powerful vision fully shared inspires everyone.

Understanding Your Shared Mission, Vision, and Values

It is important to distinguish the differences among *missions, visions,* and *values*. All three play significant parts in providing a sense of direction for employees and physicians.

Your organization's mission clarifies what kind of business it is in and why it exists. Missions also tend to be highly stable over time. A small rural hospital might have as its mission: To provide the very best care to the people of our community. A large teaching

Figure 4-2.   Vision Statement: Tallahassee Memorial Regional Medical Center

---

Because Our Hands Are Different

There is a mission hospital located in the mountains of a very poor country in South America. The country is largely populated by native Indians who live in small, primitive villages, and who speak no English. Medical care is limited to a few mission hospitals located in various mountain villages.

An international organization reviewing the health care of this country's natives found, to their amazement, that natives would walk for days, often carrying sick loved ones on their backs, to get to one particular mission hospital located in one of the country's more inaccessible mountain ranges.

On asking why they came to this particular hospital when they could have gone to one much closer to their village, the natives would answer, "At this hospital, the hands are different."

The study team found that in spite of cultural differences, language barriers, and the great distance over rough terrain, this particular mission hospital had gained the reputation that, above all else, they truly cared for the natives in everything they did. Thus, the native explanation was that "the hands are different."

Likewise, we want people to come to Tallahassee Memorial Regional Medical Center because "the hands are different." As one of the largest hospitals in the state of Florida, Tallahassee Memorial caters to the needs of patients from north Florida, south Georgia, and southeast Alabama. We think that patients from these areas, as well as the ones from within our own city, choose us because our hands are different.

And what makes our hands different is a reflection of our employees.

Reprinted, with permission, from Tallahassee Memorial Regional Medical Center, Tallahassee, Florida.

hospital might have a three-part mission: To provide teaching, research, and patient care all in the service of advancing the short-term and long-term health of the community.

Your organization's vision presents an image of what the organization's mission would be if it were completely fulfilled. Visions change with time, with technology, and with imagination. Visions spell out how you want to be perceived by patients, the kind and scope of service you want to provide, the relationships and partnerships you want to develop with stakeholders, and the culture you want to create.

Values provide guidelines for behavior, decisions, and relationships. They spell out *how* you want everyone to act to achieve your vision and mission. Terms such as *compassion*, *professionalism*, *quality*, and *teamwork* appear in different forms on the value statements of most health care organizations.

Shared mission, vision, and values encourage teamwork. People work from shared assumptions about what is appropriate behavior; they know what is expected of them and what to expect from one another. You can comfortably allow room for personal initiative and commitment when the criteria for success are clear, for example:

- My individual actions and behavior are moving us toward our vision.
- Our plans/decisions are *congruent* with or *in alignment with* our mission, vision, and values.

Because most health care organizations have clear missions and statements of their core values and far fewer have articulated their visions of service excellence (even before launching a service strategy), our discussion here focuses on the development of a vision. The process of developing a service vision can be a powerful opportunity for clarifying direction and improving unity and relationships within the organization's leadership. However, an organization's vision can never be something you borrow from another organization or find in a book on the shelf. It requires hard work and a collaborative effort.

Developing Your Vision

Developing and clarifying your vision starts with envisioning ideal service. The following techniques have been used by executive teams to help them craft their visions:

- *The nonstop writing technique:* A facilitator asks each member of the executive team to write nonstop (or to ramble on paper) for 5 to 10 minutes, with no concern for grammar, sentence structure, or organization. The idea is for the participants to envision (and record on paper) the hospital of their dreams. Participants then share the key points of their writings, capturing them on a flipchart, and brainstorm together looking for patterns and themes.
- *The guided fantasy technique:* A facilitator asks the participants to relax with eyes closed and to mentally take a guided tour through their organizations three years into the future, after the service strategy has achieved wonderful results. For 5 or 10 minutes, participants picture walking through the front door of the facility, hearing patients and families talking, observing the admissions process, riding the elevators, walking the hallways, feeling the atmosphere on patient floors and in offices, and more. The participants then share their images and look for ideals they have in common. The organization's vision statement is then built around these images.
- *Round robin of mutual interviews:* A facilitator or executive leader identifies the group of administrators and medical leaders who are to play a part in developing the organization's service vision. Each participant, or group of participants, receives a research question, for example:
  —In our ideal hospital, what service qualities would patients see?
  —In our ideal hospital, what service qualities would impress our physicians?
  —For employees, what would be the most sustaining events in a typical day?

—For physicians, what would be the quality of interactions with other staff?

—What would a visitor's experience be like?

—What would happen when a patient complained?

The facilitator arranges for each person or group to interview others so that every person or group asks the assigned questions of several others and answers every other question once. Afterward, the people who asked question number one convene, synthesize the results, and prepare to report them to the whole group. And so on with appropriate groups assigned to each of the other questions. After the reports, the entire group identifies the key elements in its service vision by drawing on the composite results of all of the interviews.

Figure 4-3 provides an example of a service vision statement.

Deciding Who Creates the Vision

There are several schools of thought about who should create an organization's service vision. In some organizations, executives create the vision, believing that this is their responsibility and prerogative as leaders. In other organizations, executive teams involve physicians, trustees, managers, and sometimes frontline staff in the process. The first option tends to solidify ownership at the top. The leaders assert their vision and take responsibility for carrying it out. The problem created by this approach is that leaders then have to "sell" the vision to others. In the second option, executives involve other stakeholders in defining the vision. This way, they don't need to "sell" it because everyone had a part in its creation. However, members of the organization who have been sold someone else's vision are sometimes less likely to advance the vision with the driving force of personal commitment that comes from having played a role in its creation. Each organization has to pick the option that will work best for it.

Sharing Your Vision

Regardless of which approach is taken, the resulting vision needs organizationwide ownership and support. Some hospitals accomplish this by communicating the vision to staff and physicians at all levels, eliciting their reactions with a technique called force-field analysis. They ask people to generate the forces working for and against the vision and to identify ways to strengthen the driving forces and weaken the restraining or opposing forces. This helps to engage everyone in perceiving the gap between the current reality and the vision and allows them to feel the stretch necessary to achieve the vision. Some organizations create visual images and maps of the vision or succinct verbal descriptions that all managers then communicate to and discuss with staff.

Figure 4-3. "People First" Strategy: MetroHealth System, Cleveland

- We, employees of the MetroHealth System, will do whatever it takes to anticipate and satisfy the needs of everyone who comes in contact with us.

- We will listen to everyone we meet in a polite, friendly, helpful, understanding, and caring way.

- We will continue to improve the hospital environment to make it more pleasant, clean, safe, quiet, comfortable, and easy to use.

- We will continuously review our systems, policies, and procedures to make sure they are convenient and responsive to those we work with and serve.

- We will work together and treat everyone as we would like to be treated ourselves.

Reprinted, with permission, from the customer services department of MetroHealth Medical Center, Cleveland, Ohio.

Generating Commitment to Your Vision

Crafting and sharing the vision is only the first step. The next step involves generating commitment to the vision—wanting the vision so much that you can taste it! The leadership team must personally embrace the vision and help everyone else in the organization to do the same. Every leader needs to identify what the organization has to gain from a wholehearted focus on excellent service. After all, it will take substantial time, attention, money, and energy to move from your current service reality to your vision.

☐ Practice What You Preach

Once your vision has been clarified, management's job is to foster organizational alignment with it. In a condition of perfect alignment, organizational practices and people's behavior and decisions all contribute to your service mission and vision. To foster alignment, then, managers must lead the charge by examining their own actions and decisions first and bringing them into alignment with the organization's service mission and vision. For example, if outsiders analyzed your budget, would they be able to detect your quest for service excellence and continuous improvement? If outsiders examined the content of management-structured staff meetings (for example, department head meetings), would your commitment to service excellence be glaringly apparent? If they followed managers around and witnessed their behavior with others—would the priority on service quality be impossible to miss?

Executives, managers, and physician leaders need to walk the walk. They must align themselves with the organization's vision and be role models of service excellence. Once the vision has been boldly communicated, management needs to translate this vision into specific standards that they exemplify through their own behavior. When employees talk about administrators, common themes emerge. Many employees see executive managers as people who are detached and out of touch with what's really happening in the organization, people who are concerned only with the bottom line. Administrators are often accused of exempting themselves from the standards they set for others—in other words, of failing to practice what they preach.

Exactly what should administrators do to set appropriate examples? Administrators need to put four primary behaviors into practice by:

- Moving close to customers
- Modeling excellent customer relations
- Modeling collegial support
- Becoming visible

Moving Close to Customers

Leaders need to devote attention to and demonstrate concern for all of the organization's customers. They can do this by personally taking steps to understand customer expectations and perceptions, by installing systems that monitor customer satisfaction and perceptions of performance, and by inviting complaints. For example, administrators might call on at least one patient, physician, or employee every day. Not only would this build goodwill, it would also create a direct feedback channel between the administrator and the customers who are the end users of the system. Such feedback is the most powerful information source available. Going to your customers shows your employees and your customers that you care about the people on the other end of your services.

The best way to keep customer needs fresh in your mind is to talk with customers, not read reports about them. Consider developing a plan that keeps your leadership team in touch with customers and prods leaders to check in with customers about their experience with your services. Here's an example of such a plan:

- Each week, call two family members of patients to find out about their experience with your hospital and employees.
- Once a week, talk with two patients (for example, over lunch) to ask them about their experience with your hospital.
- Call two physicians a month to touch base and find out how your hospital is treating them.
- Once a month, hold an employee breakfast. Invite a small group of employees (randomly selected by your human resources manager) to share their views about quality of work life, current organizational strategies, and problems.
- Once a month, call two referrers and encourage them to share their perceptions of your hospital and its treatment of them as referrers.

Ask your customers simple questions such as:

- How are we treating you lately?
- What do we do that works well for you?
- Where do your frustrations lie?
- Any suggestions?

All you need to do is listen, listen, listen, and then thank the individuals for speaking up. Although this takes time, managers who follow this plan spend at most nine hours each month systematically listening to customers. If you think about your organization's service mission and believe in the primacy of customer needs and expectations, it's a worthwhile expenditure of time and energy.

Modeling Excellent Customer Relations

Employees legitimately expect administrators to be role models and standard setters in interactions with employees, patients, visitors, and physicians. When managers demonstrate the behavior they want to see throughout the organization, accusations of hypocrisy and double standards fade.

When they are asked which behaviors matter the most, employees cite the behavior of executives in public areas. Administrators first need to be personable and welcoming in these public areas, in hallways, elevators, lobbies, and the cafeteria. If administrators do this just during their forays into public areas, they can alter their image quite significantly. Administrators need to show employees and physicians that professionals extend themselves to other people in all work situations, no matter what their mood, and especially in public areas where they contribute to the atmosphere the organization projects to customers and staff.

Try the following suggestions to move closer to your customers. In elevators:

- Make eye contact and say "hello."
- Offer to push floor buttons for people.
- Help the transporter with patients in wheelchairs or on stretchers. Open doors.
- Introduce yourself: "Hi, I'm _____. I don't believe we've met."
- Make small talk: "How do you like this weather?" "I bet you have a busy day ahead of you." "How's our hospital treating you lately?" "I see you work in the Dietary Department. How's it going?"

In hallways:

- The single most noticeable and important behavior is to establish eye contact, smile, and say "hello" to employees, patients, physicians, and visitors as you walk along instead of being absorbed in your own thoughts about the next meeting or that phone call you have to make.

- Walk at a moderate pace so that you don't appear too busy to notice the human beings along the way. Don't read memos in the hallways. Making quick contacts with people can be done without even slowing down your pace.
- Call people by name when you know them. A simple "Hello, Jim," suffices.

In quick interactions with employees, administrators can also show recognition and appreciation for excellent service behavior by sharing a compliment. For example, "I've heard good things about the burn unit lately. A woman wrote the other day about how pleased she was with the way you folks handled her son."

Employees want, need, and deserve to see administrators extend excellent service. Administrators need to find ways, in their own style, to connect with their employees and model positive customer relations toward all guests. Doing this may mean changing their behavior, but administrators ask that of employees all the time.

Modeling Collegial Support

Another administrative role that gets scant attention is the exchange of mutual support among administrators themselves. Few administrators are truly aware of their staff's perception of top-level management as a group. Typical comments about administrators include statements like these: "They just go about their business, rushing around, sitting in endless meetings, handling crises, prodding people to do their jobs, and acting more important than we are." Or, "Up there, one hand doesn't know what the other hand is doing. They don't know which end is up on the administrative floor!" Would any administrator's heart be warmed by such employee perceptions? Would any administrator consider them fair?

Administrators endure tremendous stress because they are responsible for the overall experiences of patients, the quality of life of physicians and staff, and the financial viability of the whole organization. To work successfully in a stressful environment, administrators need to support one another. They should not put one another down or fail to appreciate one another's accomplishments. When they fail to show collegial support for each other, employees and physicians notice, lose confidence in the administration, and follow suit in their behavior toward their own peers.

Administrators need to take active steps to develop their team image as strong, productive, and caring individuals engaged in a *team effort* to make the organization a place that works for everyone. Here are suggestions for developing support:

- Confront administrators who point their fingers at one another. Expect your team to help and support one another. Embrace every individual's accomplishment as a team accomplishment and every problem as a team problem.
- Discuss how to handle situations in which one administrator gripes to another about a third person. Set a norm that requires confronting the person involved directly, instead of venting to a third party and feeding the grapevine.
- Practice delivering bad news to department heads without blaming another administrator. Proclaim the importance of "keeping the faith," and explore together ways to accomplish this when the going gets tough.
- Ask administrators to model teamwork, mutual interchange, and information sharing by attending one another's meetings with department heads and employee groups and working collaboratively.

Everyone wins when administrators promote one another, show respect, and acknowledge one another publicly as effective, accomplished leaders worthy of the trust of employees and patients. This mutual support among colleagues fuels the concept of service excellence and builds confidence in management.

Becoming Visible

A contemporary management commandment proclaimed by Tom Peters and Robert Waterman is management by wandering around (MBWA).[1] On the one hand, employees need to know who their leaders are, they need to see them in action, and they need to observe their interest in frontline people and customers. On the other hand, administrators need to touch base with operational realities firsthand and assess the attitudes of their employees.

However, just getting out of the boardroom and office and strolling around the workplace is not enough. The following guidelines may help to make the visits to units and departments more noticeable and important to staff:

- Talk to people: "How are things going today?"
- Find out when most employees take their breaks or when the slower, calmer times are, and visit then so that you're less intrusive. Tell the nurse manager or department head that you'd like to visit just to say hello and talk to people. Let people know when to expect you.
- If you're uncomfortable, buddy up with an experienced colleague. One hospital formalized this type of visit as *walking-around training,* so that every administrator would be good at it and less hesitant to do it.
- *At the very least,* be sure to:
  - Smile.
  - Make eye contact.
  - Give your name.
  - Use the other person's name. If you don't know the name, ask it, and then use it.
  - Inquire about employees personally, their work, their departments, their lives outside of work.

As you walk around, remember the following:

- Don't tell anyone to do anything.
- Don't criticize anything. If you see a problem, address it through the proper channels later.
- Don't be a spy or a judge.
- Be calm and positive. If you look concerned, employees will think you're concerned with the health of the organization, and they'll lose faith, or they'll take it personally and feel judged or accused.
- Don't be distracted. Listen to what people say and respond appropriately.

Most administrators express a desire to increase their visibility, but they don't seem to get around to doing anything about it. Their only hope, many claim, is to develop a schedule for wandering around in a time-limited way, in effect to make *short* excursions designed to increase their visibility. The key is to stick to this routine religiously because visibility must stay a priority, not the first activity to eliminate when other demands arise. The following are tried-and-true methods for achieving administrative visibility:

- *Surprise welcome:* Administrators stand at a main entrance to the hospital for 30 minutes a day for one week and greet and introduce themselves to employees, visitors, and physicians. This welcoming activity should be done at different entrances at peak times of day so that the administrator can meet as many different people as possible. Administrators need to speak only briefly to each person: "Good morning. I'm not sure we've met. My name is Lee Weston. I'm an administrator. And you, where do you work? Very nice meeting you."

- *Administrative grand rounds:* Employees often say that administration is out of touch with the real life on patient floors. Administrators can make rounds, visiting different units and work areas, greeting employees, introducing themselves, asking how things are going, and showing an interest in learning what different jobs are like. One idea that works well is to have a different administrator "on call" each week—this administrator makes daily rounds to a sampling of units and departments and talks with staff and patients.
- *Administrators as tray delivery squad:* To get to know about people's jobs and to touch base with patients, administrators can deliver food trays to patients for 30 minutes each week. This way they can spend a few minutes with each patient, introducing themselves and asking, "How have we been treating you?" Then the administrator should provide feedback to staff on any praise or problems mentioned by patients. Perhaps the administrator can write a positive piece for the employee newsletter based on the experience.

Employees look to management for leadership and to set standards. They also use nonexemplary behavior by management as an excuse for nonexemplary behavior on their part. As Will Rogers once said, "People learn more from observation than they do from conversation."

☐ Talk Service Passionately

Managers need to communicate their unambiguous commitment to service excellence and the organization's service strategy. If they communicate mixed feelings, they leave others feeling uncomfortable rather than charged up and motivated. The following examples demonstrate ways in which administrators might present their thoughts about service excellence. Read each example and ask yourself, "what's wrong with this picture?"

Example 1: "I just came back from the administrator's meeting where we discussed the service excellence strategy that the corporation is endorsing. It sounds to me like the executive team really is serious about this. They made it clear that we had to come back here and tell you they mean business, so that's what I'm telling you."

This administrator is taking no personal responsibility for initiating the service excellence strategy. The idea came from corporate, and it's clear that the administrator feels no ownership. If the administrator does not convey passion and conviction, why should anyone else?

Example 2: "I'm sorry to pull you away from your work today. I know that each one of you is incredibly busy, but I'd like to discuss service excellence with you quickly. We're doing a program here to help us look for ways we can improve the service we deliver. Now I know how hard everyone is already working and how much pressure everyone is under; nonetheless, even though I know how stressed everyone is, I'd appreciate anything, even little things, that would make a difference."

This administrator goes overboard with empathy, apologies, and begging. Administrators must take a firm stand and clearly state a position of strong commitment to creating a service-oriented culture. Also, the idea that a meeting to discuss service issues "pulls people away from their work" instead of being critical and inherent to their work sends a destructive message.

Example 3: "Folks, we are initiating a service improvement strategy in our organization and it's about time. I'm delighted. I know how good we are in this hospital. I think this service strategy will make other hospitals look at us and want to be as great as we are. So that's what's happening. I thought you'd be interested."

If everything is so great, why should anyone bother to do anything differently? It's hard to get people excited about a strategy they have been told they don't need!

Example 4: "I have a very strong message to deliver. I've just come back from an administrative team meeting that dealt with the way service is delivered throughout our hospital. We talked about something I've known for a long time, and that is we must improve the quality of the service we deliver. And I'm pleased to say that everyone agrees. Service is critical, we must work for and support excellence. It's the direction this hospital must take. Our patients deserve it, the hospital depends on it, and, frankly, if you want to be with the organization next month, it is something you'd better support. I simply won't tolerate anything less than excellence from you or you're out of here."

Motivation by fear and intimidation does not work with service excellence. People need to feel good about the strategy and want to be involved in creating a better organization. Most will get on board if you avoid fear tactics.

Following are four groups of questions that administrators and managers can use to clarify their commitment and prepare to educate successive layers of people about service excellence:

1. What does "excellent service" mean to me?
2. What would this organization be like if we were truly "customer/service oriented?"
3. What do I want to change at this hospital regarding service quality?
4. Why is service excellence important? To us in particular? To me personally? To staff? To our physicians? To our community? What's in it for senior management? Why should we care about service excellence and take on the ambitious long-term strategy to improve service and create a culture of continuous improvement?

Once each team member has answered these questions, individuals on the team need to go a step further to formulate and practice articulating a *personal* commitment statement for repeated use with others throughout the organization. The following questions will help you formulate the personal commitment statement:

1. What do I want to see happen? (Summarize your service mission.)
2. *Why* do I want to see this happen? What are the benefits for patients? family members? quality of work life? ourselves (for example, integrity, self-esteem, and pride)? the organization (for example, bottom line)?
3. *How* will we make this happen? (a brief summary of service excellence strategy)
4. Express a pinch of empathy (for example, "This will not be easy in our atmosphere of lean staffing . . .").
5. My own statement of commitment—with feeling (for example, "I'm excited about this venture. I'm going to give it my all").

Who needs to hear your personal commitment to service quality improvement? Everybody, starting with senior management, medical leadership, department heads, supervisors, and all employees. Use a mix of vehicles and opportunities:

1. Make a bold statement about your service commitment and put it in writing. Post it in prominent places where a wide range of employees will see it.

2. In meetings with your management team, department heads, board, and medical staff, discuss your personal vision and commitment and invite discussion to make sure others in leadership positions understand *why* service excellence matters. Prepare a kickoff commitment speech. Follow it up at future meetings by weaving your commitment to service excellence into various remarks and speeches.
3. Look for opportunities to verbally reiterate your service commitment. When giving feedback and appreciation, make comments like: "The way you handled that doctor was great. You certainly demonstrated our commitment to service excellence." Or, "I really appreciate the way you're helping this hospital become known for great service." Other opportune moments include reward and recognition events, session for complaint handling, interdepartmental meetings, staff meetings during reports of accomplishments and plans, and introductions of new policies and procedures.

Every day, managers can find opportunities to verbalize their commitment to service in brief, one-line messages to staff and colleagues, *if* they look for these opportunities. How and how often managers share their passion for service excellence influences your employees' willingness and ability to carry out your vision.

☐ Listen and Communicate with Your Employee Customers

Engage in and encourage direct two-way communication with employees. Ask, listen, and communicate. The discussion of pillar 5 (on communication) in chapter 8 provides strategies that are key to communicating with your employees (internal customers). In this section, we emphasize the importance of creating an arena in which you invite employees to discuss their concerns and perceptions and listen nondefensively to them.

Set up open forums—or "sound-off" sessions—for employees at least quarterly, preferably on all shifts. Some administrators call these "rap sessions" or "talks with Jim." Define a time and place for constructive venting, where you encourage people to express frustration, worry, resentment, ambivalence, and so forth, and where you and others can open yourselves to whatever people think and feel. Invite employees to sound off about positives and negatives in the organization and their work life in particular. Then follow up.

☐ Hold People Accountable

How accountable should your administrators be for employee and customer relations? Unless you consider administrators accountable, you're in an unworkable bind. Administrators, consciously or subconsciously, set the tone and standards for employee behavior. Employees watch the behavior of administrators and listen to their rhetoric. When an administrator is not committed to excellent service, employees get the message.

Administrators may seem like bigger-than-life figures to employees. Their behaviors are watched and talked about. They set expectations as well as the tone and culture of the organization. They set the internal accountability mechanisms, and they set the rules and establish the systems. If a rude person is allowed to be rude year after year, how can you not point to administrative tolerance as the source of the unenforced standards? To escape the reality of administrative accountability is to negate the tremendous power of authority figures in organizations.

When an organization's strategy is aimed at service improvement, administrators must pay determined attention to accountability. Specifically, they need to shape middle-management behavior so that the internal accountability mechanisms of the organization help middle managers internalize higher standards and engage in behavior that supports, enforces, and reinforces this behavior throughout the work force. The top people must hold each other and middle managers accountable; otherwise, the middle people will not hold the frontline people accountable.

Consider an example from the airline industry. Under President Jan Carlzon, Scandinavian Airlines went from an $8 million loss in 1981 to a $71 million profit in less than one year. Carlzon's strategy was to transform the organization's focus from its internal production capabilities to an obsession with customer needs and desires. The company emphasized high standards of courtesy and service during every flight and in all peripheral services related to travel.

After its initial tremendous success, standards at Scandinavian Airlines started to slide. Planes started being late, employees were less cheerful, and service in general seemed to get sloppy. To try to learn what was wrong, Scandinavian Airlines conducted an organizational critique. They concluded that the quick change, with its emphasis on closeness to the customer, had bypassed middle management. Frontline people got more attention and rewards and more authority and resources to solve problems. Because middle managers felt left out, they resisted the changes. They continued to defend their own turf and operate according to their own individual ideas. This tug-of-war between top management's stated values and middle management's ideas created a motivational problem among frontline employees.

The problems at Scandinavian Airlines show that top managers need to do several things during the implementation of service improvements:

- Consider carefully the role of middle managers in service excellence.
- Set explicit expectations for middle managers.
- Communicate these expectations to middle managers.
- Monitor middle-management performance and enforcing and reinforcing the expectations set.

Many top executives assume that middle managers know what to do. Perhaps that's true when it comes to their overall roles. However, based on the authors' experiences with hospital middle managers across the country, it is certainly not true in the area of service excellence. Some middle managers consider service excellence to be less important than the specialized tasks their departments perform. Other middle managers have long had problems with rude employees and have made excuses for not handling the problem: "There are always a few bad apples" or "You can't win 'em all" or "He's been here for so many years that it's too late now." The thought of raising standards and enforcing them is seen as just another external pressure that will go away eventually. Still other managers perceive no blatant problems in their departments, and therefore they feel that they needn't do anything about service excellence. They've become accustomed to mediocrity or, in many cases, don't recognize the missed opportunities for their people to move beyond mediocrity to excel and impress their customers.

When executive management is really serious about achieving service excellence, new and serious expectations must be set for middle management. Preferably these expectations would also apply organizationwide to all employees. For example:

- Middle managers exemplify excellent service in interactions with patients, visitors, physicians, and employees and serve as positive role models.
- Working with individual subordinates, they develop job-specific expectations that lead the employees toward service excellence.
- Middle managers hold regular meetings with subordinates to inform them of institutionwide issues, events, and priorities and to identify and solve departmental problems.
- They monitor service-oriented behavior among employees; they ask about it, comment on it, reinforce it, and reiterate its importance.
- They confront employees who violate service expectations, and they use established disciplinary processes to counsel, coach, and, when necessary, terminate

employees who do not fulfill service standards. Service-oriented managers never tolerate mediocrity.

- Middle managers develop and sustain open lines of communication with employees. They listen to employees' concerns and respond in a timely, caring fashion.

When faced with complaints about the rudeness of frontline employees, administrators should investigate and hold the department heads accountable for the behavior of the people in their department. Incidents cannot be allowed to pass unnoticed.

☐ Take Risks

For most health care organizations, advancement toward consistently excellent service and an obsession with satisfying customers means change, and change triggers severe allergic reactions in most organizations, especially in health care. An enhanced emphasis on customer satisfaction, the concept of the patient as a customer, pressure on employees to achieve customer satisfaction despite how hard they are already working—all of these involve cultural change and changed behavior on the part of individuals.

To trigger such change, top management must first decide how it wants to change the organization. It has to make daring decisions. It has to follow through and not back off. It has to take *risks*.

In *Managerial Courage: Revitalizing Your Company without Sacrificing Your Job*, Hornstein said:

Managers become leaders by going beyond what is . . . and seeking what might be. Leaders ask fundamental questions about the appropriateness and effectiveness of established practice. They jeopardize their own welfare, since they're rocking everyone's boat. Managers who ascend the corporate ladder because they're compromising, cautious, and conforming are essential to the successful maintenance of day-to-day organizational functions. They keep the system running smoothly and predictably. They become leaders only if they find the courage to question the system and risk shaking it up.[2]

When you consider the culture of health care organizations, does the image of a turtle come to mind? Slow as the turtle is, it makes progress only when it sticks its neck out. The same is true for health care administrators. Risk taking by top management is a necessity in launching and sustaining any service improvement strategy. Administrators are rarely popular when they press for higher standards. One reason is that even they can't be sure that their best-laid plans will actually work.

The key to success, then, is keeping an experimenter's mind-set. No recipe guarantees service excellence. The best administrators can do is help to research the possibilities at each juncture, follow hunches, build on successes, and learn from mistakes. If your administrative people do not want to make a move until they have guarantees, they will sit forever on the dime and your organization will stagnate as it pays lip service to service excellence.

Franklin Delano Roosevelt said it best: "It is common sense to take a method and try it. If it fails, admit it frankly and try another. But above all, try something."

☐ Go for the Long Haul, Not the Quick Fix

Don't start up unless you plan to follow up. Service excellence only works as a long-term business strategy, as a continuous thrust that drives your organization.

Don't let your organization start until it is committed to continue year after year. If your service excellence effort is short-lived, the frustrated employee who prejudges it as "just another flash in the pan" will be painfully correct and understandably resentful. Set objectives and plan for the future. Don't undertake change just to keep up with the Joneses. Know why you're doing what you're doing, and set objectives in terms of quality, costs, and risks.

In your organization, is service excellence rhetoric or reality? Does a long-term commitment to service excellence show up in management's annual budget as an operating expense line item that continues year after year, like salaries? Or are expenditures for service excellence an afterthought? Consider these words of Flip Wilson: "Don't let your mouth write a check that your body can't cash." Commit dollars to service excellence. It's not a frivolous expenditure; it's a crucial and astute investment in quality.

If top management develops myopia about the benefits of a continued service commitment, try some of the following methods:

- Call in an outside expert on service improvement to talk about the necessity of follow-through. An outsider can describe the false starts other hospitals experienced when they let up on their efforts. An outsider does not have to mince words. Also, administrators often are more likely to listen to an outside expert.
- Create a diagnostic tool that pushes your administration to look at components of a long-range strategy and to identify the missing links. Sometimes they realize they'll lose the hard-won gains they've achieved if they don't continue to attack weaknesses.
- Look at data about customer satisfaction, and interview patients, visitors, physicians, and employees. Find out what's going well and what still needs to be improved. You can then use the survey to show your administration that more work is needed.
- Scrutinize the patterns of complaints identified by your patient representatives.
- Collect published material that discusses what makes a service excellence or guest relations strategy successful in the long run. Channel the material to administrators through the people who influence them.
- Convene a group of people who are opinion leaders in the organization. Use any of the preceding strategies to convince them of the need for follow-up. Then brainstorm with them about how to get the necessary support from top management.
- Develop an explicit, specific plan for follow-up. Perhaps you can bring in a consultant to conduct a stock-taking retreat. Present your concrete plan to your management team. Administrators often resist follow-up because they can't visualize it.

Management philosophy and practices are a critical underpinning of your service improvement strategy and are worth dwelling on up front—before you find your edifice crumbling.

☐ Final Suggestions

Consider that certain myths can doom a service excellence strategy to failure. If you hear any of the following statements made in relation to your strategy, take action:

- *"They either have it, or they don't!"* This statement is not true about leaders. When it comes to service excellence, administrative support and leadership lies on a continuum. Administrators, like other real people, vary: some are supportive, some skeptical, others cynical, and many changeable in their views. Although their rhetoric is a prerequisite to launching your strategy, you can still succeed even when they aren't perfect role models or gung-ho service champions. In a persistent, carefully wrought strategy, peer pressure and upward pressure from your savvy frontline people can gradually shape and strengthen administrators' behavior.

- *"I can't confront my administrator."* When a lack of resource commitment is eroding your efforts, you have to confront the administrator. Middle managers who have a stake in and responsibility for service excellence should creatively and persistently confront (or bring in an outsider to play the heavy) top management about what the organization needs to do to make its service strategy deliver the hoped-for results.
- *"Administrators are just too busy. We shouldn't bother them."* Administrators are indeed incredibly busy. However, service excellence only takes hold if it's an organizationwide priority. Delegating it entirely just doesn't work. Also, if service excellence does not live in the minds and hearts of top management, they will not think, feel, and act in ways that advance it.

Management vision and commitment set the stage and enable the key players—every employee and physician—to move in the same direction: toward customer satisfaction. Starting with a vision of service excellence, the top brass and every other layer of managers and supervisors need to set the tone through their own behavior; to build responsive, user-friendly systems that enable caregivers to serve their customers; to communicate openly to build understanding, commitment, and investment; and to enforce and reinforce inviolable high standards.

References

1. Peters, T., and Waterman, R. *In Search of Excellence.* New York City: Harper & Row, 1982.

2. Hornstein, H. *Managerial Courage: Revitalizing Your Company without Sacrificing Your Job.* New York City: John Wiley and Sons, 1986.

Chapter 5
Accountability

- A nurse manager interviews and hires an extremely competent nurse with impressive credentials. After she's been on the job for a while, however, it becomes obvious that she has a severe attitude problem. "I can't understand it," the manager wonders in dismay. "After all we went through to hire the best person."
- A maintenance worker sees a film on customer relations and thinks, "That's nice. But what does it have to do with me?"
- Many people wonder why a notoriously rude employee who's been a blemish on the hospital's image for years is allowed to continue this behavior unchallenged.
- When told of an employee's lack of service orientation, the employee's supervisor says, "I know he's very difficult, but we can't afford to lose him."

These situations reveal gaps in an organization's accountability systems, gaps that impede service improvement. These situations are not unusual in hospitals and are symptoms of weakness in the organization's culture that will affect service improvement. They also typify organizations that are usually disappointed in the results of their strategies.

Accountability systems need to support your service strategy. In the situations mentioned, training is not the answer. The groundwork for accountability needs to be laid in revised human resource practices that support excellent service performance and provide coaching and counseling for people who do not perform in line with service standards. In the first situation, a nurse with an attitude problem was given the job because hiring practices targeted technical competence at the expense of service skills. In the second example, the new-employee orientation process did not help the maintenance worker understand his or her role in customer satisfaction. In the third example, a problem employee's continued rudeness, year after year, demoralized and angered coworkers and no doubt turned customers off. Human resource practices failed to put "teeth" into the organization's service standards. And in the fourth example, the supervisor shirked responsibility for ensuring that employees meet service standards, apparently believing that service behavior is optional and not a realistic expectation of all staff.

In these examples, managers and supervisors did not insist on conformance to service standards. Most likely, human resource practices existed to help managers hold employees accountable, but the managers did not use them and were not themselves held accountable by their own supervisors for following them.

How well do your current human resource policies support service excellence? To find out, take the self-test in figure 5-1. If you are able to answer true to every question, your accountability systems support your service commitment. The more false answers, the more you need to strengthen accountability so that your practices support consistent conformance to high service standards among managers and staff. Employees may recognize the value your organization places on service quality, but without accountability mechanisms, you can't expect conformance to improvement-related standards. For example:

- Can people get a better raise for being exemplary in service quality?
- Will employees who violate service standards experience any consequences?
- Will disciplinary actions related to service behavior stick?

Unless there are solid "teeth" in your service strategy, negativity and mediocrity may continue to be tolerated.

Managers and supervisors need to know that they are responsible for achieving excellent service within their domains and that their everyday practices and goals must align with the organization's service vision. They must be able to clarify service expectations for all staff and to obtain backup support in confronting service offenders. They need to know that they are *expected* to hold employees accountable to high service standards and that the system will support them when they do. Finally, managers and supervisors must call on the organization's coaching, performance improvement, and disciplinary processes to help employees improve their service behaviors or risk the consequences—including termination. The remainder of this chapter is devoted to an exploration of the

Figure 5-1. Self-Test

Current Human Resource Policies and Service Excellence. *Circle the appropriate answer. The more "true" answers, the better. "False" answers indicate areas that need improvement.*

1. Courteous, respectful, and compassionate behavior toward patients and other customers is a *requirement* in our organization, not an option. True False
2. Managers and supervisors confront employees who demonstrate weak, even marginal, service behavior. True False
3. In our organization, managers are encouraged to coach, discipline, and, when necessary, terminate employees who persist in their failure to meet high service standards. True False
4. In new-employee orientation, we communicate the goals and shape of our service strategy. True False
5. Managers have established specific service improvement goals for their departments, and they are expected to engage their staff in achieving them. True False
6. Our administrators have communicated clear service management expectations to their direct reports. True False
7. New employees are oriented in their departments to the importance of customer satisfaction and the specific behaviors expected of them. True False
8. When hiring, we screen applicants for service-oriented attitudes and skills. True False
9. Service performance has a prominent place in our performance appraisal process. True False
10. We train and support our managers and first-line supervisors in ways that equip them to use our human resource practices effectively. True False

Total: ___ ___

following approaches to strengthening human resource policies and practices in support of continually improving service performance:

- Creating a systemwide policy for service excellence
- Hiring service-oriented people in the first place
- Developing and communicating service management expectations that apply to all the managers and supervisors in the organization
- Developing explicit service expectations that apply to all the employees and physicians in the organization
- Developing service standards and protocols
- Building specific service expectations into job descriptions
- Building service dimensions into the performance appraisal process
- Getting new people off on the right foot through the new-employee orientation program
- Installing a commendation process that rewards service excellence, not just technical and clinical excellence
- Providing training and support so that managers are able to implement accountability policies

☐ Create a Systemwide Policy for Service Excellence

By issuing an overall hospital policy on service excellence, you can establish, in one simple action, that service excellence is an organizationwide priority and job requirement. Such a policy serves two purposes:

- It shows employees clearly that excellent service is required of everyone no matter what their job or status and forewarns employees that service problems can result in disciplinary action.
- It strengthens the likelihood that disciplinary actions related to service violations or mediocrity will stick. If an employee being disciplined claims to be unaware of the importance of service quality, the existence of the policy, with documentation about its distribution, discredits this excuse.

Figure 5-2 shows an example of a hospitalwide policy.

☐ Hire Service-Oriented People

When you hire service-oriented people in the first place, you experience the benefits down the line, avoiding frustration, excessive demands on supervisors' time, and the expense of training, retraining, and customer complaints.

The first step is to make sure you recruit people who have a service orientation. Figure 5-3 reproduces an advertisement for a manager run in a local newspaper by the McMaster-Carr Supply Company. As you can see, this company states outright that its priority is customer service in the hope of attracting applicants with the inclination and skills that match this priority. In recruitment efforts, it's important to reveal your organization's commitment to service excellence.

Second, make sure the person who screens applicants (for example, your employment manager) personifies service excellence. The screener must be skilled, knowledgeable, and service-sensitive and be able to recognize service skills and instincts in job applicants. Applicants will spread the word about your institution; do all you can to ensure that the word they spread is positive. Even if they don't get the job, they should leave feeling that your institution is a place they'd like to work at. Leave them thinking, "If

I needed a hospital, I'd come here" and *not* "If their personnel office is any indication of what the rest of the place is like, I'll never go there."

To check out your human resources department, evaluate it in terms of the following questions:

- Do staff model service excellence by being courteous, friendly, and responsive?
- Do staff greet applicants warmly and quickly and treat them as customers, not as nuisances or strangers?
- Do office procedures demonstrate that the organization values service excellence?
- Is the office a comfortable, attractive spot where applicants can complete their application and wait?
- Does someone provide applicants with coffee or tea and offer to hang up their coats?

Third, design interviews so that they generate all the information you need to make an intelligent choice among alternative candidates, including information on the service orientation of the candidates. The key is in the *design* of your employment interviews.

Figure 5-2. Example of a Hospitalwide Service Excellence Policy

---

A. Purpose

This policy provides guidelines for attitudes and actions by employees and physicians on the staff that foster favorable relations between employees and patients, patients' families, visitors, fellow employees, and the medical staff.

B. Philosophy

At the _____ Medical Center, we recognize that a patient's recovery is aided by sympathetic surroundings and that admissions to our hospital are affected by interpersonal relationships and by the image that our hospital projects. Further, we place a high degree of importance on establishing and maintaining an atmosphere of friendliness, courtesy, and concern for each patient, visitor, physician, and coworker so that all of these people have a favorable perception of and experience with our hospital.

C. Policy

It is the policy of _____ Medical Center to encourage and expect that each person connected with the Medical Center will at all times:

1. Be aware of and concerned about how his or her attitude and actions affect patients and other individuals, including coworker relations, within the institution.
2. Demonstrate excellent service performance as described within this policy and as contained within the Service Excellence House Rules (behavioral expectations).

D. Responsibilities

1. It is the responsibility of each employee and physician to:
   a. Ensure that his or her attitude and actions are at all times consistent with the standards as described within this policy and as contained in the Service Excellence House Rules.
   b. Remind a coworker when his or her attitude or actions are inconsistent with these standards.
   c. Compliment a coworker when his or her actions comply with this policy.
   d. Call instances of excellence or noncompliance to the attention of the appropriate supervisor or department head.
2. It is the responsibility of each department head and supervisor to:
   a. Ensure that each employee under his or her jurisdiction upholds these standards.
   b. Investigate reports of and document instances of violation of these standards and take appropriate corrective actions, especially when behavior is shown to repeatedly or seriously contravene the standards of demeanor described above. Such appropriate action may include counseling and other levels of discipline, including discharge.
   c. Commend an employee under his or her jurisdiction whose attitudes and actions consistently exceed these standards. Such commendation should include the issuance of a letter of commendation for placement in the employee's personnel file.
   d. Evaluate an employee's compliance with these standards as part of conducting regularly scheduled and special performance evaluations.
   e. Bring to the attention of the appropriate supervisor or department head instances of behavior contrary to or consistently far in excess of these standards by an employee under the jurisdiction of another supervisor or department head.

Figure 5-3. Advertisement Written by the McMaster-Carr Supply Company

---

Fanatics Wanted

Fanatic/fe-nat¹ik: Marked by zeal, enthusiasm, and intense devotion.

At McMaster-Carr, we're a bunch of fanatics. We're fanatics about customer service . . . about the pursuit of excellence . . . about hands-on operational management.

We're intensely devoted to our customers. With 140,900 products, we provide our customers with the world's most comprehensive line of industrial hardware and supplies. We use the latest in computer technology and inventory management techniques to provide same-day shipment to 90 percent of our orders.

We're intensely devoted to the vision of our founders to never settle for less than perfection. We zealously pursue inefficiencies to drive them out of our operation.

We're intensely devoted to the principle that the best managers know what they are managing through intimate involvement with their operation.

This approach has resulted in 87 years of solid performance, culminating in our rapid growth and market leadership during the 1980s. If you share our devotion to these principles, we want to teach you our business so you can move into a management role and help lead our company into the next decade.

Reprinted, with permission, from McMaster-Carr Supply Company, Elmhurst, Illinois.

Most applicants can spout service-oriented rhetoric, but can they behave in service-oriented ways in concrete situations?

Four methods have been shown to help predict an applicant's future job performance:

1. Watching the applicant's behavior during the interview
2. Asking behavior-based, open-ended questions
3. Using short simulations
4. Asking the applicant to react to the value of excellent service

All four are grounded in the belief that past and current *behavior,* not *philosophy,* predicts future behavior.

Method 1: Watching the Applicant's Behavior during the Interview

Don't just listen to the content of an applicant's answers. Carefully watch behavior. For example, when applicants fail to listen to you, maintain eye contact, and/or communicate warmth during the initial icebreaker, that's probably an indication of how they behave with other people in general. Figure 5-4 presents a checklist of applicant behaviors to note during the interview.

Method 2: Asking Behavior-Based, Open-Ended Questions

By asking behavior-based, open-ended questions, you can draw forth specific job-related experiences in the applicant's past and use these experiences to predict future performance. This method assumes that, although personality is certainly important, the person's ability to perform the service aspects of the job and his or her attitudes toward internal and external customers (as reflected in past behavior) are indicators of future performance.

Behavior-based interviewing begins with an analysis of the job you want to fill. List the performance skills needed to excel at service in this job—for example, communicating with impatient physicians, verbally presenting technical information to customers, buying time with a customer when you need time to investigate a problem, saying no to customers skillfully, and handling a complaint.

Figure 5-4. Applicant Behaviors to Observe during Interviews

Traits Desired	Behaviors Observed
Friendliness	Smiles both with mouth and eyes Takes active part in conversation Actively listens or reflects back words and gestures of the interviewer Uses humor appropriately Pleasant tone of voice Firm handshake Smiles, greets, and makes eye contact with office staff
Courtesy	Lets interviewer finish talking before responding Uses courteous words ("Please," "Thank you," "Nice meeting you") Makes appropriate small talk while waiting Uses appropriate courtesy words in meeting receptionist and interviewer ("Pleased to meet you" and "Good to have met you")
Responsiveness	Uses no long "uh's . . ." before answering Goes beyond "yes" and "no" answers Volunteers information without interviewer having to prod Answers the question asked; does not evade difficult questions
Empathy	Listening behaviors include: • Head nodding when appropriate • Overall slight muscle tension, indicating alertness and energy associated with caring • Slight leaning forward • Eye contact • Paraphrasing to show understanding • Communication of feelings when substance warrants it
Assertiveness	Asks for what he or she needs in interview (clarification, information, time) Volunteers pertinent information not asked for Discloses negative information truthfully Sounds confident and forthright in voice and words

After analyzing the service skills needed for the position, *design* open-ended interview questions that will help you determine whether the person has experience handling these key service elements and *how* (in specific detail) he or she has handled situations that call for each key skill. Following is a format that might be helpful in designing these questions: "Have you ever had a situation in which _____? Tell me about it. What's the most difficult situation you ever handled of this type, and how did you handle it?" Following are other examples:

- "Was there ever a time you violated organizational policy in order to better serve a customer? What happened and how did you handle it?" (*Bending the rules when they unduly interfere with a customer need*)
- "Tell me about a time you had to handle a difficult customer complaint. What happened and how exactly did you handle it?" (*Handling a customer complaint*)
- "Tell me about a time you went the extra mile for a customer. What were the circumstances and what did you do?" (*Doing more than was called for*)
- "When did you have something happen unexpectedly that interfered with your ability to do your job? What happened and how did you handle it?" (*Rolling with the punches*)
- "Can you think of a time a miscommunication occurred between you and a customer? What happened and how did you handle it?" (*Communicating with customers*)
- "Can you describe a time you were in conflict with a coworker? What happened and how did you handle the situation?" (*Cooperating with coworkers*)
- "Can you tell me about a time when you acted professionally even though it was tempting to act otherwise?" (*Professionalism*)

If your department or organization has service standards in place, you can structure your interview questions around those elements of the job description. If the applicant answers with generalities rather than specifics, probe further rather than move on. An example of a helpful probe might be, "Play a movie in your mind and tell me exactly what you did." The further along the interview proceeds, the easier the probing technique becomes, because the applicant gets accustomed to the pattern.

Method 3: Using Short Simulations

Ask the applicant to *show* or *enact* his or her way of handling typical moments of truth with customers. For instance, "I [the interviewer] would like you to *show* me how you'd handle interactions with customers. I'll play the customer by approaching you [the employee] with a situation. I want you to react as you would on the job." Then, encouraging the applicant to *show*, not *describe*, his or her behavior, describe several situations. For example:

- "Pretend a customer approaches you and asks why your department has kept him waiting more than 30 minutes. I'll be that patient; you handle my question in the best way you can."
- "A physician calls requesting information you don't have at your fingertips. The physician is annoyed because he or she expected to get this information immediately—during the phone call. I'll be the physician; show me how you'd handle the situation."

Simulations allow an interviewer to experience firsthand an applicant's verbal and nonverbal behavior. As a result, the interviewer will be in a much better position to evaluate it.

Method 4: Asking the Applicant to React to the Value of Excellent Service

Toward the end of the interview, explain your organization's service priority and the expectation that staff consistently demonstrate not only excellent technical skills but excellent behavior in their interactions with customers and with each other. Then invite the applicant to react to this expectation by explaining what he or she brings to a service-oriented culture like yours and whether he or she would fit. This kind of explicit exchange discloses a great deal while giving applicants information they can use to evaluate for themselves whether they will fit into your environment. If their interest wanes because they don't like what they hear, you'll be more likely to find that out *before* making the selection.

Making the Best Choice Possible

Once you generate information about applicants by using these four methods, you then need to evaluate the applicants. Ask yourself, "How do they *fit*—with the service demands of the job and with our service-oriented culture?" As part of your service strategy, emphasize the importance of hiring the right people the first time. Afterall, the people chosen make or break your service reputation, and it's difficult—sometimes impossible—to help the wrong person become the right person without great cost to the organization.

Once an applicant is hired, the probationary period needs to be used to test his or her interpersonal skills. During the hiring process, interviewers should clarify that the purpose of probation is to assess not only technical skills, but also service skills. Probation also gives new employees a further chance to decide whether your institution is appropriate for them; that is, whether their values and standards match yours. Interviewers need to make it clear that the organization's standards are nonnegotiable and that only those who can meet established service standards fully are qualified for the job. Once the new employee joins the team, don't relax standards during the probationary period.

☐ Develop and Communicate Service Expectations for All Managers and Supervisors

Some department directors and supervisors consider service excellence to be peripheral, that is, less important than the task specialties they hired people to perform. Others have long tolerated rude employees, rationalizing that "there are always a few bad apples" or "they've been here for so many years that it's too late now." Some managers and supervisors think that raising and enforcing service standards is just another pressure that will go away if ignored. Still others perceive no blatant problems in their departments, having become accustomed to inferior service quality. In many cases, they don't recognize the missed opportunities their people and departments have to excel in service and satisfy their customers.

Management and supervisory behavior can be strengthened by establishing and communicating explicit service performance expectations for managers and then building these expectations into their job descriptions and performance appraisals. The question that should drive identification of service management expectations is "What do employees need from their managers or supervisors in order to excel at service?" The HCA Holly Hill Hospital in Raleigh, North Carolina, uses 16 standards that are associated with certain behaviors (see figure 5-5). These standards are used as the basis for their management performance appraisal system.

Standards like those in figure 5-5 can be developed by executives with input from managers, supervisors, and frontline staff. Once the standards are crystallized, most organizations use a mix of the following methods to communicate them and to ensure that every manager and supervisor is clear about the expectations:

- Hold a leadership retreat at which administrators present explicit expectations and help managers and supervisors explore and embrace them.
- Have each administrator meet with direct reports, individually or as a group.
- Follow up with a one-on-one discussion between administrator and direct report:
  - Beforehand, ask the manager and the administrator to evaluate himself or herself and each other on each expectation. Make it clear that they shouldn't feel bad about conformance or worry about the results because the expectations have just been made clear for the first time.
  - Arrange a meeting between administrator and manager in which they discuss each expectation and do a low-key assessment of where the manager stands on it, the barriers, and the priorities for development. This needs to be done in the spirit of coaching, not evaluation. Because the expectations are *newly* explicit, managers should not be reprimanded for nonconformance.
  - End the meetings with clear goals for the coming year and a clear sense of what the senior management person needs to do to support the manager, and vice versa.
  - Discuss the results at an administrators' meeting to identify the kinds of support mechanisms needed to help managers and supervisors meet expectations.

Figure 5-6 provides some guidelines on planning the above-mentioned meetings, and figure 5-7 shows a sample format for rating the manager and, through discussion, comparing the administrator's perceptions of the manager with the manager's self-rating. Through this process, they reach agreements that will help the manager excel in meeting expectations.

Because administrators are managers, too, make sure that they go through a parallel process assessing their own alignment with these management expectations and developing improvement priorities for themselves. At a special administrator's meeting, discuss the administrative team's strengths and weaknesses and use the management expectations to assess your own team's effectiveness. Chapter 16, on departmental alignment,

Figure 5-5. Management Position Standards

1. Set Clear Expectations

   a. Develops job-specific service expectations and behaviors for each position supervised
   b. Clearly communicates to each employee the House Rules and job-specific expectations, and establishes these as both job requirements and performance evaluation components

2. Hold People Accountable: Holds self and employees clearly accountable for meeting high standards of service toward all customers

   a. Works with individual employees to set specific behavioral goals that move employees to "excellent"
   b. Conducts performance evaluations on a regular and timely basis
   c. Confronts employees who do not abide by House Rules
   d. Gives ongoing feedback, as needed, and counsels for service improvement; does not focus solely on technical competence
   e. Uses progressive disciplinary process when necessary, terminating people who, after appropriate intervention, do not uphold high standards even if technical performance is acceptable

3. Take Risks/Initiative

   a. Actively identifies problems and opportunities for improvement
   b. Generates new ideas, alternatives, and solutions
   c. Follows through and, as appropriate, involves others in implementation
   d. Accepts uncertain outcomes in making changes
   e. Uses "mistakes" as opportunities for change
   f. Seeks feedback and support from supervisor for solutions and innovations

4. Serve Your Customer

   a. Works with staff to identify customers and assess needs
   b. Takes action and allocates resources to best meet customer needs
   c. Solicits feedback on department service effectiveness from customers
   d. Shares results with staff and follows up with appropriate action

5. Build Your Team: Effectively builds employee morale and esprit de corps to facilitate problem solving, productivity, and service excellence

   a. In addition to technical competence, consistently screens job applicants to seek information and impressions about service orientation and people skills; hires people with strong interpersonal skills and service orientation
   b. Treats employees with respect and sensitivity
   c. Facilitates and teaches effective problem solving
   d. Shows concern for group morale, and engages team in group problem solving and constructive discussion to improve morale
   e. Initiates formal/informal activities with employees to develop departmental cohesion and collegiality
   f. Considers service and interpersonal skills when making decisions regarding promotions and other special opportunities

6. Think Organization

   a. Regularly communicates the hospital's mission and strategies and lets employees know how they contribute to the big picture
   b. Positively represents the organization to management, employees, physicians, and patients

7. Take Responsibility

   a. Holds self accountable and responsible to both supervisor and own employees for standards of behavior and service excellence
   b. Actively seeks information necessary to remain informed; asks for what is needed without complaining about lack of communication

8. Empower Others

   a. Within established policies, encourages and enables decision making closest to customer
   b. Initiates action to create policies that support decision making closest to the customer
   c. Works with employees to clarify decision-making authority
   d. Clearly delegates responsibility/authority to subordinates wherever possible

(Continued on next page)

Figure 5-5. **(Continued)**

9. Listen and Respond

   a. Is accessible
   b. Actively seeks input
   c. Listens without defensiveness to customer/employee concerns
   d. Acknowledges customer/employee concerns
   e. Actively follows up in response to concerns

10. Role Model: Acts as an effective, consistent role model of service excellence, exemplifying courtesy, compassion, and responsiveness toward all customers

   a. Talks "service" routinely: speaks to employees often about commitment to service excellence in order to reinforce service-orientation mind-set
   b. Consistently demonstrates behavior and decision making that reflect House Rules
   c. Speaks and makes eye contact frequently with persons in hallways, elevators, and public areas
   d. Speaks frequently with employees and demonstrates interest in them as people
   e. Introduces self and coworkers to patients, visitors, physicians; calls people by name
   f. Handles complaints by recognizing concerns, apologizing for any inconvenience, and taking active steps necessary to address the complaint
   g. Initiates action/assistance for customers in need
   h. Handles phone calls with promptness, courtesy, and helpfulness

11. Coach, Encourage, Support

   a. Coaches new employees on specific service skills and service behavior during initial employment period and as needed
   b. Invites individual discussion of achievements and problems in supportive manner
   c. Looks for instances of missed opportunities in which employees could have better met customer needs; constructively brings such to their attention and coaches on ways to improve
   d. Provides opportunities for employees to discuss problems in constructive, understanding atmosphere
   e. Identifies training and staff development needs for employees as related to service skills
   f. Advocates for and allocates resources to best meet employee development needs

12. Recognize and Reward

   a. Frequently recognizes positive behavior and contributions to the organization; uses praise, appreciation, and reward often
   b. Develops and implements formal and informal ways to recognize individual achievements (public recognition, letters, awards)
   c. Makes recommendations for and participates in hospitalwide recognition activities

13. Explain What's Happening

   a. Holds regular and timely meetings with staff to communicate information from administration and other sources
   b. Clearly explains reasons for decisions made
   c. Effectively utilizes a variety of techniques (verbal and written) to ensure clear and timely communication

14. Remove Barriers

   a. Identifies obstacles to optimal customer service by getting input from employees
   b. Actively works to change or modify policies, systems, and resource allocations in order to remove barriers
   c. Communicates and advocates with administration/supervisor on behalf of employee needs

15. Know Where You're Going

   a. Develops service mission/vision with staff
   b. Communicates service vision to employees and other customers
   c. Provides staff with clear sense of strategic direction

16. Be a Team Player

   a. Initiates communication and problem solving with peers in organization
   b. Facilitates cross-departmental communication and collaboration
   c. Actively participates in and contributes to hospital/department functions, activities, and events
   d. Listens nondefensively and considers others' points of view
   e. When disagreements occur, negotiates solutions in the best interest of the customer and hospital

Figure 5-6. Expectations Discussion: Administrator's Guide

We agreed to follow through on our recent retreat by meeting with each manager reporting to us for a face-to-face discussion about the new expectations we presented. The objectives of this "Expectations Discussion" are:

- To review our new expectations and make sure that each one is clear
- To discuss the manager's current performance
- To identify strengths to build on and areas that need attention and development
- To discuss and negotiate a plan for growth, development, and support so that the manager can successfully meet all 10 expectations successfully in the near future

How to Proceed

1. Arrange an appointment with each manager reporting to you.
2. Ask managers to come prepared to discuss their own performance in relation to each of our expectations, including their strengths, needs, and concerns about meeting these expectations. Promise to do similar thinking ahead of time yourself. Give each manager the format for ratings (see figure 5-7), which is helpful for profiling their strengths and needs.
3. At the meeting:
   - Explain that this is *not* a performance appraisal, but rather a discussion meant to clarify the new expectations, take stock of where the manager is in relation to each expectation, and together identify plans for meeting these expectations successfully and immediately.
   - State and reiterate your commitment to helping the manager fulfill these expectations and entertain his or her ideas about how you can help.
   - Use the format for ratings to guide your discussion. Discuss each expectation and share perceptions of this manager's strengths and needs. This is an important opportunity to identify and discuss discrepancies in perception. Don't shy away from them, for such discussions inevitably help both of you become clear on the expectations and what you need to do to see that they are fulfilled.

Figure 5-7. Format for Ratings and Performance Discussion (on One Expectation)

Manager _____ Date _____

Administrator _____

Expectation: Remove Barriers

A. By getting input from employees, identifies obstacles to optimal customer service
B. Actively works to change or modify policies, systems, resource allocations, etc., in order to remove barriers
C. Communicates and advocates with administration/supervisor on behalf of employee needs

Strengths:

Development Needs/Improvement Opportunities:

Action Plans Needed to Meet Expectation:

- Actions needed by *manager* (for example, read, experiment with new behavior, consult a suggested mentor)
- Actions needed by *administrator* (for example, coaching, feedback, communication about big picture, timely responses, removal of barriers)
- Actions recommended for *organization* (for example, training, support groups, team building, policy changes, chartering of teams, expanded responsibilities)

Time we agree to meet for follow-up discussion:

Comments about this process (for example, its value; loose ends or unfinished aspects):

Follow up by including these expectations in your performance evaluation system.

spells out in greater detail the role middle managers play in developing departmental service improvement plans and taking steps to align departmental practices with service mission.

Beyond the critical foundation established by making service management expectations explicit, department heads and supervisors must be held accountable for excellent service and continuous improvement within their departments. In the face of a complaint about a frontline employee's rudeness, for example, administration should investigate and hold the department head accountable for the behavior of people in his or her department.

☐ Develop Explicit Service Expectations for Employees and Physicians

"What do customers (internal and external) want from employees? What criteria do they use to judge employee service quality?" These questions should drive the identification of service expectations and standards for employees. Beginning with employee behavior, a generic set of behavioral expectations for all employees—regardless of position, tenure, or status—should be included in your service excellence policy and be considered requirements of every job. The complex behavior involved in health care service delivery should be detailed. The following list is an example of some "house rules" developed by The Einstein Consulting Group and used by many hospitals:

- *Break the ice.* Make eye contact, smile, introduce yourself, call people by name, extend a few words of concern.
- *Stop and offer help.* If someone looks confused, try to get the person back on track.
- *Show courtesy.* Kind gestures and polite words make people feel special.
- *Explain what you're doing.* People generally are less anxious if they know what's happening.
- *Anticipate needs.* Often you'll know what people need before they have to ask, so act promptly.
- *Respond quickly.* When people are worried or sick, every minute is like an hour.
- *Protect privacy and confidentiality.* Watch what you say and where you say it. Show respect; for example, knock before entering a room and close a patient's bedside curtains before an examination.
- *Handle with care.* Slow down. Imagine you're on the receiving end.
- *Preserve dignity.* Treat a patient as if he or she were your child, spouse, or parent. Respect patient autonomy, and see the person behind the patient.
- *Take initiative.* Just because a task is not your job doesn't mean you can't help or find someone who can. Pitch in; make suggestions; take the initiative to improve service.
- *Communicate with patients appropriately.* Your words and tone should not be insulting.
- *Listen.* Don't be defensive about a customer complaint. Try to learn from it.
- *Help each other.* By helping colleagues, staff, and physicians, you ultimately help a patient.
- *Keep it quiet.* Excessive noise annoys patients and workers. It also shows a lack of consideration.
- *Use phone skills effectively.* When you're on the phone, your facility's reputation is on the line. A pleasant, helpful, and understanding demeanor goes a long way.
- *Look professional.* You're part of a long, proud medical tradition.

With the help of The Einstein Consulting Group, Luther Hospital in Eau Claire, Wisconsin, went one step further, translating each house rule into more specific behavior. For example:

1. Breaking the ice
   - Make eye contact when greeting a person, smile, say hello, address him or her by name (if possible), and extend a few words of concern.
   - Be warm and friendly; introduce yourself by name and job function when appropriate; wear name tag.
2. Noticing when someone looks confused
   - Stop and try to help by offering statements such as: "Can I help you find . . . ," or "Let me show you . . .".
   - Direct or take customers to where they need to go.
   - When directing people, walk them part of the way, then point the rest of the way or ask a passing coworker to show them the way.
3. Taking time for courtesy and consideration
   - Use "please" and "thank you."
   - Take the time to stop and help someone.
   - Apologize for delays.
   - Respond to requests in a cooperative and responsive manner.
   - Treat others as you would like to be treated.
4. Keeping people informed
   - Remember, people coming to the hospital are often anxious and frightened.
   - Explain, in easy terms, what is expected of the individual (in filling out forms, doing a procedure, or directing them in some way).
5. Anticipating needs
   - Offer before being asked.
   - Pay attention to the "little things," the small touches that let a customer know you want them to be comfortable. (Offer an extra pillow, point out rest rooms, waiting areas, or coffee shop.)
   - Offer an explanation for the purpose of policies, procedures, and interactions before being asked.
   - Update patients or visitors regarding delays, changes, or expectations.
   - Go the extra mile; extend that special Luther Touch.

Based on information from your customers, you can develop your own service expectations. Ask, "What should employees do to convey their compassion and respect for every one of our key customer groups?" Hold focus groups with patients, visitors, physicians, and employees in which you ask them to identify behaviors that affect their satisfaction with employee (or coworker) behavior. Push focus group participants to identify behavior that would irritate, satisfy, and delight them. Distill all of this customer input into a list of behaviors. Using employee focus groups, invite reactions to your list, listening to suggestions related to missed items, unclear or potentially offensive wording, and the like. Then issue the resulting list as generic service expectations that apply to every member of your team.

☐ Develop Service Standards and Protocols

Many people believe that consistently excellent service interactions are hard to maintain because such exchanges are "soft," elusive, and a matter of style. These beliefs endure because leaders have not done the hard work of defining standards and *designing* service delivery so that these standards are real and therefore achievable.

Beyond defining generic behavioral expectations for all staff, you also need to design and communicate service standards and protocols that achieve a level of excellence even in routine service transactions. Such standards and protocols should be applicable hospitalwide (for example, "answer the phone within three rings") and some should be department and/or job specific. Others apply to specific service processes.

Which standards and protocols should be targeted? One hospital's Service Excellence Committee generated a list of functions committee members felt merited standardization in an effort to upgrade service quality and make service performance more consistent from person to person and customer to customer. Their list included the following:

1. Service protocols related to the admissions process
   a. First contact: How should patients and family be greeted? What questions should be asked and what information given in order to get the customer off on the right foot, thinking well of the hospital? What is/should be done to set a positive tone about the hospital stay—and to build confidence in staff?
   b. The process: What are all the steps in the admissions process and the customer's quality criteria for successful completion of each step?
   c. Time frames: What should the maximum waiting time be during each phase of the process?
   d. Last contact/sendoff: How should staff complete their contact with patient and family? What behavior will leave people with positive impressions and confidence that they will be in good hands when they reach the next phase of their visit?
2. Service protocols related to phone use
   a. How people answer the phone (words and tone to be used in greeting, ending conversations, transferring calls, putting people on hold, taking messages)
      • On outside lines
      • On internal lines
   b. How people return calls
      • Time frame
3. Service protocols related to clinical assessments
   a. Time frames
   b. Mechanisms for reporting results
   c. Behavior of people involved
4. Lobby behavior
   a. How to greet people and help them find their way
5. Other public area behavior
   a. Elevators
   b. Hallways
6. Other important turnaround times that affect customer perceptions of service quality (for example, turnaround of lab results, callbacks when family calls)
7. Confidentiality at front desks
8. How to handle inquiry calls
9. Complaint-handling process by every employee
10. The "good-bye—we wish you well" interaction upon discharge
11. Follow-up phone calls to discharged patients

In your organization, start by finding answers to the following questions:

• What service standards already exist?
• Whether written standards already exist or not, what do people think *should* be the standard for that function in order to satisfy customers?
   —Exactly what should the process be in order to exemplify excellent service?
   —What words should staff use?
   —What time standards should be established (for example, maximum turnaround time, maximum permissible waiting time)?
   —Are there any other aspects of this function that should be standardized?

After you identify areas where standards are needed, ask your customers (for example, in focus groups) what they expect. Engage committed staff in considering the extent to which the customer expectations can be met given your current work process. Are they achievable? If not, how can you rework the process so they become achievable? In the meantime, set standards that are as high as possible within the capability of your work process. Then make sure all relevant managers and supervisors are well aware of the standards and have had a chance to identify those that apply to people or process steps within their span of authority.

Service standards and protocols can then be documented in writing and translated into brightly colored, handy job aids (for example, laminated cards, posters) for appropriate employees. Figure 5-8 presents an example of telephone performance standards developed by MetroHealth Medical Center in Cleveland. If you think they are too rigid, consider the alternative—employees who behave as they or their supervisors see fit; that is, according to the "normal curve" of behavior. That means that some small percentage of people are terrific, another small percentage of people are awful, and most people are somewhere in the middle. The variation is too great to ensure customer satisfaction, because you have not *designed* the process to meet customer expectations at every key juncture.

By designing service protocols, you can raise the average level of behavior and also reduce the variation around this average so that *most* people are functioning in line with a higher standard. If rigidity is the price you pay, it's worth it.

☐ Build Specific Service Expectations into Job Descriptions

Beyond these required service standards, managers and supervisors should also think through the service aspects of *each position* within their realm of influence and identify job-specific service expectations for each position. Once the manager or supervisor develops and communicates the job-specific service expectations, he or she should include these in the job description for the relevant position or summarize them in a memo that becomes an addendum attached to the job description. (Chapter 16 on departmental alignment spells out processes department managers can use to develop job-specific expectations for or with staff.)

You can build service dimensions into job descriptions by using broad, generic statements that apply to all employees or by developing job-specific statements. Broad generic statements are much easier to institute because they apply to every employee regardless of position. Here are examples:

- For supervisors, managers, and administrators: Exemplifies excellent service toward patients, visitors, physicians, and coworkers; holds staff accountable for conformity to the "house rules."
- For nonsupervisory employees: Exhibits excellent service to patients, visitors, physicians, and coworkers; shows courtesy, compassion, and respect; conforms to the "house rules."

Job-specific expectations take more work but are more likely to elicit the desired behavior. They spell out the unique opportunities for service excellence inherent in a particular position. Here are examples:

- Admissions officer: Welcomes patients and visitors to the hospital and to the department; introduces self, calls patient and family members by name, explains what patients/families can expect (whens, whys, and hows); takes action to make patients comfortable, invites and responds to their questions.
- Tray deliverer: Knocks before entering a patient's room; greets the patient in a friendly and positive manner, introduces self, calls patient by name, places the tray within reach of the patient, offers assistance in opening packets of silverware,

Figure 5-8. "People First": Telephone Performance Standards

Purpose: To ensure that MetroHealth Medical Center callers receive courteous and efficient telephone service.

1. Telephones will be answered within three rings—five rings if staff is covering more than their assigned lines.

2. The employee will provide appropriate identification when answering calls.
   a. *Main Switchboard and Information*
      Outside Call—"MetroHealth Medical Center"   Inside Call—"Operator"
   b. *Nursing*
      Nursing Unit, first and/or last name, and job classification. "Twelve South, this is Mrs. Green, Ward Clerk."
   c. *Department*
      Department, first and/or last name, and job classification as determined by the department. "Admitting, this is Barb Doe speaking."
   d. *Private*
      Department and/or name. "Mr. Jones's office, this is Terry."

3. Tone of voice will be alert, pleasant, distinct, and expressive (answer with a smile in your voice). The caller's name will be used if it is known.

4. Telephone users will not eat, drink, or chew gum while on the phone.

5. Transfer calls promptly.
   a. Every effort will be made to assist callers before transferring or terminating calls. "Mrs. Jones isn't here, may I help you?"
   b. Announce to the caller what you are going to do, and give the transferring number, if known.
   c. After dialing the transfer, identify yourself and announce the caller and/or reason for transfer when transferring to another MetroHealth employee.
   d. On telephones that have the capability, connect the parties and announce "Go ahead please, sir/ma'am."

6. Calls will be screened, when requested, using the phrase: "May I ask who is calling?" or "May I tell Ms. Smith who is calling?"

7. Caller's name will be used (when known) by person receiving the call, and receiver will also give his/her name. "Hello, Mrs. Jones, this is Ms. Smith."

8. If a caller waits, the hold button will always be used if the telephone is so equipped.
   a. Ask the caller if he/she can hold. Then *wait* for a response before doing so.
      "If you will hold, I will get that information for you."
      "If you will hold, I will see if Mr. Jones is available."
      "Can you please hold? I will be right back."
   b. Every 30 to 40 seconds, progress reports will be given to callers on "hold" or offer option to phone back.
      "Mr. Jones's line is still busy; will you continue to hold?"
      "Mr. Jones's line is still busy; would you like to leave a message or call back?"
   c. Thank callers for holding.

9. Messages will be taken accurately and legibly. All messages will be written and include:
   a. The name of the caller, date, time, telephone number, appropriate instructions for receiver, and name or initials of the person taking the message.
   b. Messages will be delivered promptly.
   c. Message response should occur within 24 hours when possible.

10. When placing a call, identify yourself when an individual answers. "This is Mary Jones from Pathology calling for . . ."

11. Sincere regrets will be directly expressed (verbally or by tone of voice) whenever you are unable to help the caller. Also, offer to take a message. "Mr. Smith, I am sorry, but Mrs. Jones is not available. May I take a message?"

12. Employees should be familiar with the available features of the system and their phone (call pick-up, forwarding, paging, etc.).

13. Terminate the call courteously with a simple "Good-bye," "Bye," or "Thank you," and let the caller hang up first.

14. Basic words and courteous phrases will be used:

Use		Avoid		
"Please"	"Will you please hold?"	"Hold on"	"What?"	"You have to"
"Thank you"	"I would be glad to"	"Hang on"	"Hold on"	"You must"
"Good-bye"	"If you will"	"Yeah"	"Honey"	
"May I help you?"		"Who's calling?"	"Huh?"	

15. When initiating phone calls, identify yourself and your department when your call is answered. "Hi, Mary. This is Theresa Jones in Medical Records."

16. Notify the receiving person or department prior to call-forwarding your telephone lines.

17. To provide personalized service, answering machines should be used only when telephones are unmanned or already in use.

Reprinted, with permission, from MetroHealth Medical Center, Cleveland, Ohio, 1988.

salt, milk, bread, and the like; asks if patient needs further assistance; assures patient that he or she will take action or inform appropriate persons if additional help is needed; wishes patient a good day upon departing from the room.

• File room clerk: Greets physicians and other staff with a friendly hello/good morning; calls them by name; asks "How can I help you today?" or "Which chart may I find for you?"; responds quickly to customer requests, sets aside other tasks to give full attention to customer; handles complaints by listening and being nondefensive; takes action to correct problems; apologizes for delays or difficulties in meeting customer needs; quickly acknowledges additional customers waiting in line to be helped by letting them know they'll be with them shortly.

It's also important to derive job descriptions that (1) make the organization's and department's service mission explicit and clarify for employees where they fit in and (2) connect job *activities* to *customer needs and expectations* so that employees not only see what they're supposed to be doing, but also *to what purpose*. Figure 5-9 is an excerpt from a job description for a patient education coordinator that was rewritten to include the customer focus. The worksheet in figure 5-10 provides a format to help managers do the thinking involved in developing a customer-based job description.

☐ Build Service Dimensions into the Performance Appraisal Process

Deming has created quite a stir about the sacred cow of performance appraisal, calling it one of the "deadly sins" that impedes continuous quality improvement.[1] The reasoning is that processes, not people, are largely responsible for customer dissatisfaction and employee performance problems. Following this logic, a heavy burden should be placed on managers because managers have the lion's share of the power to improve processes.

Because of Deming's assertions, many health care organizations are experimenting with alternative approaches to performance appraisal. On the radical end of the

Figure 5-9. Job Description: Patient Education Coordinator

Primary Function:

Develops, implements, and evaluates patient and family education program in order to help patients and their families become knowledgeable about the patient's condition, treatment options, and follow-up care and in order to support caregivers in their education of patients and families.

Duties and Responsibilities:

Establishes priorities for patient education programs by collaborating with Nursing and selected ancillary departments in order to ensure that patients benefit from their knowledge of patient needs and in order to support and complement their patient care roles.

Develops patient education programs congruent with accepted educational methods and effective in communicating important information to patients and families so that they absorb and act on this information.

Identifies appropriate materials for each unit. Maintains, lists, and updates patient education materials being used so that nurses and other caregivers can easily learn, access, and support our education protocols.

Consults with Division Chairperson and selected individual physicians for approval of teaching programs in order to ensure quality and agreement with program content and in order to expedite their advocacy for and use of these programs with physicians and other caregivers.

Evaluates the effectiveness of each patient/family teaching program using effective evaluation methods and makes continuous improvements in order to better achieve our goals of informed and knowledgeable patients and families who are aware of their choices and who take as much responsibility for their health as possible both during their hospital stay and postdischarge.

Figure 5-10. Worksheet for Developing a Customer-Based Job Description

Position Title: _____

The organization's service mission:

The department's service mission:

Customers	Their Main Requirements	Your Role
External		
1	• • •	• • •
2	• • •	• • •
3	• • •	• • •
Internal (other departments)		
1	• • •	• • •
2	• • •	• • •
3	• • •	• • •
4 Coworkers	• • •	• • •

continuum is the system being tried by a client of Innovation Associates in Framingham, Massachusetts. This performance evaluation process consists of only four questions:

1. What do you want to do this year?
2. What do you need from us to do it?
3. What is management doing that gets in your way?
4. What is your failure pattern, and how can we recognize it early?

The employee is asked the questions early and receives an across-the-board salary increase no matter how the evaluation turns out.

On the other end of the continuum are enhancements to traditional performance appraisal systems. Organizations look at their current systems and figure out the best way to incorporate their service dimensions hospitalwide and on an individual employee job-specific basis.

Using Traditional Performance Appraisal Systems

Each of the four most common types of traditional performance appraisal systems focuses on a key area. These areas are traits, on a person's major job requirements, on objectives for the year, and on performance standards:

- *Traits:* This type of performance appraisal includes service as a trait to be evaluated. For example, if the system already has a trait called "attitude," replace it with "service" or whatever name you use for your program (for example, at Einstein it's *hospita*lity).
- *Major job requirements (or key tasks):* This system includes a service statement (either generic or specific) as one of a job's key tasks. The statement can be the same as the one recommended for job descriptions discussed previously.
- *Objectives for the year:* An objectives-focused system provides supervisors with sample objective statements related to service. You can use job description statements or more specific goal statements. The following are sample objectives for the year:
  - For a receptionist: To welcome patients and visitors in a consistently friendly, cooperative, and helpful manner.
  - For a unit clerk: To improve service behavior toward doctors (greet them by name, move quickly to obtain their charts, and exhibit friendly and professional nonverbal behavior).
- *Performance standards:* With this performance appraisal system, you must back up the series of dimensions (such as quality of work and attendance) with *standards* that define each possible rating. Include service as a dimension and spell out standards related to it. Be careful to define *high* standards. Mediocre service should be in the unacceptable category because, as pointed out earlier, your standards should push people beyond mediocrity to excellence.

What will work for your organization? Consider a hybrid approach. Employee performance matters and responsibility for that performance need to be treated, in large measure, as the employee's responsibility. Employees working within the same process vary in their performance. An enlightened performance appraisal system that is oriented toward "performance development" instead of evaluation, reward, and punishment makes the most sense.

Start by separating performance appraisal and development from your system of rewards and punishments. In this way, you can eliminate an atmosphere of fear and encourage nondefensive receptivity to feedback and personal improvement planning. Performance evaluations become communication opportunities. The reward system can then focus largely on managers and teams, because they need to be held accountable for desired outcomes and continuous service improvement. There are various ways to build service dimensions into performance development, including 360-degree performance evaluations and team appraisal systems.

Following the 360-Degree Approach

The premise underlying the 360-degree approach is that several people have a perspective on a given employee's performance, not just the employee's supervisor. Consequently, employee performances need to be rated by the cluster of people with and for whom they work: their supervisor, their customers, their staff (if applicable), and their peers.

In a 360-degree approach, all employees are evaluated and all employees are evaluators. This aligns with the fact (stated earlier in this book) that all employees are both suppliers and customers of other employees. Rating one another from both viewpoints is critical. As employees rate each other, their awareness of service criteria that are important to them and their customers becomes heightened. The rating process in itself becomes an educational intervention that pushes employees toward improved service quality. Also, because the role of managers in a customer-driven organization is to empower and support their staff to serve customers, ratings by employees become particularly important.

Figure 5-11 provides some key instructions and five questions from three viewpoints (employee, supervisor, peer) of a 360-degree evaluation survey. Use this format to create tools tailored to your own service performance expectations. The employee version of

Figure 5-11. Employee Service Performance Inventory: Employee, Supervisor, and Peer Versions

---

Employee Version

This inventory helps you assess your performance in a number of key areas relating to the service you provide to your organization's customers (patients, visitors, physicians, other departments, and your coworkers).

- Think about how you interact with the people you come into contact with throughout your workday.
- Select the number that best describes your response to each statement.
- Enter your response next to the corresponding item on the Answer Sheet.
    1 = "Rarely"
    2 = "Occasionally"
    3 = "Often"
    4 = "Always"
- Please respond to ALL items.

1. When people enter my work area, I greet them in a friendly manner.

2. I go out of my way to help people reach their destinations.

3. I thank people when they do something for me.

4. I tell customers what I'm going to do before I do it.

5. When I'm finished doing something for a customer, I ask if there's anything more I can do for him or her.

Supervisor Version

This inventory helps you assess the performance of one of your employees on a number of key areas relating to the service the employee provides to your organization's customers (patients, visitors, physicians, other departments, and your coworkers).

- Think about how this employee interacts with the people he or she comes in contact with throughout the workday.
- Select the number that best describes your response to each statement.

The employee's name _____ (the person being rated)

1. When people enter the work area, this employee greets them in a friendly manner.

2. This employee goes out of his or her way to help people find their destination.

3. This employee thanks people when they perform a helpful service.

4. This employee tells people beforehand what he or she is going to do.

5. When finished with a patient, this employee asks if there's anything more he or she can do for the patient.

Peer Version

Your coworker _____ is interested in knowing your perceptions of his or her service behavior toward the organization's customers. Your frank responses will help. You need not sign your name on this Evaluation. Your coworker will not see your individual Evaluation. We will tally the results about this coworker based on *all* evaluations completed. Your coworker will see only the *group* score. Thus, your ratings will be confidential.

- Think about how your coworker acts with the people he or she comes in contact with throughout the workday.
- Select the number that best describes your response to each statement.
- Please turn in your completed inventory in the attached envelope to your supervisor.

Thank you very much.

1. When people enter the work area, this employee greets them in a friendly manner.

2. This employee goes out of his or her way to help people find their destination.

3. This employee thanks people when they perform a helpful service.

4. This employee tells people beforehand what he or she is going to do.

5. When finished with a patient, this employee asks if there's anything more he or she can do for the patient.

the assessment (or self-assessment) invites an employee to rate himself or herself on conformance with the house rules. The supervisor version asks the employee's supervisor to rate the employee's conformance to the house rules. The peer (or internal customer) version allows coworkers to provide one another with feedback about the extent to which they perceive each other as acting in accordance with the house rules.

Supervisors can use this inventory in a discussion to clarify service expectations of employees or to evaluate their performance. The supervisor and employee share and compare their perceptions of employee behavior and then discuss development needs and goals in the context of performance appraisal or discussion designed to clarify job expectations.

This inventory can also be used to sharpen employees' awareness of their own behavior and other people's perceptions of their behavior. This is best done after employees are made aware of the house rules and the role everyone in the organization is expected to fulfill. The inventory then becomes a chance for employees to take stock of their own performance and assess their strengths and weaknesses.

Implementing an Integrated Approach

The self-rating and ratings by the supervisor, customers (internal and external), and peers help provide perspective on the individual's performance, especially when similarities and differences in perception are examined. Building on this principle, Shawnee Mission Medical Center in Shawnee Mission, Kansas, developed an impressive integrated approach to performance appraisal called the Personal Development Process (described in figure 5-12). The approach integrates customer, peer, self, supervisor, and subordinate feedback in a positive, forward-looking personal development plan. Employees begin their year with a planning meeting among the employees (or associates) and their supervisors (or reviewers). At these meetings, employees:

- Identify the primary customers served by the employee
- Review the hospital's four values of "respect, integrity, service, and excellence"
- Identify three to six key service areas (KSAs) to become the employee's performance focus
- Set individual self-improvement and educational goals
- Pinpoint several "challenge opportunities" that would stretch the employee's skills, abilities, and contributions

At least twice a year, supervisors invite feedback about the employee from the employee's coworkers and customers and hold "coaching sessions" to take stock with the employee of the employee's progress toward the self-selected goals. At year's end, there is a wrap-up meeting in which the supervisor and employee discuss the extent to which the employee achieved his or her goals. An employee who achieved his or her goals receives the same percentage "contributory" increase (raise) as others. The session also is an opportunity to consider some kind of superstar reward system to supplement the system described.

Using the Team Approach

Another approach that some health care organizations are currently experimenting with is team evaluation. Work teams establish service targets and goals, as well as install measures for monitoring the team's performance. Rewards are dispensed based on team, not individual, achievement. The premise is that if the team suffers as a result of individuals who do not contribute their fair share, peer pressure will provide continuous feedback and performance improvement assistance.

Figure 5-12. Shawnee Mission Medical Center Guidelines for the Personal Development Process (Excerpts)

The Personal Development Process is designed to support our Vision and Values and empower associates to become peak performers. Communication provides the framework for performance development and it is important that each associate be involved in the process.

Personal Development Planning Discussion

At the beginning of each personal development cycle, the associate and the reviewer will complete the following steps:

1. Identify Primary Customers—Each of us has contact with a variety of customers as we do our jobs. In Section 1 identify the associate's three or four primary customers—remember to consider both internal and external customers.

2. Review the Medical Center's Key Service Areas—In fulfilling our mission and serving our customers, there are certain behaviors that are expected of all associates. These are identified in Section 2 as Shawnee Mission Medical Center Key Service Areas (KSAs) and are included in each associate's personal development plan. It is important that each of these KSAs and the accountabilities be discussed, and if appropriate, job-specific examples can be added.

3. Develop or Update Job-Specific Key Service Areas, Accountabilities, and Projects—These KSAs should reflect the most important responsibilities of the job, the job description, and customer needs. It is recommended that there be no more than 3–6 KSAs. Accountabilities/Projects are functions, activities, or special projects that should be discussed throughout the personal development cycle. Identify primary customers for each Job-Specific KSA. Projects should include a target date for completion. Write Job-Specific KSAs, Accountabilities, and Projects in Section 3.

4. Establish Individual Goals—Identify personal goals and objectives. This may include a variety of areas such as skills development, continuing education, or cross training. (Note any action plans with target dates agreed to in the recent performance review.) Record in Section 4 and refer to throughout the year.

5. Identify Challenge Opportunities, If Appropriate—These projects or goals represent significant challenges. If a Challenge Opportunity is accomplished it will be evaluated favorably, but if it is not achieved, it will not be negatively reviewed. A Challenge Opportunity should not be performed at the expense of other KSAs. It should be recorded in Section 5.

6. Give the Associate a Copy of the Associate Accomplishment Form—Explain that the associate can use this form to record his or her accomplishments throughout the year.

7. Set a Date for a Formal Performance Coaching Session—The personal development plan provides a road map for the year. However, it is important that the plan be reviewed regularly. At least once during the year, approximately six months into the cycle, the associate and the reviewer formally will review the plan. Choose a date for this session and record it on the front of the form under Performance Coaching Session.

Performance Coaching Session(s)

Throughout the year, there should be frequent coaching on an informal and formal basis, including:

1. Hold Informal Meeting—Share positive feedback about accomplishments, identify obstacles, and work together to problem solve. Record comments about positive performance and opportunities for growth in the spaces provided in each KSA.

2. Conduct a Formal Performance Coaching Session—Approximately six months into the performance year, the associate and the reviewer will formally identify strengths, stretches, and targets in Section 6, the S-S-T a preliminary S-S-T form as a basis for discussion. To ensure a positive outcome, the reviewer and associate collaborate in a two-way exchange focusing on the present and the future.

3. Review the Personal Development Plan, If Appropriate—We recognize that there may be a need to revise a personal development plan during the year. Revisions should be agreed upon by both the associate and the reviewer. Whenever possible, changes should be made at least three months before the performance review. The associate and the supervisor should each receive a copy of the revised plan.

Initial Employment Review

1. Complete Initial Employment Review (if appropriate)—All associates new to the Medical Center should receive a progress review at 30 days, 60 days, and 90 days in their initial employment period. Record comments and action plans in the Coaching Notes in each KSA. Associate and reviewer should sign and date the form on the cover sheet after each discussion. If the initial employment period is to be extended, the reviewer should note the extension date and contact Personnel.

Figure 5-12. (Continued)

Coworker Feedback Process

At any time during the year, the reviewer will:

1. Offer the Associate the Opportunity to Receive Coworker Feedback—In the spirit of teamwork and recognizing each associate's contribution, associates will have the opportunity to receive feedback from their coworkers. A coworker is any associate of SMMC who is familiar enough with an associate's work to provide meaningful feedback. The decision to gather coworker feedback will be done, will be made jointly by the associate and reviewer. We suggest gathering it prior to the mid-year formal coaching session and discussing it at that session.

2. Gather Coworker Feedback—The associate will provide the supervisor with the names of two to three coworkers to be asked for feedback. The reviewer will choose one to two additional coworkers. The reviewer will send the selected coworkers the Coworker Feedback Form two to three weeks before the agreed-upon discussion date. When the forms are received, the reviewer will compile the comments from the coworkers on a blank copy of the form to maintain confidentiality. The original feedback forms submitted by the coworkers will be destroyed.

3. Discuss the Coworker Feedback—At the agreed-upon date, the associate and reviewer will discuss the summary Coworker Feedback Form. At the end of the discussion, the summary form will be given to the associate unless he or she decides it should be placed in the department personnel file.

Annual Performance Review Discussion

In preparation for the annual review, the reviewer will:

1. Schedule the Performance Review with the Associate—At least six weeks before the actual review, select a date, time, and place, and encourage the associate to complete the Associate Accomplishment Form.

2. Draft Comments on the Personal Development Process Form—Review the Associate Accomplishment Form if submitted. Use notes, records, and input from other sources to draft comments on the Personal Development Process Form. Record comments and results in the appropriate spaces for each KSA in Sections 2 and 3 and for Individual Goals in Section 4 and Challenge Opportunities (if applicable) in Section 5.

3. Conduct the Review
   - Review each KSA and discuss the reviewer's comments and the associate's comments.
   - Review the Individual Goals in Section 4. Record status or results of the Individual Goals.
   - Review the Challenge Opportunities in Section 5, and discuss results.
   - Discuss the Associate Accomplishment Form and any differences from the reviewer's evaluation. Make adjustments if pertinent information surfaces during the discussion.
   - Offer the associate the opportunity to write comments on the cover sheet of the form about his or her performance or thoughts about the Personal Development Process.
   - Indicate whether associate will receive contribution increase.

After both the reviewer and the associate have signed and dated the form, both will retain a copy for his/her personal records and forward the original copy to Personnel.

The Personal Development Process is a cycle. The annual performance review discussion signals the end of one year and the need to plan for the upcoming year. The associate and the reviewer will establish a time to develop a new personal development plan (it may be at the same discussion). Reviewing the Medical Center and Job-Specific KSAs provides a good starting point for developing the plan.

Reprinted, with permission, from Shawnee Mission Medical Center, Shawnee Mission, Kansas, 1991.

Team accountability systems are new and full adaptation to them will take time, because they reflect a radical departure from the health care tradition of holding individuals, not teams, responsible for outcomes. One thing, however, is very clear: to foster service attitudes and empowerment, performance reviews must feel like development opportunities, not performance autopsies. The new methods need to do the following:

- Focus on setting service improvement goals.
- Make sure that selected goals will improve service processes and/or increase internal and external customer satisfaction.
- Urge managers to coach staff frequently around critical incidents—positive or negative events that present opportunities for reinforcement, learning, or improvement.

- Encourage frequent informal discussions (perhaps daily) and formal discussions at least twice (preferably four times) a year.
- Prompt input from the employee's customers and coworkers.
- Include explicit service dimensions stated in behavioral (concrete, discussable) terms.

Adapting the Disciplinary Process

Whatever disciplinary process you have can be adapted for use with service dimensions of behavior. However, in the spirit of development-oriented performance coaching, consider the exciting improvement on progressive discipline called Positive Employee Discipline. Tested at the Children's Hospital of Boston, among other places, Positive Employee Discipline has the following elements, according to Ann Lang, Esq., vice-president of human resources:

- This system emphasizes improving behavior and eliminates, to the extent possible, an emphasis on punishment.
- It involves four steps:
  (1) Counseling notes summarize discussions in which the manager gave the employee feedback and suggestions about performance (no prescribed number needed before moving to a performance improvement agreement).
  (2) Performance improvement agreements are negotiated between manager and employee. They clearly articulate expectations of the employee, specific improvements needed, and methods for making these improvements.
  (3) The employee is allowed to take a decision-making leave, a paid day off (not a punishment) for the purpose of deciding whether to try to live up to the agreement or resign.
  (4) Termination (which should be used only as a last resort) results when the employee chooses to return and then violates the performance agreement.
- The manager acts as a coach and is responsible for helping the employee change his or her behavior.

This system is nonpunitive and more constructive than most progressive discipline processes. It is, therefore, more aligned with the spirit of partnership between managers and staff, which is required in service efforts.

☐ Get New People Off on the Right Foot

From day one, new employees must know the value your organization places on service excellence and the precise expectations you have for their behavior. Depending on osmosis to slowly take its course is a mistake. Your new-employee orientation program should communicate the difference between service excellence in your organization and in any other service settings in which the new employees may have previously worked. Before a new employee is allowed to fall back on any negative proclivities (inattentiveness, impatience, or indifference toward service, for example) in this new environment, set the record straight so that he or she starts off on the right foot.

New-employee orientation presents a golden opportunity to convey the mission and values sacred in your organization's culture. In this orientation, you should:

- *Give the big picture about your organization's mission, challenges, and strategies for success.* Emphasize that each employee has his or her own customer base.
- *Encourage interaction among new and veteran employees.* Structure orientation so that people get to know one another. Stress the value you place on the human

ingredient. For example, some organizations institute a buddy or mentor system—pairing an experienced, positive employee with each new employee.

- *Set clear expectations about what constitutes excellent job performance.* Your explanation of the generic expectations that every employee in your organization is expected to meet should be lively, anecdotal, and illustrative. Communicate assertively that these standards are part of every person's job.
- *Explain your organization's service strategy.* Enumerate all the things your facility does to make continuous service improvement a daily fact of life.
- *Touch people's emotions.* Using films, anecdotes, or small group exercises, emphasize that for staff at the patient's bedside, in the laundry room, or at a computer terminal, the patient is each employee's primary concern.
- *Allow the theme of service excellence to take prominence during orientation.* Do this by:
  - Allocating time to service excellence in proportion to its value. How much of the orientation is spent on service? Twenty minutes? A full day? Do you leave it out if you're running late?
  - Positioning your service excellence component in prime time, and not as a filler.
  - Making sure that an advocate of service excellence conducts the orientation session. The CEO, an enthusiastic administrator, or a frontline worker are natural candidates. Your service excellence facilitators, human resource professionals, and training professionals could also conduct this portion, but only if they are effective communicators and true service proponents.
  - Following through after the initial orientation. For instance, two months later, have an administrator reconvene new employees for breakfast to find out about their first months on the job.

☐ Install a Commendation Process That Rewards Service Excellence

Consequences hold a powerful influence over human behavior. Too often supervisors emphasize negative consequences for negative behavior but neglect positive consequences for positive behavior.

When a negative emphasis is allowed to prevail, your strategy for service excellence is tinged with a punitive, watchdog overtone, which is demoralizing to employees and fails to shape the behavior you want. It does not energize workers or call attention to stellar performers.

To counteract this tendency toward negativism—and to fuel your service excellence strategy—strengthen your organization's methods of focusing on the positive with praise, recognition, and shows of appreciation. Consider using the following tactics:

- *Use your performance appraisal system to formally reinforce positive behavior.* Once you build service into your performance appraisal system, use the system to demonstrate that excellent service can result in high ratings, which can translate into merit increases.
- *Encourage verbal and written feedback.* Supervisors should be encouraged to increase their *daily* use of verbal and written positive feedback to employees.
- *Incorporate recognition systems.* In addition to Employee of the Year or Employee of the Month programs, consider methods that recognize *more* people *more* often. (See chapter 11 on rewards and recognition for a smorgasbord of approaches.)
- *Implement a formal commendation system.* Most organizations include disciplinary documents as part of their human resource function. A commendation form issued by supervisors could also serve as a standard human resource practice. One copy could be awarded to the employee, and the other placed in his or her file as part of the permanent employment record.

☐ Provide Training and Support for Managers

To accomplish your service excellence goals (no matter what policies are in place), managers and supervisors need special training and support if they are to skillfully discuss service behavior with employees within the context of performance development. Excellence-oriented policies and procedures would have no value if your supervisors and managers failed to *use* them at all or used them ineffectively.

Service-focused organizations need to provide training and support for managers so that they can effectively set, support, and enforce standards. Most managers benefit from help with following human resource policies and procedures and applying the disciplinary process. Human resource departments employ specialists who can help managers choose the language and approach they will use in counseling employees. Some departments sponsor training programs on accountability skills and monthly clinics that provide a forum in which supervisors and department directors share their frustrations over problem employees and help each other prepare their approaches. Many hospitals provide workshops on accountability skills and subsequent support groups that accomplish these goals:

- Strengthen managers' behavior as service role models
- Build skills for clarifying and communicating explicit behavioral, job-specific expectations to staff
- Improve skills in providing feedback, coaching, managing problem employees, documenting problems, negotiating performance improvement plans, and so forth

Describing Service Behavior Problems in Behavioral Terms

Too often, managers and supervisors fail to document marginal service performance because they find it so difficult to describe service behavior, whether it's good or deficient. Consequently, behavior-related problems come back to haunt you as the employee darkens your department's image and your customers' satisfaction. That's why it's so important to learn how to describe negative service behavior. Following are some general guidelines:

- Service performance problems are best described by contrasting required or expected performance to the actual performance observed. Supervisors need to use specific examples to illustrate violations and also document when they occurred.
- Descriptive behavioral language should be used that avoids labeling or attacking the person.
- Talking or writing about "attitudes" should be avoided; instead, focus on observable behavior. Most people think they have good attitudes. If you imply otherwise, employees may become defensive and matters get worse.

Consider this example of contrasting a required service performance expectation to observed behavior:

Service expectation: Lee Stevens, an admissions clerk, is required to welcome patients and visitors to admissions in a friendly, positive manner and demonstrate a willingness to respond to all of their admissions needs.

Actual performance:

- *Inaccurately identified:* "Your attitude is poor; you're cold and indifferent."
- *Accurately identified:* "I'm concerned about how you're coming across to patients. Over the past two weeks, I've mentioned to you three complaints from patients

who said your manner was cold and indifferent. Yesterday, I observed your interaction with patients up close so as to see the behavior that might have given patients that impression. You barely spoke when patients and visitors entered the office. You failed to say hello or introduce yourself, instead scowling, rolling your eyes, and sighing when asked how long they had to wait. Your manner came across as abrupt and impatient."

Thus, an event is documented and described in terms of behavior rather than attitude.

Giving Feedback Skillfully

Supervisors inevitably need to confront certain problem employees by offering direct feedback. Effective feedback describes the employee's undesirable service behavior and its consequences and at the same time communicates respect for the employee and acknowledges his or her good intentions. The result is better communication, less defensiveness, and more likelihood that the employee will find the feedback helpful in guiding his or her future behavior decisions. One effective model for delivering face-to-face feedback includes five steps:

1. *State your positive intention.* For example, "I want to be sure our customers are satisfied with service quality, and I need your help."
2. *Describe the behavior in performance terms.* For example, "I'm concerned about your failure to meet the service standards required of every employee in our department. I'm talking specifically about the incident this morning with Dr. Blakely. I was in my office and I couldn't help overhearing the words exchanged between you and observing the interaction. It was evident he was waiting to talk to you about his incomplete charts, yet you failed to acknowledge his presence, continuing instead to talk on the phone in what sounded like a personal conversation. Once you hung up, you didn't look up, and in a flat monotone said, 'what do you need?' You didn't address him by name, nor did your voice tone or actions demonstrate a willingness to help him with his needs."
3. *Describe the effects or consequences of the behavior.* "This lack of attention and rude treatment angered Dr. Blakely and created a conflict. We work hard to get the doctors to complete their charts properly. This behavior antagonizes doctors and makes it hard for us to obtain their cooperation."
4. *Express a touch of empathy and/or acknowledge employee's positive intention.* "I recognize that not all doctors are easy to work with and that Dr. Blakely can be difficult. And I realize you want to work harmoniously with physicians."
5. *Make an "I expect" statement.* "So, next time Dr. Blakely or any physician approaches your desk, I expect you to put aside whatever you're doing, including bringing personal phone conversations to a close. I want you to look up, smile, make eye contact, address the person by name, and ask what you can do to help—in a positive upbeat voice. In addition, I expect you to respond as quickly as possible to all requests."

Documenting Service Problems with Extreme Care

Supervisors need to document performance discussions so both employee and supervisor are clear about what was discussed and how it was resolved. The supervisor will need this documentation if problem performance persists and disciplinary actions need to escalate. Figure 5-13 provides a suggested outline for a memo documenting service performance problems and corresponding expectations.

Managers and supervisors need to embrace their critical role in holding employees accountable while using accountability tools that give employees maximum respect and

Figure 5-13. Suggested Outline for Documentation Memo

I. Purpose of Memo
   A. To provide a written summary of the discussion with employee
II. Background of Problem
   A. Prior discussions
   B. Incidents/problems leading up to meeting with employee
III. Problem Identification
   A. Identify problem areas
   B. Cite examples
   C. Give impact of problems
   D. Get employee's assessment
IV. Expectations/Standards
   A. State and/or clarify performance expectations/standards
V. Action Plan
   A. What employee will do
   B. What supervisor/others will do
   C. Changes in work methods, procedure, etc.
   D. Feedback process
   E. Agreement reached
VI. Closing
   A. Optimism/confidence in employee
   B. Make the statement that the "memo represents my summary" and give employee opportunity to alter it so that both parties agree about what happened
   C. Have employee sign copy to acknowledge receipt of documentation

responsibility for their own development. This is a difficult tightrope to walk, and managers often need support and help.

☐ Final Suggestions

Consider the following suggestions as you align your organization's accountability practices with your service mission:

- *Avoid talking about attitude.* Instead, talk about behavior. Define for employees the behavior you want and set inspiringly high standards. People think they have good attitudes, and if you imply otherwise, they may become defensive and accuse you of having an attitude problem yourself. You're at loggerheads because attitude is debatable, subjective, elusive, invisible, arguable. Demand and expect appropriate *behavior* and define what that behavior is in no uncertain terms.
- *Mean what you say.* Devising elegant human resource practices is pointless unless you inform people about them and enforce the practices. An excellent human resource policy that is not enforced simply reflects double standards and failure to follow through. If employees do not meet your standards, you have to be ready to enforce disciplinary action up to and including termination of employment.
- *Have written job descriptions.* Written job descriptions should include performance expectations and their intended effects on customers. Job descriptions help employees embrace service expectations instead of being focused solely on routine job-related activities. Problem employees can use a lack of explicitness as an excuse for inappropriate behavior by asking, "Where's it written?"
- *Provide accountability training for executives, managers, and supervisors.* Even the best human resource policies fail to achieve their purposes if supervisors are ill equipped or disinclined to use them. Training sessions on accountability skills are a necessity in most health care organizations, where there has traditionally been ambivalence toward accepting serious accountability. According to one health care executive

frustrated at supervisors' tolerance of service offenders, "I think we're here to provide our customers with a consistently high level of service, but many of our supervisors think we're a halfway house for dysfunctional employees." (The irony was that the executive did nothing about service atrocities among his own direct reports, thus promoting a culture of mediocrity.) Once you have human resource policies that support service excellence, confront nonconformance at every level or expect your service standards to break down.

- *Don't worry that human resource policy changes might foster unionization.* Many hospitals have revamped their human resource practices in the ways described. The changes recommended herein do not stimulate unionization, and in organizations where unions exist they have not been found to create problems with the unions. Unions value explicit performance standards and appreciate clear practices. The premise underlying all of the changes recommended in this chapter is that problems are solved, not created, by making the implicit explicit.

Accountability, or lack of it, can make or break your service strategy. As is true in most organizational change strategies, policies and practices require reexamination and revision. Hiring customer-oriented people prevents later regrets and the ongoing need for excessive retraining. Policies and practices that clearly hold managers, staff, and teams accountable for achieving your higher standards make success achievable in the long run.

Reference

1. Deming, W. E. *Out of Crises.* Cambridge, MA: MIT Center for Advanced Engineering Study, 1986.

Chapter 6
Measurement and Feedback

Before reading this chapter, consider your organization's current practices related to measurement and feedback by taking the self-test in figure 6-1. The self-test will help you gauge your organization's customer satisfaction as revealed by more than management and staff opinions of success or failure. The test data, while assisting your facility with monitoring customer satisfaction and operational processes that are key to achieving customer satisfaction, can also drive service improvement initiatives.

Figure 6-1. Self-Test

Measurement and Feedback. *Circle the appropriate response. The more "true" answers the better. "False" answers indicate areas that need improvement.*

1. Our organization has systems in place for monitoring key operational processes that have an impact on customer satisfaction.	True	False
2. We routinely assess patient satisfaction with attributes of service important to patients.	True	False
3. Managers here regularly track their department's actual service performance on service attributes most important to their customers.	True	False
4. We have a system for listening to physicians' concerns and suggestions.	True	False
5. Departments here consult one another as internal customers to find out how they can better serve each other.	True	False
6. We regularly assess *employee* satisfaction with coworkers, managers, the work environment, and hospital systems.	True	False
7. Our organization has a regular system for measuring interdepartmental or internal customer satisfaction.	True	False
8. We have systems in place to invite customer and employee suggestions.	True	False
9. Every department here measures customer satisfaction and operational performance.	True	False
10. We have designed and implemented a process that ensures our using measurement data to identify improvement needs and priorities.	True	False
Total:	____	____

Listening to customers is a prerequisite to meeting customer needs, and a number of approaches are available for collecting customer satisfaction information (for example, surveys, interviews, audits, and focus groups). Do you have ongoing, effective methods of evaluating patient, visitor, physician, employee, and payer satisfaction? Are you confident that the information you collect is reliable enough to provide an accurate picture? Do managers use such tools as logs, checklists, histograms, clocks, trend charts, and control charts to monitor key operational processes? If you answered "false" to one or more of these items, consider broadening your evaluation strategies to track customer satisfaction and operational performance so that you can use data regularly and rationally to drive service improvement.

How you measure the effectiveness of your strategy for service excellence and how your organization goes about obtaining information from key customer groups so as to make course corrections are critical to your service improvement efforts. Traditionally, systems for obtaining information from customers on a regular basis have not been at the top of most organizations' priority lists. This chapter will provide specific guidelines for designing and implementing a data-driven measurement and feedback system.

□ Why Data Drive Improvement

People generally want to know "How am I doing?" Sound feedback methods provide constructive and reliable answers to this question, thereby providing information that can be used to confirm or change actions. By showing you what does and does not work, empirical testing allows you to revise your strategy midstream. Those who succeed in their service improvement efforts tend to think and act like experimenters—proposing and testing hypotheses, learning from the results of their testing, and then revising their tactics to achieve even better results. Without measurement, the effectiveness of these "experiments" is left to opinion.

Strategies with little or no measurement become activity driven, not results driven, and the mere performance of activities will not necessarily ensure positive results. In their article "Successful Change Programs Begin with Results,"[1] Schaffer and Thomson point out that many multifaceted change strategies mistake means for ends and processes for outcomes. Completion of training does not mean that improvements are under way. Only meaningful measurement tied to desired outcomes provides the hard evidence that your efforts are paying off. Meaningful *ongoing* measurement provides you with formative information that helps you shape your strategy incrementally, based on what happens at the previous phase. Simply put, you can keep doing what does work and stop doing what does not work. Therefore, it takes discipline to develop meaningful measures of service improvement, and this discipline has the result of making your vision specific, concrete, and, ultimately, more achievable.

Documentable progress energizes your service improvement process, building confidence and optimism about expanded possibilities of improvement. Furthermore, the Joint Commission on Accreditation of Healthcare Organizations (JCAHO) now requires customer satisfaction measurement as a key indicator of quality in health care institutions. When you allow data to drive improvement, you tend to advance service by introducing changes and new activities *for a reason*—with a clear purpose.

Advancing Service

To advance service, you need to regularly identify the discrepancies between current reality and your vision and then take action to bridge the gap. To assess and improve your service strategy and to drive service improvement at every level of your organization, you must have systematic access to specific sources of information from each of your key customer groups, sources that are both quantitative and qualitative. These old adages speak volumes:

- Until you measure, you don't control.
- People respect what management inspects.
- You can't manage it unless you measure it.
- You can't tell if you're winning without a scorecard.
- What gets measured gets done.

Recall from chapter 2 the five key customer groups to be targeted:

1. Patients
2. Visitors
3. Physicians
4. Employees
5. Payers

How well your organization currently assesses the satisfaction of these key customers depends on how you answer these questions:

- What exactly are your current assessment methods, both formal and informal?
- How helpful are your current methods?
- To what extent are results effectively fed to people who can act on them to improve service both at job function levels and across function lines?
- To improve your systems for assessing satisfaction, do you focus on identifying priorities? identifying customer groups? identifying which evaluation systems or methods work best?
- How effective are your methods for measuring performance at critical control points in service processes?
  - Which processes have the greatest impact on customer satisfaction?
  - What are critical control points in those processes?
  - What methods need to be installed to monitor these processes so that you have the data needed to identify improvement priorities and monitor progress?

Once you've established the service advancement parameters needed, your next step is to identify what should be measured.

☐ What to Measure

Figure 6-2 shows the spectrum of roles that measurement can play in a quality or service improvement strategy. Although all of these measurement roles are important, this chapter explores the measurement activities that have the greatest impact on service improvement, particularly those related to customer and employee satisfaction.

Measurement activities need to focus on *your customers'* criteria for judging service quality. First, you need to identify the service attributes that are important to your customers and then measure their perceptions of these attributes in the services you deliver. This should be done for all five groups you identified as your primary customers.

Your customers' perception of the quality of service attributes that are important to them is crucial. Even when your measures indicate that, for example, you are 98 percent on time in your service delivery, if a customer doesn't perceive your service as timely, you have not succeeded. A central objective of service strategy should be to improve customer *perceptions* of the quality of care—whether it is courteous, compassionate, respectful, or convenient—extended to them by employees.

Emphasis here is on *perceptions*, not actual behavior. Of course, changes in employee behavior and changes in your organization's processes lead to changes in customer perceptions. However, measuring changed behavior directly is often difficult. You can use observation techniques to count the frequency of certain behaviors. For example, you can station observers in the admissions waiting area and have them watch admissions

Figure 6-2. Measurement Model for Total Quality Management

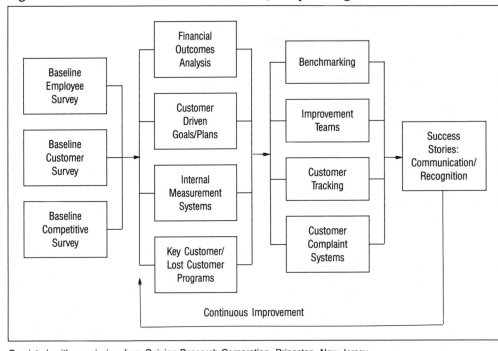

Reprinted, with permission, from Opinion Research Corporation, Princeton, New Jersey.

staff and count the number of smiles, words of concern, or times a person's name is used, but such observational techniques are cumbersome and time-consuming. And even if these behaviors were found to increase, your strategy falls short of the expected results if patients and visitors don't *perceive* the improvement. Again, perceptions, not necessarily the facts as you know them, influence the decisions your customers make and the word-of-mouth impressions they spread about your organization.

As mentioned above, when you measure perceptions of service attributes, you are measuring perceptions of service attributes that are *important to your customers.* Figure 6-3 shows the relationship between the *importance* of a service attribute and the *performance (or satisfaction) rating* of that attribute, as perceived by the customer. To plot a result, find the point at which the performance rating (along the *x* axis) intersects with the importance rating (along the *y* axis). You can then plot many service attributes and look at the results to help you identify improvement priorities. For example:

- *Quadrant 1 (high importance/low performance):* Data points that fall in quadrant 1 where importance to customers is high and employee performance is low demonstrate competitive weakness. This weakness provides improvement opportunities.
- *Quadrant 2 (high importance/high performance):* The data points that fall in quadrant 2 are your strong points. You need to maintain and defend them.
- *Quadrant 3 (low importance/high performance):* The points in quadrant 3 don't deserve your focused attention because, although they are strengths from a performance viewpoint, your customers don't value them much; some call this the area of "irrelevant superiority." You might consider reallocating resources you're devoting to improvement here.
- *Quadrant 4 (low importance/low performance):* The points that fall in quadrant 4 don't require much attention. Even though performance is weak, it has little effect because it has little value to the customer; some call this the "area of relative indifference."

Figure 6-3. Importance–Performance (Satisfaction) Matrix of Service Factors

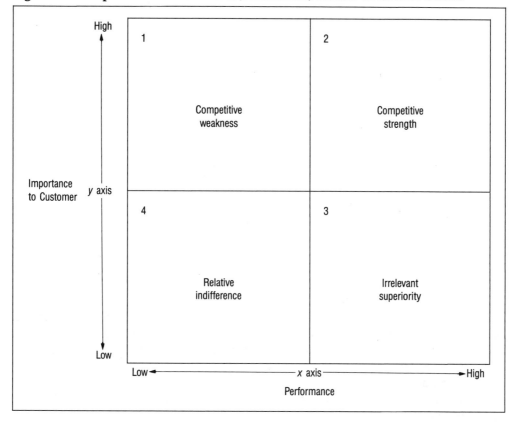

You need to know both ratings in order to make sense of customer feedback. For instance, if you conduct a survey and find that food receives very low ratings, you might be inclined to devote considerable attention to the quality of food. However, this effort might be futile if the quality of food *doesn't matter all that much* to the customer. The attributes you need to fix first are those that are indeed important to the customer, but rated low in satisfaction.

Once you know how customers define service quality, you can design three types of measures: (1) measures of overall customer satisfaction, (2) measures of customer perceptions of important service attributes, and (3) measures of performance of key elements in your service processes. This means measuring both processes and outcomes. Ask these questions:

- *Processes:* Which elements in our service delivery system are key to fulfilling our customers' criteria for judging service quality? How can we measure our performance related to each of these criteria so that we can control and improve them?
- *Outcomes:* How do our customers judge quality? What criteria do they use? Which of their criteria are most important to them?

Taking Organizationwide Measures

To create a context for discussion and show how your department measurement plan connects with your organization's overall measurement plan, let's first look at the three components as they are measured throughout the organization. The pyramid in figure 6-4 shows a three-part customer-oriented measurement system for your organization as a whole.

Figure 6-4. Sample Customer-Oriented Measurement Pyramid (Organization)

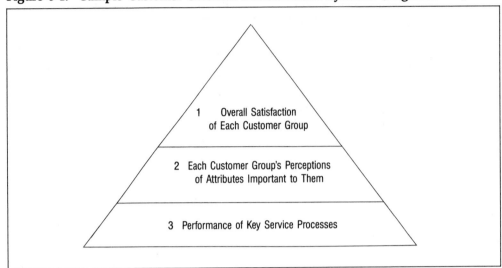

Overall Customer Satisfaction

At the top level, your organization might survey patients, family members, physicians, payers, and community members to determine their level of overall satisfaction with your organization compared, perhaps, with your competitors. Questions to patients might include, for example, "How likely would you be to choose our organization again if you need health care services?" At this level, other organizational measures of overall satisfaction might be the ratio of compliments to complaints, employee turnover, and dollars spent on rework.

Customer Group's Perceptions of Attributes Important to Them

At the middle level, your organization would monitor each customer group's perceptions of the attributes of service quality important *to them*—attributes that enter into overall satisfaction. You might survey "timeliness of service," "courtesy of service," "staff competence," and "communication quality," because patients tend to select these attributes as key to their satisfaction. For physicians, you might ask about the turnaround time of laboratory and radiology test results, the overall "user-friendliness" of the hospital, the quality of nursing care, and the responsiveness of the organization to the physician's needs. These tend to be the specific criteria physicians cite as important to their satisfaction.

Performance of Key Service Processes

At the lower, more specific and detailed level, the organization would measure the performance of key cross-functional service processes that have a great impact on customers' perceptions. For example, because patients value timeliness of service, the organization might measure the timeliness of several key processes such as admissions, discharge, and nursing services.

Taking Department-Level Measures

At the department level, the measurement pyramid might look like the one shown in figure 6-5. For example, the director of maintenance and engineering might survey nursing, one of its key customers. At the top level (1), maintenance might survey nurses monthly about their satisfaction. At the middle level (2), maintenance might ask nurses for feedback about performance on specific service attributes most important to them, such as response time to regular work requests, response time to stat requests, and staff courtesy when nursing calls with a question or complaint. Finally, at the lower, more

Figure 6-5. Sample Customer-Oriented Measurement Pyramid (Department)

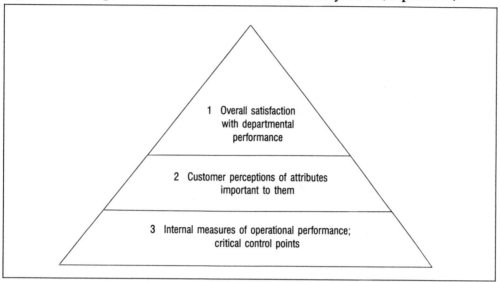

1 Overall satisfaction with departmental performance

2 Customer perceptions of attributes important to them

3 Internal measures of operational performance; critical control points

detailed level (3), maintenance might measure its own response time to stat and routine maintenance orders, monitoring critical control points, including the time from request to order submission, from dispatch to onset of service, and from onset of service to completion of service.

Technical or internal measures of service quality alert you to performance inconsistencies and problems that need attention. Without internal measures, you lack clues as to where your service process broke down. Internal measures also enable you to compare satisfaction with operational experience so that you can set customer-driven service standards.

Consider the example in figure 6-6 provided by Opinion Research Corporation based on aggregate data from studying problem resolution waiting time in many organizations. This figure examines the relationship between satisfaction ratings and the time customers wait for their problems to be resolved. As the figure shows, problems resolved within the first day hardly affect satisfaction. After that first day, satisfaction declines sharply. By seeing this relationship, the organization would appropriately set a standard for resolving all problems within one day and redesigning their internal processes and resources to make this possible. Such action should prevent the predictably sharp decline in customer satisfaction and its costly consequences for customer retention.

Inviting Complaints

In addition to measuring these levels of performance, it is also necessary to dig for complaints, which present a tremendous opportunity—a second chance to make things right. As stated by Fairchild in *Quality Letter for Healthcare Leaders*, "A complaint isn't bad; it's free market research and a hidden treasure—an opportunity to exceed expectations."[2] Instead of discouraging complaints, your feedback systems should encourage your customers to share their frustrations, dissatisfactions, resentments, and suggestions.

Perhaps you think that by inviting—and getting—more complaints, the executive management in your organization will conclude that your strategy for service excellence is failing. Convince them otherwise. An increase in complaints is rarely a sign of failure, just as a reduction in complaints does not signal success. The number of complaints is largely a function of the organization's openness to complaints and to self-improvement.

Figure 6-6. Chart Showing Relationship between Satisfaction and Problem Resolution

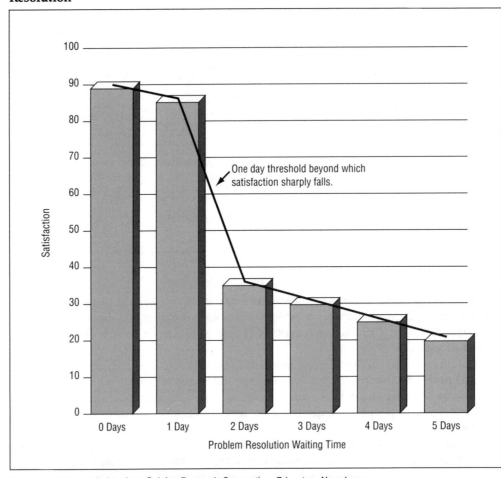

Reprinted, with permission, from Opinion Research Corporation, Princeton, New Jersey.

☐ How to Measure

There are many methods for measuring service quality, both in fact and in perception. To monitor customer *perceptions*, surveys and face-to-face or telephone interviews work well. To monitor *facts* about timeliness, accuracy, rework, or other attributes of your work processes, simple check sheets and logs work well. To evaluate and enhance your organization's mix of measurement methods related to service quality, consult the internal professionals who are most experienced in measurement, including those in quality assessment and improvement, marketing, customer service, management engineering, computer services, risk management, and research.

Most hospitals already have *live* data collectors—their patient representatives—many of whom already have in operation excellent systems for tracking complaints and identifying patterns that merit attention. Enlist them in your efforts to measure customer satisfaction.

Measuring Patient Satisfaction

Patient satisfaction can be measured in a number of ways. The following sections specifically discuss satisfaction surveys, postdischarge interviews, and focus groups. A combination of these is ideal.

Patient Satisfaction Surveys

Many hospitals survey their patients before and after discharge. This kind of survey may be the best tool for measuring customer perceptions of staff behavior. However, in order to provide the best data, the survey should do the following:

- Combine ratings of service performance on key attributes with "importance" ratings so as to prioritize improvement opportunities (see figure 6-7 for an example)
- Allow trending of performance in departments, units, and specialties
- Contain items or dimensions specific to service quality; for example, courtesy, concern, attention, responsiveness, explanations, and friendliness
- Yield an ample response (10 percent is low, 40 percent is too good to be true, and 30 percent is achievable)
- Be comprehensible to users and thus easy to fill out
- Provide enough responses to allow reliable conclusions
- Be designed to ask openly for opinions, instead of being a public relations ploy designed to elicit smiling faces and hype that influence the respondent
- Ask about specific areas (for example, nursing responsiveness) so that you can identify and act on problem areas
- Produce actionable results that are circulated to people in the right positions to review and act on
- Be supplemented by qualitative methods, such as focus groups, to delve more deeply into patient perceptions and values

Many satisfaction measurement systems, some of which are commercially available, provide information that compares your organization's performance with that of other relatively similar organizations. However, the most helpful approaches are ones in which you compete against yourself by trying to improve on your own past data. If you develop your own survey systems, tailor them to *your* customers in *your* geographic locale and change some of the questions so as to collect information that will help you make *specific* informed decisions.

The patient satisfaction measurement system developed at The Thomas Jefferson University Hospital in Philadelphia is a state-of-the-art approach. Over several years, a very sophisticated approach (the Cadillac model) was developed, refined, and implemented at Thomas Jefferson. Developed by Trevor Fisk, past senior vice-president for marketing and planning, this Patient Satisfaction Management System (PSMS) is grounded in five essential components:[3]

1. Patient surveys that are accurate, repetitive, and useful and that highlight priorities
2. Committed leaders who can mesh patient satisfaction issues with quality assurance mechanisms

Figure 6-7. Sample Survey Question Measuring Importance and Performance

	How important is this to you?	How good are we at this?
When I called to make appointments, phones were answered promptly.	VI IM N UI VUI 5 4 3 2 1	VG G N NG VP 5 4 3 2 1

Key:

VI = Very important	VG = Very good
IM = Important	G = Good
N = Neutral	N = Neutral
UI = Unimportant	NG = Not good
VUI = Very unimportant	VP = Very poor

3. Attention to complaints and their relationship to satisfaction issues
4. Guest relation efforts that are universal and focused on responsiveness to prioritized patient needs and concerns
5. Measurable goals for patient satisfaction and loyalty

The challenge at Jefferson was to combine these components into a scientifically sound and administratively practical system. Figure 6-8 shows a graphic summary of the Jefferson approach. The developers of this methodology consulted several corporations—including Procter & Gamble, Whirlpool, Disney World, Campbell Soup, Maytag, and several hotel chains—having a reputation for effective approaches to customer satisfaction. Although they adopted certain features of each approach, they did not find any overall models to be sufficiently applicable to health care and therefore built their own model.

The Jefferson approach is based on the following research findings:

- Total satisfaction can be related meaningfully to satisfaction with the individual components of service[4-6]
- Individual service features differ in their contribution to total satisfaction. An effective satisfaction management system does not treat all factors as equally important. It must reveal their relative contributions to total satisfaction if managers are to set valid priorities for action.[7,8]
- Aggregate satisfaction with a service is the principal determinant of subsequent brand loyalty and intent to reuse and recommend.[9,10]
- Not all satisfied consumers remain brand loyal through postusage evaluation of their service experiences. Further, brand loyalty tends to be lowest for services like health care, perceived to be major decisions and used infrequently.[11,12] Therefore, health care organizations must attain extremely high levels of service satisfaction to minimize the extent of this subsequent erosion of brand loyalty.
- Dissatisfied consumers share their discontent with many more people than do satisfied consumers.[13] For that reason, health care organizations need to achieve very close to 100 percent satisfaction for word-of-mouth to be more positive than negative.
- Regarding survey layout, survey response rates are more a function of layout and consistency of question format than questionnaire length.[14]
- The semantic differential questioning format lowers risk of positive bias and produces more subtle insights into the nature of satisfaction.[15]

Figure 6-8. The Jefferson Method for Measuring Patient Satisfaction

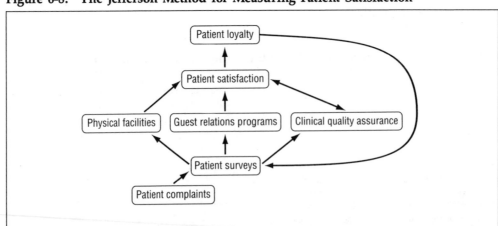

- The principal purpose of attitude measurement is not so much to produce absolute measures as to produce usable and comparable measures that highlight problems and afford before-and-after comparisons.[16]

The features of the model are as follows:

- Jefferson selected a common survey format that has been adapted to a wide range of satisfaction measurement needs. This format is used with inpatients at Jefferson, two associated community hospitals, and a rehabilitation hospital; with outpatients; with same-day surgical, laboratory, and radiology patients; and with medical office patients in their faculty practices and referring physician practices. They find it advantageous to use the same format for all evaluation needs, because they can make improvements in their method and also because managers become more familiar and comfortable with the format.
- Although the questionnaire is long, ranging from 40 to 90 questions, its length does not affect response rate.
- The instrument relies largely on the semantic differential format, which has been shown to protect against response bias (see figure 6-9 for an example).
- Scores are reported in easy-to-grasp composite form, making them easy to "eyeball" by the end user. The marketing staff also examines distribution of the data so as to identify situations where a reasonable average score disguises a sizable dissatisfied minority. Scrutiny of distributions allows for identification of service features that work most of the time but break down occasionally, with costly consequences for patient satisfaction, repeat business, and reputation of the organization.
- Jefferson developed software that allows them to determine the importance ratings for particular service features *implicitly* (by figuring gamma correlations of service features with overall satisfaction), instead of *explicitly* (by asking patients to rate the importance of each feature).[17] Research shows that explicit ratings of importance by patients are valid only when patients are asked to rate fewer than 10 features.[18] The implicit ratings method does not rely on patients' differential abilities to do this mental sorting. Instead, it is based on observable patterns of correlation between ratings of specific features and overall satisfaction using a large sample of respondents.
- Jefferson calculates two types of importance-to-satisfaction correlations: First, nurse responsiveness is correlated with overall satisfaction with nursing to yield the importance of a service feature (nurse responsiveness) to the overall service category (nursing). Second, nursing satisfaction is correlated with overall satisfaction with Jefferson to yield the importance of an overall service category to the overall hospital experience. Being able to see both correlations helps managers set priorities for action.
- Another unique feature of the Jefferson system involves the establishment of "target scores" for key service features. Jefferson wants to achieve and maintain at least a 95 percent level of patient loyalty (intention to choose Jefferson next time and willingness to recommend). To achieve this level, Jefferson derived target levels

Figure 6-9. Semantic Differential Format

Your nurses were:						
Responsive	Very	Somewhat	Neither	Somewhat	Very	Unresponsive

for individual service features as follows: "very important" features must score above 90, "somewhat important" features must score at least 75, "less important" features must score at least 65, with no particular target for "unimportant" features.

- The PSMS software calculates the margin of error so that users of the data can tell whether falling below target could be attributed to sampling error.
- The surveys provide enlightening information about subgroups (ages, gender, severity of illness).

Jefferson executives report that the survey has proven both reliable and helpful in practice. When identified problems have been addressed, increase in satisfaction and loyalty result.

The effectiveness of the Jefferson approach can be attributed to its scientific soundness and to the commitment by administration to integrate it into the organization's ongoing management decisions and service improvement systems:

- Jefferson's president and chairman of the board declared that "customer satisfaction is one valid measure of quality."
- A formal Medical Staff Patient Service Committee was instituted to review survey results and report to the Executive Committee (including all clinical chiefs), which is key to change in academic medical centers.
- A system has been developed that integrates complaint handling with the survey system, as shown in the algorithm in figure 6-10.
- A patient service department was developed to handle not only patient representation activities but also a wide range of guest services.
- On the first day of their orientation, all house staff are educated about the survey system and its uses.
- Results are reviewed at all key administrative meetings.
- Marketing staff who are experts on the survey methodology and results are included in meetings on quality assurance, strategic planning, and in other arenas where survey results are used to inform decisions.

The Jefferson experience yields important lessons:

- Your organization's leaders must be committed to optimizing patient satisfaction and loyalty to the extent that they are willing to be inconvenienced by changes that satisfaction measurement dictates.
- Patient satisfaction needs to be measured systematically if you want meaningful, reliable, and usable results.
- To tap the full potential of satisfaction measurement, your customer satisfaction measurement systems need to be complemented with a far-reaching service commitment; a system for soliciting, recording, and responding to complaints; and formal service improvement tactics.
- Customer satisfaction must be a high priority and continuous focus of health care leaders. Measurement systems need to demonstrate reliability and practical value for leaders to use them in decision making.
- Although it takes time, people, and money to manage a top-notch satisfaction measurement and management system, the benefits outweigh those of other marketing activities.
- To make the most of satisfaction measurement, you need to attend to the details.

For further information about patient satisfaction measurement, see *Measuring and Managing Patient Satisfaction*, by Steven Steiber and William Krowinski,[19] and *Measuring Patient Satisfaction for Improved Patient Services*, by Stephan Strasser and Rose Marie Davis.[20]

Figure 6-10. Patient Complaint-Handling Algorithm

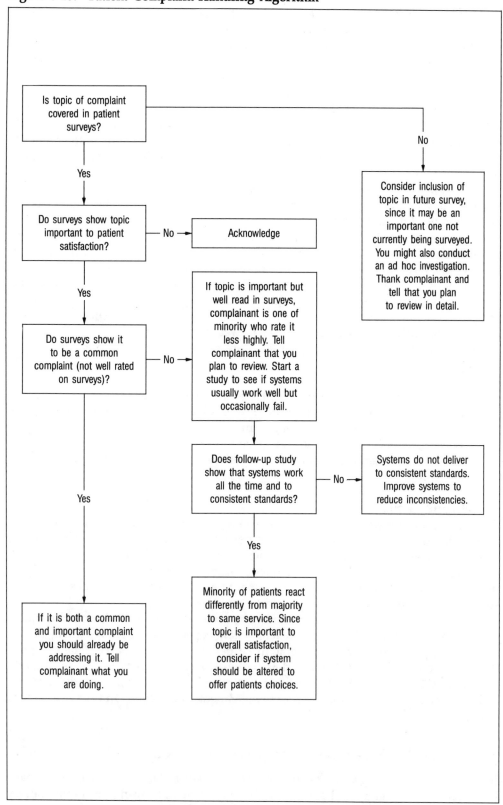

Postdischarge Interviews

Postdischarge interviews, a wonderful source of feedback, involve talking to randomly selected patients or to all former patients within two weeks of discharge. These interviews can yield both quantitative and qualitative data.

Strasser and Davis[21] tout the advantages of telephone follow-up methods for soliciting qualitative information about problems to supplement information produced by surveys and also for achieving service recovery. For example, at the Ohio State University Hospitals, patients who included their name on the patient survey and rated satisfaction below a targeted level received follow-up phone calls by hospital managers. The benefits were grateful patients, rich and actionable information about the nature of the problems encountered, and managers forced to intervene quickly and effectively across department lines and to overcome departmental myopia.

At Aultman Hospital in Canton, Ohio, a patient callback system gives the emergency department valuable information about patients' experiences. According to the September 1986 issue of the newsletter *Convenience Care Update,*[22] two full-time registered nurses with emergency nursing experience share the position of 40-hour-per-week telephone communicator. A nurse phones patients 48 to 72 hours after their emergency department visit, asks questions from a carefully developed form, and responds to the patients' questions. The 687-bed hospital sees about 130 patients daily in its emergency department. Nurse communicators call more than 100 former patients a day, five days a week. Hospital leaders are convinced that the public relations, patient satisfaction, and quality assurance benefits make the callback system well worth the money.

To be sure that postdischarge interviews are effective, you need to ensure the following:

- *A sensitive person must conduct the interviews.* Some hospitals train graduate students or hospital volunteers, other hospitals have nurses make these calls, and still others divide up calls among administrators.
- *Follow-up must be conducted.* To encourage complaints, have the interviewer promise absolute confidentiality and ask the patient's permission to follow up on the complaint.

Patient Focus Groups

Focus groups, a richly informative qualitative method, are carefully designed and facilitated group discussions intended to assess perceptions held by a customer group and to test responses to new ideas and approaches. As a patient feedback device, focus groups can be used to learn about patients' experience with your organization and their suggestions for improvement. You can also use them to explore what is important to patients so that you can develop appropriate survey questions.

Linda DeWolf, director of patient and community services at St. Luke's Hospital in Cedar Rapids, Iowa, established an excellent system of patient focus groups run by patient representatives. Other hospitals prefer to use experienced focus-group facilitators or hire them to train in-house people to use state-of-the-art focus group facilitation techniques.

Figure 6-11 describes St. Luke's focus group program. For more information, see DeWolf's article, "Focus Groups: Assessing Patient Satisfaction and Targeting New Services."[23]

Measuring the Perceptions of Family Members and Other Visitors

Because of the scrutiny given to hospital services by patients' families and friends, many hospitals monitor family and friend satisfaction—sometimes using an annual survey and/or focus groups to provide qualitative insights into key satisfiers and dissatisfiers. Others use simple methods such as *visitor-in-the-hall interviews.* Conducted properly, these hallway interviews seem more like chats between concerned persons than interviews,

Figure 6-11. Focus Group Program

Patient Representative Department
Focus Groups

Purpose

To offer posthospitalized patients the opportunity to share their perceptions of their hospital experience.

Policies

1. Composition of focus group:
   A. Six to eight patients (from the same patient area and discharged within a two- to six-week time period) plus a support person of the patient's choice, if desired.
   B. A patient representative acting as coordinator and facilitator.
   C. One representative from the particular patient area, if desired.
2. Format:
   A. Patients will be invited to St. Luke's for a light supper or refreshments with group discussion of the hospital experience to follow.
3. Preparation:
   A. Food Service shall be responsible for preparing any meals or refreshments for the group.
   B. Housekeeping shall be responsible for setting up the facility.
4. Follow up:
   A. The Patient Representative Department shall be responsible for initiating follow-up on any voiced concerns.

Procedures

1. Focus group members will be selected from a random sample of former patients (using the criteria established above).
2. Persons shall receive a personal phone call extended by the Patient Representative Department and followed by a letter of invitation.
3. Feedback regarding group discussions shall routinely be provided to administration, quality assurance, and the appropriate patient areas.
4. Routine evaluations of the process shall be conducted by the Patient Representative Department.

Reprinted, with permission, from St. Luke's Hospital, Cedar Rapids, Iowa.

enabling you to see your organization from an invaluable perspective. You may learn something vital about how to make your hospital a better place for visitors and family members who too often are overlooked as a customer group.

Begin by politely excusing yourself and then asking individual visitors if they would be willing to share any comments they may have on how to improve your organization. The following is what you might say in such an interview:

Pardon me. I'm _____ from the _____ department here at the hospital. I'm trying to touch base with visitors to our hospital to see what they think of their experience with us. Would you mind if I ask you a couple of short questions on the way to your car?

- Have you been visiting someone here?
- How are they doing?
- How has your experience with us been?
- How does the patient you've been visiting feel about his or her experience with us?
- Based on your experience here and on what the patient you're visiting may have told you, what might we do to improve?

Measuring Physician Perceptions

Physicians, a key customer group, make what many people still agree is the lion's share of decisions about which hospitals and ambulatory care services consumers use. At the very least, they influence consumer choice dramatically. Therefore, the answer to the following question is vital: "How satisfied are your physicians with the people and services in your organization that influence their ability to serve their patients?"

With a systematic evaluation strategy geared to tap physician perceptions, you can:

- Measure the effects of your service strategy on physicians' perceptions of employee behavior.
- Raise physician awareness of the value your organization places on excellent service.
- Solicit input so you can stay in touch with their views of what makes it easy (or hard) to practice in your institution.
- Gain information on your strengths and problems so you can modify your strategy and focus your improvement efforts on the right issues.

Getting information from physicians is not easy, but you can do so successfully if you ask questions and *act* on what you hear. To obtain information, consider methods such as mail surveys, phone interviews, extensive surveys, or focus groups, discussed below.

Simple Mail Surveys

A simple one-page questionnaire (figure 6-12) can help raise physician awareness of your strategy for service excellence, provide you with a rough reading of physicians' perceptions of change, and obtain physician perceptions of problems that need monitoring or solving. Distribute the questionnaire to a sample of physicians before you implement your strategy and at periodic intervals later.

Figure 6-12. Physician Questionnaire on Customer Relations

Physician Survey on *Hospitality*				
	Almost Always	Often	Occasionally	Rarely
1. How often do you think our employees are courteous and helpful to patients?				
2. How often do you think our employees are courteous and helpful to physicians?				
3. What are your patients telling you about the service they receive at our hospital and the courtesy our employees extend them?				
4. What do you see as the biggest problems our employees have in their interactions with patients?				
5. What do you see as the biggest problems our employees have in their interactions with physicians?				
6. What do you see as the biggest problems our employees have in their interactions with fellow employees?				
7. Do you have any other observations or advice about problems we need to address in our *hospitality* effort?				
We've provided a return envelope for your convenience. Please return to:				

Phone Interviews

Another technique is to telephone a random sample of physicians to find out how they think your employees and your institution are faring in service excellence. You can call before you initiate your customer relations strategy if you do not already have a functioning strategy, and at regular intervals—perhaps quarterly—thereafter.

At Albert Einstein Medical Center, we called 20 physicians from different departments on a quarterly basis. We stratified our sample of callees so that we could reach "high," "medium," and "low" admitters. We asked each callee 5 to 10 minutes' worth of questions about their perceptions of our *hospital*ity program.

In our baseline interview, we told them about our plans to conduct the *hospitality* effort and asked them to describe from their point of view the strengths and weaknesses in employee behavior to date. We also asked them to compare employee behavior in our hospital with that in other hospitals. They were also asked to describe the kinds of comments their patients make about employee behavior and service at our hospital and to include compliments and complaints.

Three months after our initial *hospitality* workshops, we conducted another round of telephone interviews with physicians. In these interviews, we asked physicians the extent to which they had perceived changes in employee behavior toward their patients, toward one another, toward visitors, and toward the physicians themselves.

Extensive Survey of Physician as Customer

In their role as *users* of your organization's services, physicians deserve and expect excellent service from staff and systems, calling it *ease of practice*. Thus, physicians tend to be more cooperative with staff and more emotionally available to patients if they are not constantly frustrated in their interaction with systems and people. They want what you want: a user-friendly hospital.

Survey questionnaires, typically mailed annually or biannually, help raise physician awareness of your service commitment and strategy, provide you with a reading on physicians' perceptions of change, and show physician satisfaction levels and problems that need attention. These surveys ask about the overall quality of care; the breadth, depth, and quality of services offered to them and their patients; their perceptions of the competence of staff; the efficiency of systems; and the quality of relationships.

The key is to identify the criteria your physicians use to judge service in your institution and to focus your survey on these criteria, stated in actionable form. Many hospitals use the "Hospital Quality Trends: Physician Judgments System (nicknamed "HQT:MD"), developed and validated by the Hospital Corporation of America, the Rand Corporation, the Harvard Community Health Plan, and the New England Medical Center, to obtain physician feedback about hospital services (available from Quality of Care Research, Hospital Corporation of America, Nashville, Tennessee). After extensive research identifying factors of quality that are important to physicians and actionable by hospital administrators, the HQT:MD measures the following areas:

- Nursing staff
- Administrative staff
- Medical records and clinical information
- Efficiency in scheduling patients
- Treatment of family
- Staff to manage emergencies
- Medical equipment
- Selected features of the hospital
- Discharge process
- Medical staff's attention to quality
- Overall hospital quality
- Willingness to use or recommend hospital

- Quality of hospital-based medical staff
- Quality of hospital departments

Users of this tool prefer to rely on professional researchers to do their data collection and reporting, allowing the hospital leadership to focus their time and energy on using the results to improve performance.

The questionnaire includes 89 items focusing on "workplace quality" and "patient care quality." It includes fixed-response items and open-ended questions. An excerpt from the questionnaire is shown in figure 6-13. According to Nelson and others, the HQT:MD works as follows:[24]

1. *Sampling:* A 100 percent sample of the most active members of the medical staff and a representative sample of less active physicians are identified, and their names, addresses, and phone numbers are sent to research headquarters.
2. *Data collection:* Questionnaires are distributed to physicians for completion at a convenient time and returned to headquarters.
3. *Nonrespondent followup:* Physicians who don't return the questionnaire are urged through their office staff to participate.
4. *Data analysis and report production:* The research service tallies the results and produces graphic trend reports, as illustrated in figure 6-14.
5. *Consultation:* The research service helps the hospital interpret and make use of the results within their quality improvement and strategic plans.
6. *Education:* Hospital leaders attend a workshop to learn ways to disseminate the findings and make wise use of them to improve hospital performance from physicians' perspectives.

To develop your own physician survey, use focus groups to identify physicians' criteria for service quality; that is, determine what they expect of your organization in the way of service. Once you identify these requirements, you can build a survey around them to find out quantitatively their relative importance levels and physician ratings of performance related to each.

Physician Focus Groups

Focus groups are particularly helpful in identifying key service factors as a basis for survey design or for soliciting feedback about a specific aspect of service, like one clinical program or one hospital support service. Alliant Health System in Louisville, Kentucky, conducted a series of focus groups targeting particular specialties and then followed up with mail surveys. The two central questions in the focus groups were "How important is this service?" and "How are we doing?" As with patient focus groups, physician focus groups can yield rich, qualitative results. If you want to know how user-friendly your organization really is, just ask physicians these questions:

- What about a hospital encourages you to admit patients?
- What discourages you from admitting patients?
- What encourages you about the way our hospital operates?
- What discourages you about the way our hospital operates?

A focus group works best with targeted, or homogenous, groups. For example, a group can be composed of physicians who are low admitters, medium admitters, high admitters, nonadmitters, former admitters, or residents, but not combinations of these physicians.

Ideally, an outside disinterested party with focus-group facilitation skills should conduct the group. Physicians may be more comfortable with a facilitator who has no vested interest in the outcome and therefore will maintain confidentiality. Usually the session

Figure 6-13. HQT:MD Questionnaire (Excerpt)

HOSPITAL-BASED MEDICAL STAFF QUALITY

Evaluate the quality of each of these hospital-based medical specialties regarding:

- **Communication with Attending Physicians:** specialists' communication skill & ability to answer questions
- **Availability of Attending Physicians:** adequacy of numbers & types of specialists on staff
- **Skill & Efficiency:** specialists' technical ability; they perform the job right the first time

SPECIALTY	COMMUNICATION WITH ATTENDING					AVAILABILITY TO ATTENDING					SKILL & EFFICIENCY				
	Excel.	Very Good	Good	Fair	Poor	Excel.	Very Good	Good	Fair	Poor	Excel.	Very Good	Good	Fair	Poor
48. Anesthesiologists	$\square_5$	$\square_4$	$\square_3$	$\square_2$	$\square_1$	$\square_5$	$\square_4$	$\square_3$	$\square_2$	$\square_1$	$\square_5$	$\square_4$	$\square_3$	$\square_2$	$\square_1$
49. Pathologists	$\square_5$	$\square_4$	$\square_3$	$\square_2$	$\square_1$	$\square_5$	$\square_4$	$\square_3$	$\square_2$	$\square_1$	$\square_5$	$\square_4$	$\square_3$	$\square_2$	$\square_1$
50. Radiologists	$\square_5$	$\square_4$	$\square_3$	$\square_2$	$\square_1$	$\square_5$	$\square_4$	$\square_3$	$\square_2$	$\square_1$	$\square_5$	$\square_4$	$\square_3$	$\square_2$	$\square_1$

HOSPITAL DEPARTMENTS' QUALITY

Evaluate the **overall performance** of each department. Base your rating on these factors:

- skill, efficiency, morale, and the extent to which the department treats physicians like valued customers.

After evaluating each department, indicate with an "X" whether or not you are a regular user of this department.

Please "X" the last column (i.e., "No Department") if this hospital does not have the department.

COMMON CLINICAL DEPARTMENTS	Excellent	Very Good	Good	Fair	Poor	Regular User	No Department
51. Anesthesia	$\square_5$	$\square_4$	$\square_3$	$\square_2$	$\square_1$	$\square_1$	$\square_9$
52. Maternity	$\square_5$	$\square_4$	$\square_3$	$\square_2$	$\square_1$	$\square_1$	$\square_9$
53. Medical	$\square_5$	$\square_4$	$\square_3$	$\square_2$	$\square_1$	$\square_1$	$\square_9$
54. Pathology	$\square_5$	$\square_4$	$\square_3$	$\square_2$	$\square_1$	$\square_1$	$\square_9$
55. Radiology	$\square_5$	$\square_4$	$\square_3$	$\square_2$	$\square_1$	$\square_1$	$\square_9$
56. Surgery	$\square_5$	$\square_4$	$\square_3$	$\square_2$	$\square_1$	$\square_1$	$\square_9$

SELECTED DEPARTMENTS & AREAS

	Excellent	Very Good	Good	Fair	Poor	Regular User	No Department
57. Med/Surg Unit(s)	$\square_5$	$\square_4$	$\square_3$	$\square_2$	$\square_1$	$\square_1$	$\square_9$
58. Intensive Care Unit	$\square_5$	$\square_4$	$\square_3$	$\square_2$	$\square_1$	$\square_1$	$\square_9$
59. Cardiac Care Unit	$\square_5$	$\square_4$	$\square_3$	$\square_2$	$\square_1$	$\square_1$	$\square_9$
60. Neonatal ICU	$\square_5$	$\square_4$	$\square_3$	$\square_2$	$\square_1$	$\square_1$	$\square_9$
61. Pediatrics In-patient Unit	$\square_5$	$\square_4$	$\square_3$	$\square_2$	$\square_1$	$\square_1$	$\square_9$
62. Psychiatry In-patient Unit	$\square_5$	$\square_4$	$\square_3$	$\square_2$	$\square_1$	$\square_1$	$\square_9$
63. Operating Room	$\square_5$	$\square_4$	$\square_3$	$\square_2$	$\square_1$	$\square_1$	$\square_9$
64. Recovery Area	$\square_5$	$\square_4$	$\square_3$	$\square_2$	$\square_1$	$\square_1$	$\square_9$
65. Physical Therapy	$\square_5$	$\square_4$	$\square_3$	$\square_2$	$\square_1$	$\square_1$	$\square_9$
66. Respiratory Therapy	$\square_5$	$\square_4$	$\square_3$	$\square_2$	$\square_1$	$\square_1$	$\square_9$

Reprinted, with permission, from Nelson, E., Rose, R., and Batalden, P. Measuring and improving physician satisfaction. *The Quality Letter for Healthcare Leaders* 2(2), Mar. 1990.

Figure 6-14. Sample Page from HQT:MD Report

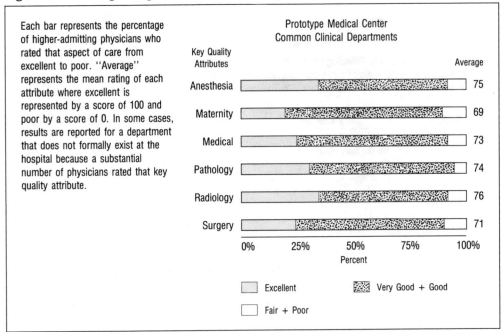

Each bar represents the percentage of higher-admitting physicians who rated that aspect of care from excellent to poor. "Average" represents the mean rating of each attribute where excellent is represented by a score of 100 and poor by a score of 0. In some cases, results are reported for a department that does not formally exist at the hospital because a substantial number of physicians rated that key quality attribute.

Prototype Medical Center
Common Clinical Departments

Key Quality Attributes	Average
Anesthesia	75
Maternity	69
Medical	73
Pathology	74
Radiology	76
Surgery	71

Excellent   Very Good + Good   Fair + Poor

Reprinted, with permission, from Nelson, E., Rose, R., and Batalden, P. Measuring and improving physician satisfaction. *The Quality Letter for Healthcare Leaders* 2(2), Mar. 1990.

is taped, or someone takes extensive notes for later analysis. (Be sure that the participants understand beforehand that the proceeding is being taped or that notes are being taken.)

Sometimes hospitals hire a focus-group professional to conduct two or three focus groups and tape the sessions. They then use the tapes to train a local, less expensive facilitator to conduct groups on a regular basis. If you don't want to use outsiders, choose skillful, open-minded, and trusted staff members.

Other Methods
An increasingly popular method for obtaining feedback from physicians is through *physician liaisons.* Usually full-time staff members, physician liaisons visit with physicians and their office staffs several times throughout the year to take the pulse of their relationship with the hospital and identify ways the organization can serve them better.

At Memorial Health System in South Bend, Indiana, *senior administrators pay annual visits to physicians* in their offices for structured one-on-one interviews. Having found that their physicians do not like to give numerical ratings to hospital services, the administrators ask open-ended questions like, "How does turnaround time on lab results compare to last year?" The administrators compare notes and identify trends and improvement opportunities. These administrators also rely on physician feedback gained from informal contacts, such as chats over lunch, management by walking around, and discussion with employees who have repeated contact with physicians.

Smaller organizations rely more often on *informal and face-to-face methods,* such as talk during sports or social events and discussion at medical staff–administrative meetings. Yet another technique is to telephone a random sample of physicians to find out how they think your employees and your institution are faring in service quality.

Assessing Employee Perceptions and Satisfaction

The group having the most firsthand experience with your organization's people, systems, customers, and outcomes is made up of your employees. Do not overlook the perceptions and experiences of this group; they are a top-notch source of information. Furthermore, failure to ask their views devalues employees and dims their commitment and sense of ownership in your organization. These internal customers are the key to service excellence and, consequently, to the organization's image in the professional and patient community; in other words, employees are the key to your organization's success.

By focusing evaluation techniques on employees as caregivers and as customers, you can accomplish several things:

- Identify the effects of your service strategy on employee behavior, morale, and pride in the organization.
- Target strengths and weaknesses that help delineate your future tactics.
- Welcome employee participation in identifying strengths and achievements that deserve acknowledgment as well as problems that cry for attention.
- Focus on ways to help employees feel better served and more satisfied as recipients of service by coworkers.
- Identify ways your organization can help employees feel recognized, appreciated, and cared for.

A variety of methods, used singly or in combination, can serve to measure employee perceptions and satisfaction. Some of these are summarized briefly below.

- *Behavior self-report:* If your service strategy promotes specific behaviors, you can ask employees how often they and coworkers exhibit these behaviors. Administer such a survey before the strategy is instituted and at periodic intervals later. At Albert Einstein Medical Center, we used a "Taking Stock" survey to tap employee perceptions of their behavior (figure 6-15). The survey asks employees to comment on the frequency of each of our *hospitality* "House Rule" behaviors, both their personal behaviors and those of coworkers.
- *Workshop evaluation:* Every service-related workshop you sponsor is an opportunity to collect valuable employee perceptions. Incorporate questions on pride and loyalty, for example.
- *Internal customer survey:* Employees are each other's customers across functional lines. An enlightened service strategy raises employee awareness and builds skills that should translate into better service extended by one department to another, one employee to another.

  Consider a survey like the one in figure 6-16 to assess interdepartmental perceptions of perhaps 10 departments at a time. Within a month, all departments should be subjected to peer evaluation.
- *Focus groups:* Focus groups tend to win the evaluation method popularity contest. Ask people to talk about what they think and feel, and they'll do so frankly and constructively. A focus group should have anywhere from 6 to 15 participants. Begin by explaining your intention to make organizational improvements with their help. Post and explain a Customer-Service Matrix, as shown in figure 6-17. Ask people to form groups of three or four and to identify specific strengths and weaknesses in what they consider to be the most important boxes on the matrix. Reconvene the entire group and invite a sharing of each group's results. Then—and this step is key—explain what will be done to improve the problems that the group thinks are important.
- *Perception surveys:* You can find out employee perceptions of the degree of external customer satisfaction and identify discrepancies between what employees tell you and what customers actually think—discrepancies important to address so as to improve service. You can monitor employee satisfaction with their own ability to meet customer expectations. You can also identify employee perceptions of key factors that affect employee satisfaction, such as communication, organization goals,

Figure 6-15. "Taking Stock" Survey Form (Excerpts)

Taking Stock: Your impressions of *hospital*ity

I. What's your sense of how often *employees* show the following behaviors?		Hardly Ever	A Little	A Lot	Almost Always	Not in a Position to Do This
A	Employees smile at patients, visitors, and one another.					
B	Employees make eye contact with patients, visitors, and one another.					
C	Employees introduce themselves to patients.					
D	Employees call people by name.					
E	Employees help people who look confused.					

I. What's your sense of how often *you* show the following behaviors?		Hardly Ever	A Little	A Lot	Almost Always	Not in a Position to Do This
A	I smile at patients, visitors, and coworkers.					
B	I make eye contact with patients, visitors, and coworkers.					
C	I introduce myself to patients.					
D	I call people by name.					
E	I help people who look confused.					

Reprinted, with permission, from the Albert Einstein Healthcare Foundation, Philadelphia, Pennsylvania.

Figure 6-16. Survey to Assess Interdepartmental Perceptions

Department Name: _____

very low   very high

Responsiveness to "rush" needs:

1   2   3   4   5   6

Telephone courtesy:

1   2   3   4   5   6

Accuracy of tasks performed:

1   2   3   4   5   6

Comments and suggestions:

Reprinted, with permission, from the Albert Einstein Healthcare Foundation, Philadelphia, Pennsylvania.

Figure 6-17. Customer Service Matrix

Key Components	Customer Groups				
	Patients	Visitors	Physicians	Employees	Third-Party Payers
Technical competence					
Environment					
People skills					
Systems					
Amenities					

Reprinted, with permission, from the Albert Einstein Healthcare Foundation, Philadelphia, Pennsylvania.

management practices, employee services, teamwork, interdepartmental relationships, degree of participation, use of authority, reward and recognition, supervision quality, and organization support. Typically, organizations hire outside research firms to conduct perception surveys. A word of warning: don't conduct an attitude survey unless you're clear about your purpose and your strategy for following up on results. You'll take 10 steps backward if you give people a chance to let off steam and then do nothing about it. Even the employees who adopt a wait-and-see attitude gradually come to feel patronized and resentful.

- *Exit interviews:* When employees leave the organization, your human resource specialists should arrange for an exit interview. These interviews help you gain valuable information about your organization, certain departments, and quality-of-work-life issues that affect your organization's ability to achieve service excellence. Also, in that employees are considered customers, exit interviews can make an employee's departure more amicable.

Assessing Satisfaction of Third-Party Payers

Unions, employers, insurance companies, HMOs, and PPOs all want to do business with a high-quality, cost-effective, user-friendly health care provider who is responsive to their requests for service, access, and information. Focus groups can serve to identify the critical issues that affect the satisfaction of these third-party payers. You can then follow up with periodic, perhaps annual, telephone or mail surveys to keep you informed about the important perceptions and needs of third-party payers.

In your focus groups or surveys, you can ask the following questions:

- What do you look for in a hospital? What factors need to exist to attract you to do business with one hospital versus another?
- How do you view this hospital as a health care provider? What makes this hospital attractive or unattractive to you?
- What are your frustrations when dealing with this hospital?
- What do your members, constituents, subscribers, or employees say about this hospital?
- How could this hospital improve its effectiveness in your eyes and, consequently, its relationship with you?

Assessing Department-Specific Customer Satisfaction

Departments also need to solicit perceptions of their particular customers and should administer a short survey with each of their internal and external customer groups. The focus is the extent to which that department is currently meeting customer requirements. To keep such surveys manageable, they should be brief, easy to fill out and understandable to multiple users, and administered at least quarterly so they can identify trends. Figure 6-18 provides an example of such a survey developed by a pharmacy department to evaluate patients' perception of their services.

One pharmacy department talked with its users and uncovered their priorities on timeliness, attitude, quality of information, and responsiveness to procedure changes. To examine user perceptions of performance related to their priorities, the department developed a simple survey to poll perceptions, believing that low scores would point the way to problems to be tackled. The department developed a series of scales that poll perceptions held by other departments served by the pharmacy staff to identify problems that might be addressed beneficially (see figure 6-19).

Figure 6-18. Pharmacy Department Survey of Patient Perceptions

Will You Help Us Improve Our Services?

Our department is working to provide you with the pharmacy services you need while you're here. We want to improve our services and solve any problems that patients are having. Will you please help by sharing your experience with us?

1. Have you had any problems with your medications while you've been here? (please describe):

2. Have medications been:

	always			never
delivered on time?	1	2	3	4
explained to you?	1	2	3	4
correct item?	1	2	3	4
given courteously?	1	2	3	4
available when needed?	1	2	3	4

3. How can we improve our services related to medications?

Your responses will be kept strictly confidential. Please leave this completed form on your meal tray. Your response will be very helpful to us. Thank you very much.

Figure 6-19. Pharmacy Department Survey of Other Departments' Perceptions

1. In filling routine orders, the Pharmacy is
1 2 3 4 5 timely....................untimely

2. In filling stat orders, the Pharmacy is
1 2 3 4 5 quick to respond.......slow to respond

3. The attitude of Pharmacy personnel is
1 2 3 4 5 professional............unprofessional

4. Drug information supplied by the Pharmacy is
1 2 3 4 5 not useful....................useful

5. The Pharmacy's response to changing needs is
1 2 3 4 5 appropriate..............inappropriate

6. The hours of Pharmacy coverage are
1 2 3 4 5 adequate.................inadequate

7. The procedures to use Pharmacy services are
1 2 3 4 5 efficient.................cumbersome

As an indicator of future trends, Boulder Community Hospital in Boulder, Colorado, uses portable computers for *spot surveys* that ask customers just a few questions about a specific topic before or after they receive service.

Utilizing Tools for Measuring Internal Operations and Process Steps

The beginning of this chapter described the importance of including in your measurement mix regular methods for monitoring internal operations and feeding back the results in time to make course corrections. A number of quality improvement tools for measuring internal operations—for example, checklists, counts, histograms, and clocks—are described in *The Health Care Manager's Guide to Continuous Quality Improvement.*[25] The point here is that satisfaction measurement is useless unless you have a grip on the process steps that constitute the service package producing these levels of satisfaction.

In addition to the measurement tools delineated in the quality improvement literature, use of various "audits" can help ensure that service includes what you think it does and that your strategy is being implemented properly. Once you know which service features are valued by customers, you can build an audit that enables observers to walk around and take a tally of which features are present. (The ambience audit of a medical office environment shown in figure 10-7, p. 192, is an example.)

Other audits can be developed for specific services. The first step is to make a service process explicit and identify the quality specifications for completion of each step in the process. Then an auditor or audit team follows the customer or paperwork being processed through the system to see whether each step is completed with each quality specification being fulfilled.

Tailor-made audits like these help you to learn which service produced the results reflected on satisfaction indicators. Because of low satisfaction scores, health care executives often conclude that a strategy or a service process failed when in fact it was never implemented. You can also develop an audit device around the detailed plan for your service strategy. After listing each planned activity, assign an audit team the task of circulating among designated people and places to see whether indeed each step in your plan has been implemented on time.

Tracking Complaints, Evaluating Scuttlebutt, and Other Investigative Methods

Apart from the methods described earlier in this chapter that tap each major customer group, other methods can provide valuable information. Some of these are complaint tracking, suggestion boxes, outsiders' perspectives, and scuttlebutt evaluation.

When *soliciting and tracking complaints* from customers, be sure you use a solid system for doing so. Several systems are commercially available. Whichever one you choose should be able to yield specific data sets. These include the number and nature of complaints so you can identify patterns, percentages, the nature of the complaints resolved versus unresolved, and the time it took to resolve complaints.

Don't discount *scuttlebutt* as an evaluation technique. Collect anecdotes, complimentary letters, and complaints from every source in order to evaluate your strategy for service excellence. Scrutinize the comments, complaints, and suggestions to learn how people feel about the services rendered to them by your organization.

Install a *suggestion box* in a prominent place on each patient floor and major public area and encourage people to use it. To make it convenient, attach a notepad with a headline like the following: "Help Us Make Things Better." Suggestion boxes are a great way to get invaluable feedback on how you're doing and what you could be doing better.

Try an *outsider's perspective*. Citizens' groups, volunteers, peers from a sister organization, and people from businesses with a strong tradition of service can provide you with information from a unique perspective. Ask them to visit, observe, and consult with you on ways to advance toward service excellence. Consider using the expertise of hotel managers by asking them to tour your facility and answer the question: "If this were your hotel, what changes would you make?" You can also learn by visiting their hotels and examining their customer relations policies. Talk to other customer-oriented business-people, including restaurant managers, retailers, and airline personnel. Consulting firms can also provide an experienced outsider's view of your organization.

☐ When to Turn Data into Feedback through Information Sharing

Data are meaningless unless they end up in the hands of key players *and* in a form that is easy and quick to digest. These key players include you, your staff, senior management, and any teams organized to pursue service improvements.

To be effective, information sharing must become routine, not an afterthought. Posted charts, memos, meetings, and periodic reports can all be used to feed data back to managers and teams who have the power to set improvement priorities and change processes. Progress plotting is a powerful reinforcement device. Trend charts are especially powerful vehicles for communicating about performance levels. Consider decorating walls with huge trend charts that show performance trends related to key results. Also devote significant time in management meetings to reviewing service performance data and identifying improvement needs. By routinely devoting meeting time to performance results, you reinforce the value you place on service quality, continuous improvement, accountability, and ownership in improving work processes. (Chapter 8 discusses in more detail methods for communicating measurement data that drive improvement.)

☐ Final Suggestions

Consider these suggestions when evaluating your systems for measurement and feedback:

- *Measure performance on dimensions of service quality as defined by your customers; don't dwell solely on internal measures of service quality:* Some organizations measure service dimensions such as waiting time, results turnaround time, and number of rings before answering the phone. These are important to measure as internal indicators of the degree to which service delivery meets specifications. But what does the customer perceive? In your quest to develop a customer-focused organization, make sure your customers' quality criteria are the focus for your measurement system.
- *Hold your customer perceptions in esteem:* Even if quality does exist in fact, without quality in perception, you don't have satisfied customers.
- *General questions on satisfaction surveys yield general information:* The more specific the questions, the more helpful they are in setting service standards, acting on them, and motivating change.
- *Don't rule out short, specific surveys:* These can be more helpful than the more costly shotgun approach.
- *Connect survey data to tangible market damage:* Print events, such as lost customers and word-of-mouth problems, in bold type in reports to executives.
- *Select internal measures based on the service promises you make:* If you promise rapid service, measure time. If you promise courteous service, measure perceptions of courtesy. Unfulfilled promises are devastating to your service image.
- *Measure often:* Timely feedback can lead to timely course corrections instead of after-the-fact regrets.

- *Do competitive analyses:* If you can, find out how your service compares with the service of competitors in your market area.
- *Be wary of unfair criteria for evaluating your service strategy:* Ask whether a proposed indicator is influenced by factors that may overwhelm the effects of even a strong service strategy. For example, although hospitals compete for patient volume or admissions, volume should not be used to evaluate the strategy results because too many variables are in play. If you have declining hospital admissions after implementing your strategy, can you say with certainty that the strategy caused the decline? It is possible that without your strategy admissions may have declined even faster—perhaps your strategy helped to stem the tide.

    Although market share is a better indicator than admissions or patient volume, it too is influenced by variable forces. For this reason, focus your evaluation on *perceptions* of staff behavior and customer satisfaction with service. That is, *focus your evaluation on what your strategy can affect directly.*
- *Include substantive, ongoing customer surveys in your mix of measurement strategies:* Administrators who assume they know what customers think without asking them invite problems. A systematic and ongoing survey system discloses trends in customer perception and has the credibility of hard data behind it.
- *Worry if you can't get support for evaluation:* Ongoing evaluation or input from your customers is your lifeline. If administrators won't dedicate resources to evaluation, find a quiet room and meditate seriously on top management's commitment to service excellence. If top managers won't pay for good evaluation, they are only paying lip service to service excellence. If necessary, double energy to building a case for serious evaluation. Find models from other hospitals by benchmarking. Invite administrators to sit in on customer focus groups to show them that they have much to gain from listening to customer feedback.
- *Beware of dogged insistence on research purity:* Textbooks about research admonish against "dirtying" the data by impure methods. Is it really sensible to delegate the task of staying close to your customers entirely to "pure" researchers, outsiders whose stock in trade are detachment and objectivity? Consider instead the maverick view that some of your evaluation and customer-listening techniques should be *obtrusive interventions that reinforce your employees' and physicians' service orientation and keep them mindful of how they treat customers.* Such "obtrusive" methods also show that your organization cares about meeting patients' and visitors' needs.

References

1. Schaffer, R. H., and Thomson, H. A. Successful change programs begin with results. *Harvard Business Review* 70(1):80–89, Jan.–Feb. 1992.

2. Bader, B. Patient satisfaction with the quality of health care and health services. *Quality Letter for Healthcare Leaders* (published by Bader and Associates, Rockville, MD) 2(1):7, Feb. 1990.

3. Fisk, T., Brown, C. Cannizarro, K., and Naftal, B. Creating patient satisfaction and loyalty. *Journal of Healthcare Marketing* 10(2):5–15, June 1990.

4. Parasuraman, A., Zeithaml, V., and Berry, L. A conceptual model of service quality and its implications for future research. *Journal of Marketing* 48:41–50, Fall 1985.

5. Shostack, G. L. Service positioning through structural change. *Journal of Marketing* 51:34–43, Jan. 1987.

6. Solomon, M., Suprenant, C., Czepiel, J., and Gutman, E. A role theory perspective on dyadic interactions: the service encounter. *Journal of Marketing* 49:99–111, Winter 1985.

7. Bearden, W., and Teel, J. Selected determinants of consumer satisfaction and complaint reports. *Journal of Marketing Research* 20:21–28, Feb. 1983.

8. Churchill, G., and Suprenant, C. An investigation into the determinants of customer satisfaction. *Journal of Marketing Research* 19:491–504, Nov. 1982.

9. Bearden, W., and Teel, J. Selected determinants of consumer satisfaction and complaint reports. *Journal of Marketing Research* 20:21–28, Feb. 1983.

10. Reibstein, D. *Marketing: Concepts, Strategies and Decisions.* Englewood Cliffs, NJ: Prentice-Hall, 1985.

11. Frank, R. Is brand loyalty a useful basis for market segmentation? *Journal of Advertising Research* 6:27–33, 1967.

12. Kotler, P. *Marketing Management.* Englewood Cliffs, NJ: Prentice-Hall, 1988.

13. Technical Assistant Research Programs Institute. *Consumer Complaint Handling in America: An Update Study.* Washington, DC: Consumer Affairs Council of the U.S. Office of Consumer Affairs, U.S. Department of Commerce, 1986.

14. Technical Assistant Research Programs Institute.

15. Vichas, R. *Complete Handbook of Profitable Market Research Techniques.* Englewood Cliffs, NJ: Prentice-Hall, 1982.

16. Carey, R., and Posavac, E. Using patient information to identify areas for service improvement. *Healthcare Management Review* 7(2):43–48, 1982.

17. Fisk, Brown, Cannizarro, and Naftal.

18. Carey, R., and Posavac, E. Using patient information to identify areas for service improvement. *Healthcare Management Review* 7(2):43–48, 1982.

19. Steiber, S., and Krowinski, W. *Measuring and Managing Patient Satisfaction.* Chicago: American Hospital Publishing, 1990.

20. Strasser, S., and Davis, R. M. *Measuring Patient Satisfaction for Improved Patient Services.* Chicago: American College of Healthcare Executives, 1991.

21. Strasser and Davis, pp. 187–89.

22. *Convenience Care Update,* Sept. 1986, published by United Communications. (No further information available.)

23. DeWolf, L. Focus groups: assessing patient satisfaction and targeting new services. *Hospital Topics* 63(2):24–26, Mar.–Apr. 1985.

24. Nelson, E., Rose, R., and Batalden, P. Measuring and improving physician satisfaction. *The Quality Letter for Healthcare Leaders* 2(2), Mar. 1990.

25. Leebov, W., and Ersoz, C. J. *The Health Care Manager's Guide to Continuous Quality Improvement.* Chicago: American Hospital Publishing, 1991.

Chapter 7

Problem Solving and Process Improvement

To what extent does your organization have mechanisms for ensuring ongoing problem solving and process improvement? Before reading this chapter, take the self-test in figure 7-1. A high number of "true" answers indicates a well-organized effort to identify and pursue problems, make process improvements, and handle complaints effectively. A lower score provides opportunities to strengthen or enhance your practices so that effective problem solving, process improvement, and complaint management become routine.

Figure 7-1.   Self-Test

Problem Solving and Process Improvement. *Circle the appropriate answer. The more "true" answers, the better.* *"False" answers indicate areas that need improvement.*

1. We have a clear, smooth-running system for responding to patient complaints.	True	False
2. Our organization has an ongoing system for making continuous improvements in processes and systems that hamper efficiency and customer satisfaction.	True	False
3. We have a clear, smooth-running system for responding to physician complaints and needs.	True	False
4. Our administrators and middle managers respond to employee complaints and concerns, even if they cannot (or decide not to) resolve them.	True	False
5. Our employees cross department lines to solve service problems.	True	False
6. In this organization, all levels of staff recognize the ongoing need to make our services ever better, not just when service problems arise.	True	False
7. Executives, managers, and staff here know and use effective problem-solving techniques.	True	False
8. Service problems that frustrate customers are tackled here, not ignored.	True	False
9. Employees and physicians here have ample opportunities to participate in making service better.	True	False
10. We identify *priority* processes that need improvement, so we can focus our time and energy on significant problems with significant potential to improve customer satisfaction.	True	False
Total:	___	___

This chapter will discuss foundations for problem solving and service excellence, service recovery (solving problems reactively), and proactive resolution through process improvement. Focus will be on the positive benefits of inviting customer complaints and overcoming obstacles.

☐ Foundation for Problem Solving and Service Excellence

Obviously, problems interfere with customer satisfaction; unresolved problems lead to dissatisfied customers. Unsolved problems also affect employee morale and pride; employees want to do a great job and be proud of their organization. No one in your organization benefits when dissatisfied customers go elsewhere for care, and no one enjoys feeling oppressed every day by problems left unattended.

Many health care workers choose their careers because they want to help people. When they are compelled to implement processes and procedures that frustrate customers, they become disaffected and angry, perceiving that top management is unwilling to tackle problems or make changes that improve conditions for everyone. Consequently, employees' commitment to service excellence and their willingness to work hard for the organization diminish.

Does your organization make it easy for customers and staff to speak up about problems? Does your organization take service snags and problems seriously, promoting an eagerness among staff to overcome them? Does your organization initiate continuous process improvements, so that processes serve the needs of both internal and external customers? Ideally, all of your staff should be persistent in asking the following questions:

- Why are we doing this?
- Must we do it this way?
- Can we find a better way to do it?

As already indicated, problems and work processes should be viewed and expressed as opportunities to improve customer satisfaction, not as hassles created by people through their own negligence, oversight, and incompetence. Through accountability systems discussed in chapter 5, managers must make it eminently clear that service excellence is everybody's business and that improvement initiatives are expected of everyone. Managers at every level should ask each other not only how things are going, but what changes are being made to improve customer satisfaction.

Managers must recognize and reward employees and teams who make service improvements and invest time and effort in prevention-oriented process improvement, rather than fighting short-term fires that reappear as fast as they are put out. Managers also should create a supportive culture for continuous improvement and innovation by everyone and emphasize management's role and accountability for ensuring continuous improvement. What you do with the satisfaction and performance data, complaints, and suggestions from each customer group makes the difference between a responsive organization and a stagnant, defensive, and self-satisfied one that erodes customer and employee confidence.

You need reactive systems for handling the problems you hear about, but you need proactive methods for preventing them through process improvement. Ongoing systems built into daily operations help minimize the reactive frenzies that occur in the absence of proactive systems.

Your management team needs to communicate to all service providers your commitment to aggressive on-the-spot problem solving and continuous service improvement by taking these steps:

- Install *systems* for problem solving, effective complaint management, and process improvement.

- Earmark high-priority problems that must be solved and processes that must be improved if the organization is to satisfy its key customers.
- Identify and assign clear responsibility to individuals or teams who will tackle each problem or process, no matter how complex, and provide resources as needed.
- Institute a reporting system so that progress can be tracked and a problem does not fall through the cracks.
- Institute a system for evaluating managers that includes as a critical criterion their active and effective participation in efforts to make service improvements.
- Build a system of people who serve as patient representatives, who invite and listen to customer problems and expedite effective service recovery.
- Hold people accountable. Hire people who are creative, nondefensive, and aggressive problem solvers. Reward those who are active and effective in tackling problems and resolving complaints. When necessary, terminate problem employees who just don't cut it.

Many quality experts claim that at least 85 percent of the problems in an organization are the fault of systems controlled by managers. Therefore, only 15 percent (or less) of the problems stem from employee performance.

The ultimate responsibility for problem solving and process improvement lies with top management, who must actively participate in the chain of events needed to institutionalize, through hands-on leadership, aggressive complaint resolution and continuous service improvement. Instead of pointing the finger at middle managers who allow problems to go on year after year, top managers need either to successfully engage middle managers as active, responsible quality improvers or get new middle managers. If middle managers are ineffective in minimizing problems and in solving those that could not be avoided, then top management has failed to communicate that problem solving and continuous process improvement are key management (including middle management) responsibilities. Or, they've tolerated middle managers who shouldn't be there.

Although management involvement is key, so too is employee participation. How often have outside consultants been brought in to "debug" departmental procedures that the department's employees could have streamlined themselves? How many solutions have been foisted on people who do the job by people who do not, only to find that their out-of-touch solutions are unrealistic? In both cases the result is employees who feel devalued and discounted instead of appreciated and respected for their knowledge and potential to help improve the organization. That's why the quest for continuous quality and service improvement relies so heavily on employee and physician involvement in process improvement.

Most health care customers would rather not be using our services to begin with, so that their tolerance for inconvenience, delays, and perceived inefficiencies is lower than under other circumstances. No matter how well your people and systems perform, no matter how precision-coordinated your staff or how timely your procedures, inevitably you will be confronted with dissatisfied customers, including complaining patients, visitors, family members, physicians, and staff. Sometimes your organization deserves to take the heat, and sometimes it doesn't. Sometimes mistakes are real and your staff and systems are at fault; other times mistakes are perceived—a misunderstanding between customer and organization.

Whether justified or not, a dissatisfied customer presents two golden opportunities—one, to make things right on the spot, and two, to improve your services and systems so that the problem does not recur for future customers. This chapter describes several approaches to problem solving, some reactive and some proactive or preventive.

□ Reactive Problem Solving, or Service Recovery

Bless the dissatisfied customer who speaks up. Some people think that no news is good news, but it isn't, because about 30 percent of dissatisfied customers never complain to the organization that wronged them. Instead, they resentfully spread the word to their network of acquaintances and take their business elsewhere next time. If you can encourage customers to speak up, chances are most likely they'll remain loyal to your facility—especially if you can correct the matter and be empathetic in the process.

In the service sector, the process of making things right in the face of complaints is known as *service recovery*. In plain language it means doing all you can to correct a wrong perceived by the customer—and doing it in such a way that the customer's interests are protected and emotions are calmed.

Not only is it good business to develop skillful recovery systems, it is also required by the Joint Commission on the Accreditation of Healthcare Organizations (JCAHO). Since 1990, attainment of JCAHO accreditation hinges partially on a hospital's system for handling complaints. Specifically:[1]

- A mechanism must exist for receiving complaints.
- Patients must be informed of this mechanism and of their right to complain.
- The organization must respond to significant complaints and take appropriate actions.
- Patients cannot be penalized for complaining.
- All health care facilities must *document* patient complaints and their responses to them.

Although you are required to have a system for handling complaints, at the Conference "Closing the Service Gap III,"[2] John Goodman, president of the Technical Assistance Research Programs (TARP), presented persuasive arguments why you would *want to* implement a system even if you weren't required to. As shown in figure 7-2, it is important to invite complaints, because the 30 percent of dissatisfied customers who don't speak up means that 65 percent complain directly to frontline people, who consequently must be equipped with the ability and resources to handle complaints effectively.

Goodman also emphasizes the need to resolve complaints well and in a timely fashion if you want to cultivate customer loyalty. Figure 7-3 shows the degree of customer loyalty you can expect from people who don't complain, those whose complaints are not resolved, those whose complaints *are* resolved, and those whose complaints are resolved quickly.

Figure 7-2. The Tip-of-the-Iceberg Phenomenon

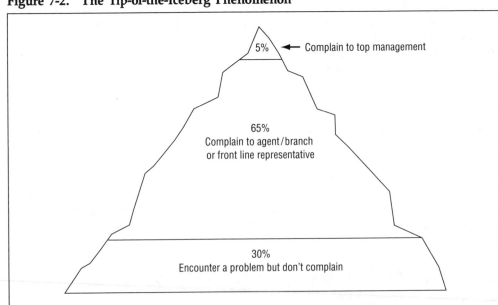

Reprinted, with permission, from Technical Assistance Research Program (TARP), Arlington, Virginia, 1990.

Figure 7-3. Customer Loyalty in Relation to Complaint Resolution

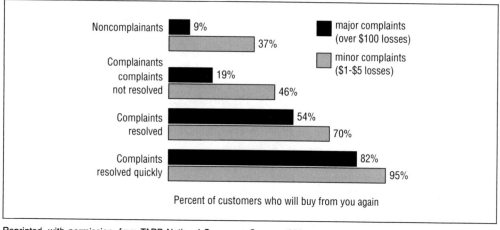

Reprinted, with permission, from TARP National Consumer Survey, 1990.

Ironically, whether your organization causes complaints or not is not the main problem. The problem is how customers *perceive your response* once they complain. As discussed in chapter 6, this perception has a powerful effect on customers' overall evaluation of your facility's services and on their willingness to choose your facility for health care the next time. Complainers are more likely than noncomplainers to do business with the organization that upset them even if the problem is not resolved. Thus staff, and not only patient representatives, should *always* be available to hear complaints. Furthermore, of those who do complain, between 54 percent and 70 percent do business again with the organization if their complaint is resolved; this figure climbs to a staggering 95 percent if the customer believes that the complaint was resolved quickly.

If you are motivated only by financial arguments, we want to emphasize that complaints also can cost your organization dearly. The TARP process for measuring the financial consequences of dissatisfied customers can be applied to health care as follows:[3]

- Let's say that 150 complaints are voiced in a year. For every complaint voiced, an additional 26 complaints are not voiced. That means there are 150 × 26, or 3,900 complaints not voiced in that period.
- Approximately one complaint in five is serious. That means that of the 3,900 complaints, about 780 are serious.
- If 50 percent of the people with serious complaints left unaddressed go elsewhere the next time they need service, that means that of the 780 people with serious complaints, 390 choose another health care provider next time. That's a loss of 390 patients.
- If the average revenue per admission is $4,000 (which is probably a conservative estimate), then your organization loses potential revenues of 390 patients × $4,000, or $1,560,000 in the next 12 months if every lost patient needs hospitalization in the next 12 months. However, it is more likely that 40 percent of them or their close family members will need hospitalization in the next 12-month period. So $1,560,000 × 40 percent, or $624,000, is revenue lost to you because these people with serious unresolved complaints chose another hospital for themselves or their families.

If, on the other hand, their complaints had been resolved quickly, your organization would have gained that $624,000. And that's only in a one-year period. The people you've turned away will probably endure *several* future hospitalizations. If you could figure out the revenue lost to you over a 10-year period because dissatisfied customers went to the hospital down the street, the figures would be staggering. In short, not only do you frustrate people you're in business to serve when you engender dissatisfaction, and not only are you required by JCAHO to have a system for effective service recovery, but failure in this regard will cost you millions of dollars in lost business.

The TARP research shows that what consumers want from an organization they patronize is "no unpleasant surprises." However, if they do encounter trouble, the key factors that will restore their satisfaction are promises kept, clear expectations, taking ownership, acknowledgment, accessibility, timeliness, and courtesy.

Although on the surface it seems that recovery should benefit everyone involved, employees often resist engaging in it for at least five reasons:

1. Some people are philosophically opposed to apologies. They feel that by apologizing they admit to having made an error.
2. Some are annoyed by what they perceive as excessively high or unreasonable customer expectations. "They want the impossible" is the catchphrase here.
3. Some people don't know *how* to recover gracefully; the situation leaves them feeling uncomfortable and immobilized.
4. Some employees *want* to make things right, but they know they cannot count on others in the organization to do their part in the corrective actions needed—and they can't make things right by themselves.
5. Some employees want to make things right and don't know whom to turn to when red tape must be cut through to do so.

These reasons explain why effective complaint management involves a multifaceted *system*. An effective system meets requirements: spreading a positive attitude toward complaints throughout your work force; helping staff educate customers about what they can reasonably expect; helping employees develop the tact, skills, and finesse needed to handle complaints skillfully and graciously, without anger or defensiveness; and creating express routes for communicating complaints and making things right, and then making sure every staff member knows how to use them.

The next four subsections will discuss four specific approaches to progressive complaint management. These are inviting customer complaints, installing a *designed* system for complaint handling, training every employee to handle complaints effectively, and establishing timeliness standards and the systems to support them.

Inviting Customer Complaints

Service recovery starts with a welcoming, positive attitude toward complaints. After all, if complaints aren't voiced, they can't be fixed. To begin, every organization needs to explicitly beg customers to complain and make it easy for them to do so.

Most hospitals find it helpful to have a team whose only job is to handle complaints and who can therefore document and track problems, see patterns, and then facilitate problem solving and actions that prevent these problems from recurring. These staff members may have various titles: *patient representatives, patient advocates, guest relations directors, physician liaisons,* or *ombudspeople*. The name is unimportant, but the job they perform is not. Patient representatives (advocates for patients' concerns) and a physician liaison (advocates for physicians' concerns) are skilled in complaint resolution and able to confront the complaint on a moment's notice. These people should be accessible at all times; invested with the clout needed to elicit cooperation across departmental lines; and allowed time for extensive full-time involvement in handling problems.

Luther Hospital in Eau Claire, Wisconsin, urges patients to express their concerns *to the staff member closest to the problem* using the card shown in figure 7-4. Some hospitals designate a phone number or complaint hotline for customer use. At one time, Good Samaritan Hospital in Cincinnati linked their hotline with their Service First Guarantee, which encouraged patients to call with complaints.

Figure 7-4. Concerns Card: Luther Hospital

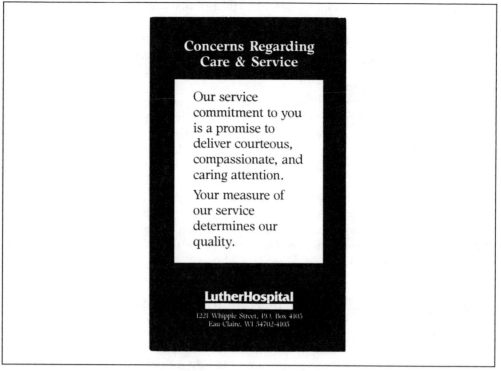

Reprinted, with permission, from Luther Hospital, Eau Claire, Wisconsin.

According to Phil Newbold and Diane Serbin Stover,[4] Memorial Medical Center in South Bend, Indiana, implemented an intense daily patient visitation program that reflected their total commitment to problem recovery. They selected two medical/surgical floors for their pilot test of the "Right Things Right" program, then assigned 30 managers and nursing personnel to specific patient rooms they were to visit daily. They were trained and mandated to probe patients gently for problems, using open-ended questions. The pilot program showed the following benefits:

- Patients feel that we care and that we're a hands-on institution.
- Managers see systems problems firsthand.
- Patients can sound off.
- Patients feel a more personal sense of importance.
- Overall communication is enhanced within and between departments.
- Staff become more proactive and recognize the value of rapid response.

As a result of their pilot, the following conclusions were drawn:

- Although some problems could be identified and solved, some required in-depth systems analysis and long-term correction to prevent recurrence. Unless the root causes of problems are addressed, heroic efforts are needed—day after day; thus, the argument for process improvement.
- Daily visits represent a powerful damage control strategy if no problem is deemed too small, if problems are reported faithfully, solved outside of a meeting structure, solved quickly, involve a number of people, and make open communication across department lines standard operating procedure.

The most innovative and exciting health care service recovery approach we've seen comes from Leslie Sabo, Director of Service Relations/TQI at Meridia Hillcrest Hospital in Hillcrest, Ohio. To extend the squad of people skilled in complaint handling beyond the scope of patient representatives, Meridia Hillcrest developed its "Service Assistance Line," which is staffed by 50 employees monthly in eight-hour shifts. These employees from diverse positions receive special training that includes role playing, problem solving, and dress rehearsals. They then take turns as "service representatives," leaving their regular positions for a few hours at a time to staff the phone lines, which are located in many areas of the hospital.

Service representatives feel honored by this training and, in the process, extend their knowledge and skills as resources in the organization. They learn to locate the right people in order to respond to different kinds of customer problems. More than 6,000 people used the line during its first 10 months of operation. More than half of all complaints are resolved within 15 minutes of receipt of the call. Within 90 minutes, virtually all concerns are resolved.

CGH Medical Center in Sterling, Illinois, makes recovery easier for staff by providing them with a tangible token of apology they can grant to outpatients who have been inconvenienced or are dissatisfied. Their policy (shown in figure 7-5) provides a complimentary meal coupon to patients (and sometimes their families) who are inconvenienced for certain reasons.

Installing a *Designed* System for Handling Complaints

A culture that supports problem solving is not enough. Formal systems are needed so that problems don't fall through the cracks. For example, what happens when your patient representatives track complaints and identify recurrent problems? When employees generate lists of problems, big and small, what do you do with the lists? When patients, visitors, or physicians complain to a frontline employee and the employee handles the complaint, does the complaint get recorded so that patterns can be identified, even if the employee can react effectively to the complaint on the spot? Listening to the patient representatives and employees is not enough; you need to take the results and feed them through a process lest valuable information "evaporates." You also generate deep resentment among employees and patients who have been led to expect responsiveness.

Thus, a designed, predictable, regular system for handling complaints is requisite. Chapter 6 provided an example of the algorithm for complaint handling followed at Thomas Jefferson University Hospital. Figure 7-6 (p. 122) provides another example of complaint handling—the Patient Response System from St. Clare's Riverside Medical Center in Denville, New Jersey.[5]

Excellent computer software is also available to help you record, follow up on, and analyze complaints for patterns. An example is FLEX/MIS, available from the National Society for Patient Representation and Consumer Affairs. This software performs complaint tracking and provides activity logs, patient survey reporting, and graphics reporting. It also provides menus of standard follow-up reports and standard complaint response letters that can be changed using the software's modified word-processing capability.

Training All Staff to Handle Complaints Effectively

Chapter 12 emphasizes the importance of equipping *all* employees to handle complaints effectively. Patient representatives should be the customer's last resort for complaints, after all else—including frontline staff responsiveness to the complaint—has failed. All staff should be trained in service recovery, which is the wave of the future. Service recovery nips complaints in the bud and achieves quick responsiveness by the people close to and responsible for service to the customer.

Establishing Timeliness Standards and the Systems to Support Them

In that *quick* resolution of complaints is the most powerful way to win back a dissatisfied customer, consider establishing a time standard by which every complaint should be resolved. Develop this standard from data about the time complaints currently take to be resolved and then create a process improvement team to study and redesign your complaint processes so that you can speed up this standard over time. Your improvement team can track the timeliness of response and focus attention on improving the complaint resolution process for the high percentage of cases that take longer to be resolved.

Figure 7-5. Complimentary Meal Ticket Policy

Policy:	It is the policy of CGH Medical Center to offer a complimentary meal coupon to outpatients (and sometimes to their family or transporters) who are inconvenienced due to a scheduling problem or oversight, an unexpected or unusually lengthy delay, equipment malfunction, or similar occurrence. This is a rather informal process and staff are encouraged to use their judgment in assessing the problem and our response.
Procedure:	1. Identify the inconvenience. It is our intention to alleviate a problem, not to find fault or to fix blame. 2. Notify Central Scheduling of the need for a coupon (or coupons when a spouse or friend is waiting as well). 3. Complete the information on the coupon including the name of the employees distributing the coupon, date, and department. (This information will assist in logging appropriate use.) 4. Complete or pass along information for the log in Central Scheduling. 5. Distribute and explain the coupon to the patient/other. A cafeteria cashier will collect coupons and pass them along to Accounting for recording.
Observation:	The program may help CGH identify areas of service needing more attention. However, some of those problems are unpredictable and simply require the courtesy of an apology, with the coupon as an added expression of same.
Coupon:	

We are sorry things haven't gone according to plan. Please accept our sincere apology for any inconvenience this may have caused you or your family.

Please use this card in the CGH cafeteria to purchase up to $5.00 in refreshments, snacks or meals.

_____
Employee name / Dept. / Date

We realize this will not solve the problem or confusion that you've had to deal with today. We simply want to let you know that you and your needs are important to us.   *Thank you for your patience.*

_____
Cashier enter amount

Reprinted, with permission, from Community General Hospital, Sterling, Illinois, 1992.

Figure 7-6. Flowchart for Complaint Handling

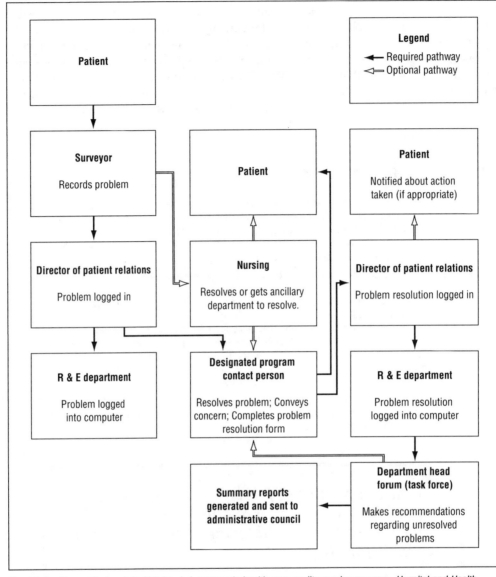

Reprinted, with permission, from Kalafat, J. A systematic health care quality service program. *Hospital and Health Services Administration* 36(4):571, 1991.

Time standards are the basis of satisfaction guarantee programs that some hospitals have installed to focus staff attention on the timeliness of response and to put "teeth" into their time standards. Although some hospitals have been very successful with these programs, you must be sure that you make only those promises you can keep. Also, ensure that systems are in place to resolve complaints quickly; otherwise, you frustrate and oppress employees in a satisfaction guarantee program, because they *want* to resolve the complaint quickly, but feel disempowered without a system to make this possible.

☐ Proactive Problem Solving through Process Improvement

As shown in figure 7-7, an essential step in customer-driven management involves making improvements once you've identified problems. After identifying improvement

Figure 7-7. Phase 2 of Customer-Driven Management Process

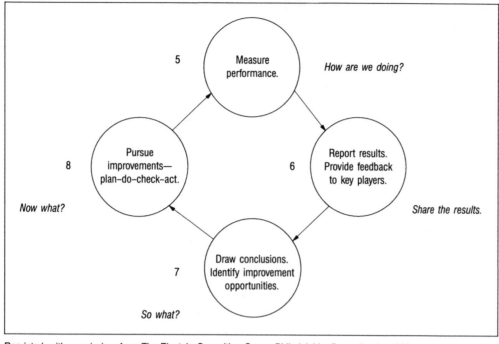

Reprinted, with permission, from The Einstein Consulting Group, Philadelphia, Pennsylvania, 1990.

opportunities, step 8 of the customer-driven management process calls for proceeding to make improvements in a rational and efficient manner.

In hospitals especially, systems problems are so critically important to service strategy that they deserve special attention. Consider the following example: Rosie started out being enthusiastic about our customer relations strategy because she entered health care to help people. She was delighted when the administrators decided to pay attention to the human ingredient in an explicit way. Rosie did all she could to ease long waits in physical therapy: she apologized for delays, kept people posted, offered tea and magazines, and apologized again when the patient was still not seen. Finally, Rosie got fed up: "Why doesn't management fix the scheduling so that people don't have to wait in the first place? Why do I have to spend all my time and energy apologizing to people who are rightfully impatient, bored, and upset because they've been sitting here for hours?" Rosie's right. She has wonderful people skills but is ready to pull the plug on the light she brings to patients because she's so angry about the systems problem that makes doing her job virtually impossible. An overt attack on systems problems or work processes has to be part and parcel of the formula to achieve customer satisfaction and service excellence.

Having performance problems means that people are *doing things wrong*. Having systems problems means that people are *doing wrong things*. Your goal is to get people to do the right things right. George Labovitz, consultant on productivity and quality in health care, points out that it costs $1 to fix a problem during the process, $10 to fix it at the end of the process, and $100 to fix it by the time it reaches the customer. He goes on to claim that the cost of systems problems in service organizations is at least 30 percent of gross sales.[6]

In health care, the cost of systems problems is probably higher because systems problems cost the organization more than the steps needed to improve them. Costs associated with damage to reputation, denied reimbursement, lawsuits, staff energy diverted into complaint handling, slow receivables, staff turnover, retraining, access barriers, lost records, and the like are notoriously expensive.

Then why don't hospitals just fix the systems? They don't because fixing them is tough. Labovitz tells this instructive joke: A police officer sees a Volkswagen going 50 miles per hour in a 40-mile zone. He also sees a Ferrari going 110. The officer stops the Volkswagen and writes out a ticket. The driver asks, "Why me? That Ferrari was going more than 100." The officer replied, "Yeah, but I couldn't catch him."[7]

Blaming customer dissatisfaction on employee behavior is like catching the Volkswagen. You can "catch" employee behavior, but "catching" systems problems or dysfunctional work processes is much harder even though systems problems are more likely to play havoc with the long-term satisfaction of every customer. If you ask your employees, your physicians, and your patients what's getting in the way of your hospital being the best it can be, they'll tell you in no uncertain terms: systems problems that go on year after year and oppress everyone.

Overcoming Obstacles to Improving Systems and Processes

Although the causes of systems problems vary from organization to organization, several obstacles to improving them seem universal, particularly among large institutions. Identifying these obstacles, some of which are listed below, is the first step in overcoming them.

- *Acquired myopia:* Recognizing that systems problems even exist is often hard. After having been with an organization for a few years, people tend to become acclimated to the environment and its ways of doing things. For example, if locating a wheelchair at a given hospital usually takes 20 minutes, a 20-minute wait becomes accepted as the norm rather than being attributed to an intolerable scarcity of wheelchairs. A fresh perspective is needed to break myopic reactions and habits.
- *Diffusion of responsibility:* By their nature, most systems problems involve several departments, not to mention many, many people. Who's responsible? Everyone involved, and that's an obstacle. If everyone has, say, a 5 percent share of responsibility for the system, and therefore for the problem, no *one* person has the authority or control to take the initiative and effect a solution.
- *Territorialism:* Because systems problems transcend departmental boundaries, a lot of finger pointing often results. People tend to see the problem and the responsibility for solving it as someone else's; and department heads tend to defend and protect their own people.
- *Complexity:* Once systems problems are acknowledged and a decision is made to address them, their sheer complexity can be overwhelming. Discerning the causes can be difficult and frustrating; implementing a one-shot cure-all can be impossible. Consequently, the commitment to solve problems often languishes because no solution solves every aspect of the problem.
- *Remote problem solvers:* When responsibility for systems troubleshooting is assumed by top management alone, solutions may be a long time coming because administrators don't have to grapple with the problems on a day-to-day basis. Also, administrators may design elegant solutions that never get refined to levels that are practical and that work. Input is needed from the people who actually implement the systems.
- *Lack of follow-through:* Early success in systems problem solving is often accompanied by a gradual abandonment of the effort. Progress may be followed by progressive complacency so that the problems get only half-solved or the solutions only half-implemented.

Selecting Strategy Options

A service culture needs *ongoing* structures and supports that encourage proactive service improvement. Six approaches are outlined below:

1. Identify and tackle breakthrough objectives.
2. Adopt and promote a step-by-step process improvement model to help people approach process improvement systematically.
3. Train all managers in effective problem solving and process improvement; expect them to involve their staff in improvement initiatives.
4. Consider suggestion programs.
5. Engage in benchmarking.
6. Institute structures and special supports for *team* improvement initiatives.

Identify and Tackle Breakthrough Objectives

In their significant study of quality improvement strategies in health care, the Healthcare Advisory Board reinforces the importance of carefully selecting process improvement priorities. One of their key conclusions is, "Strategic project selection is the single most important thing a hospital can do to leverage TQM results."[8] Figure 7-8 shows the end product of misappropriation of effort.

The Board concludes that many improvement strategies have faltered or failed because people chase problems that are not priority problems, or they chase small problems whose solutions have no cumulative impact. The Board recommends that management take steps to focus process improvement on what truly matters and "then reinforce the constant ethic of prioritization to ensure that teams expend not an ounce of energy on less than top priority projects."[9] The chart in figure 7-9 demonstrates the impact of unfocused versus focused efforts. As can be seen, the value of selecting breakthrough objectives is that many small contributions to a solution can add up to breakthroughs.

The focus of the Japanese theory of Hoshin Planning is that a breakthrough objective is one that is important to customers; one that *everyone* in the organization can play a role in achieving; and one that results in a substantial, noticeable effect even if everyone makes only small contributions to it.[10] A breakthrough galvanizes effort in a single direction. As everyone focuses on the same objective, people learn quickly and can help each other. Consider as an example "decreasing cycle time." Internal and external customers want prompt service—people don't like to wait. Patients want prompt results: they want answers to their questions quickly; they want a nurse immediately upon activating the call light; and they want their pain medication *now.* Physicians want rapid turnaround of test results; rapid scheduling of their admissions; rapid reports from physician consults; and rapid answers to their questions to pharmacy, utilization review, and the

Figure 7-8. Result of Effort Spent on the Wrong Projects

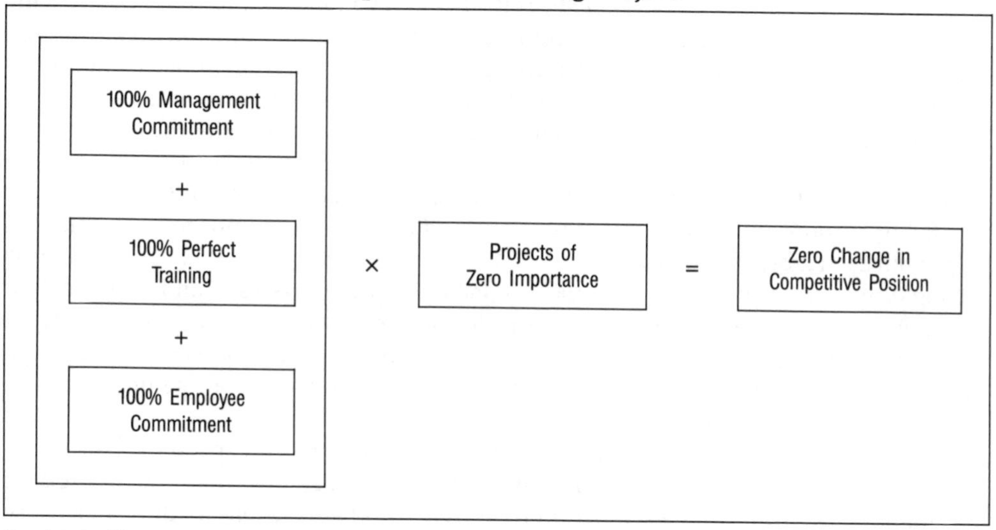

Reprinted, with permission, from the Healthcare Advisory Board, Washington, DC, 1992.

Figure 7-9. Impact of Unfocused versus Focused Efforts

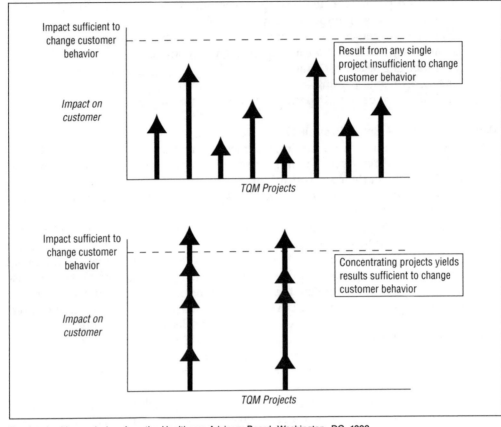

like. Each department's internal customers want quick return of phone calls, rapid delivery of requested supplies and linen, and quick response to special needs—all because they can't serve their customers until their suppliers serve them. *Time* is at a premium, and both internal and external customers judge a supplier partly by the degree of respect shown for the customer's precious time and immediate needs.

Imagine a hospital adopting "reduction of cycle time" as an *organizationwide* breakthrough objective. Imagine the *cumulative* effect of every manager and staff hospitalwide focusing on speeding things up; the cumulative effect could be phenomenal. But you won't reap a phenomenal cumulative effect in cycle time if different departments adopt different objectives. To use another example, imagine "improving communication" as a breakthrough objective. Every department hospitalwide would identify the communication needs of its customers and suppliers and devote substantial effort to filling these needs more effectively. Nursing would improve discharge instructions and ensure patient and family understanding of them. Physicians and nurses would improve their relationships with each other. The executive team would strengthen its methods of communicating the big picture to employees and physicians. Patient representatives would improve their methods for feeding back complaint patterns to staff involved. Pharmacy would improve feedback to physicians about illegible handwriting. The cumulative effect of these examples could be a tremendous improvement in communication and, consequently, the satisfaction levels of diverse customers.

If one department focuses on improving courtesy, another on speeding up service, and another on improving quality of information given to customers, each might produce important results. But from a broader perspective, the effects would be diffuse because they lack a cumulative effect.

In an ambitious and exciting service strategy, senior management identifies and persistently promotes and pursues at least one breakthrough service objective a year—and mobilizes everyone hospitalwide to tackle that objective with a vengeance. In its "perfect prioritization process" shown in figure 7-10, the Healthcare Advisory Board recommends seven screens to select a project.

Following are three steps to follow in a simple group process that employs selected quality improvement tools to identify a breakthrough service improvement objective.

1. Take your knowledge about customer needs and summarize high-priority needs on Post-it™ notes (each need on its own note). Also brainstorm every goal your group wants to accomplish based on group perception of the organization's priorities.
2. Engage the group in making an Affinity Chart. Cluster the related ideas by physically moving related Post-its™ together into a cluster. Name each cluster by finding its essence.

Figure 7-10. The Perfect Prioritization Process

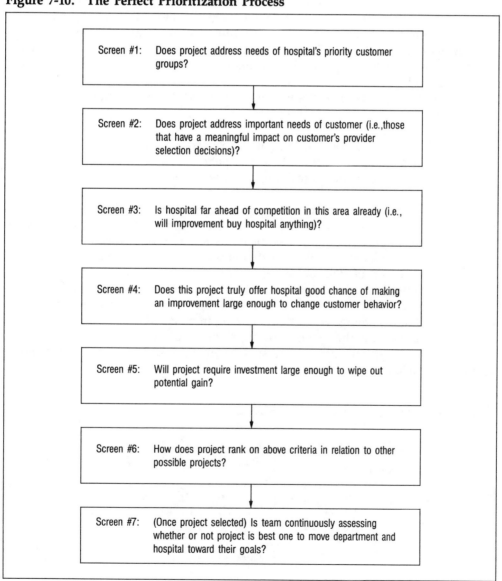

Screen #1: Does project address needs of hospital's priority customer groups?

Screen #2: Does project address important needs of customer (i.e.,those that have a meaningful impact on customer's provider selection decisions)?

Screen #3: Is hospital far ahead of competition in this area already (i.e., will improvement buy hospital anything)?

Screen #4: Does this project truly offer hospital good chance of making an improvement large enough to change customer behavior?

Screen #5: Will project require investment large enough to wipe out potential gain?

Screen #6: How does project rank on above criteria in relation to other possible projects?

Screen #7: (Once project selected) Is team continuously assessing whether or not project is best one to move department and hospital toward their goals?

Reprinted, with permission, from the Healthcare Advisory Board, Washington, DC, 1992.

3. Make a Relationship Diagram (sometimes called an "Interrelationship Digraph") with the cluster headings.
   - Identify the causal relationships (if any) between each pair of headings. Reflect these with arrows.
   - Count the number of arrows leading out of each heading. The one with the most arrows leading out of it is a root cause of many other effects you want to achieve. Because of that, the heading makes a great breakthrough objective.
   - Focus the entire organization on achieving that breakthrough objective.

(These steps are discussed fully in *The Health Care Manager's Guide to Continuous Quality Improvement*.[11])

Adopt and Promote a Step-by-Step Process Improvement Model

A number of models are available to help individuals and teams pursue process improvements systematically. We use the Model for Process Improvement described in detail in *The Health Care Manager's Guide to Continuous Quality Improvement*.[12] Like many available models, this is an expansion of the "Plan–Do–Check–Act" (PDCA) cycle (shown in figure 7-11), which was coined by Shewhart in the 1920s and since promoted by Deming. In the PDCA cycle, first, you *plan* your improvement. Next you *do* (implement) it on a trial basis. Then, you *check* to determine the consequences or results. Finally, you *act* accordingly, building your improvement into everyday operations in order to hold the gains.

Years ago, behavioral scientist Kurt Lewin described change as a three-step, sequential process:

- Step 1: Unfreezing—or thawing out established behavior patterns
- Step 2: Changing—or moving to a new pattern
- Step 3: Refreezing—or maintaining the new pattern

The Model for Process Improvement assists you in moving yourself and your staff through these sometimes painful steps. To *unfreeze*, you acknowledge a problem or opportunity for improvement and investigate its ramifications and causes. By doing so, you create a plan for making things better and you take steps to gain a commitment to change on the part of staff and other powers-that-be. To *change*, you experiment, testing out your proposed improvement in a trial run and closely monitoring the intended and unintended effects. Then, if you become convinced that the experiment worked and that the change is worth integrating into everyday operations, you move to *refreezing*—building in the changes and supporting people during what can be a disconcerting and unsettling change process. Figure 2-5 (p. 22) shows the PDCA model as a more detailed 12-step process.

Figure 7-11. Plan–Do–Check–Act (PDCA) Cycle

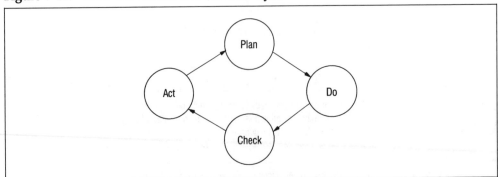

In the more refined 12-step model shown in figure 2-5, within each of the four basic phases of the PDCA cycle are important substeps. The *planning* phase has six substeps. The team:

1. *Identifies outputs, customers, and customer expectations:* What product of service is the process in question meant to accomplish? For whom—its customers? What do these customers expect? What criteria do they use to judge the process outputs?
2. *Describes current process:* To improve a process, start by understanding how the process currently works and flows (the current reality). Flowcharting the process is important here.
3. *Measures and analyzes:* Once you have a clear picture of the process, collect baseline information about current performance. Are customers satisfied? How long does performance take, and how much does it cost at each step? Who does what? Are there checks or controls on important steps along the way? Before you know how to change the process, you need to know a lot about it.
4. *Focuses on an improvement opportunity:* After getting a grip on the process, you then need to target a problem or improvement opportunity, selecting one or more aspects of the process that you want to change, eliminate, or strengthen.
5. *Identifies root causes:* Once you've identified a problem, sleuth for root causes. You get the biggest bang from your effort by tackling the root causes, not the symptoms.
6. *Generates and chooses solutions:* Having identified root causes, you then need to generate countermeasures or solutions and pick the best ones to test in a trial run.

In the *do* phase (comprised of two substeps), the team executes the improvement as an experiment. Does the proposed improvement indeed do a better job than the old process? This phase involves two substeps:

7. *Mapping out a trial run:* Work out the details for a trial run, concretely planning every step, securing the needed support and resources, and training people. Prepare every element so that you can give the experiment your best shot at success.
8. *Implementing the trial run:* Implement your experiment according to plan.

At the *check* phase (two substeps), the question is, "Did it work?" Did your process change achieve the desired results? The two substeps involved are:

9. *Evaluate the results:* Using measures you used earlier, figure out what happened. Are the outputs better? Are customers happier? What intended (and unintended) effects resulted from your experiment both within the process itself and for its customers?
10. *Draw conclusions:* With the results of measurement in hand, you need to make sense of them. Ask, "Do the results warrant standardizing the changes we made?

At the *act* phase (two substeps), if you decided to make your change standard practice, figure out how to do that by using these two substeps:

11. *Standardize the change:* Create an implementation plan that will incorporate the improvements you achieved in your trial run into your everyday process (and perhaps into other processes that might also be improved by what you learned). This substep typically involves developing a plan for integrating the change; preparing people and equipment for the change; installing it; modifying policies and procedures to reflect it; and helping those involved come to terms with the change, accept it, and conform to it.
12. *Monitor to hold the gains:* Once you've integrated the change into everyday operations, keep watch to make sure the change sticks, lest people revert to the old way.

Models like these provide blueprints to give direction to process improvement. They build on the powerful techniques of flowcharting and service blueprinting.[13]

By making the implicit explicit, by making the unconscious conscious, you gain control over your approach and *decide* what you need to do to pursue an improvement opportunity constructively. Just as a flowchart creates new possibilities for controlling and improving work processes, this Model for Process Improvement, which is a flowchart, creates new possibilities for controlling and improving your effectiveness at process improvement.

Train All Managers in Effective Problem Solving and Process Improvement

To advance process improvement in your organization, you need to train managers in particular. Chapter 9 describes a training model that includes training in process improvement. This can be supplemented with just-in-time training within the context of improvement teams, so that all team members have the same baseline education about the group's process.

Using members of your squad of problem-solving facilitators (an experienced inside person, an internal consultant, or an outside training resource), equip your managers to address problems and revamp processes alone and through teamwork—with efficiency and effectiveness. Help them learn to follow the Model for Process Improvement and equip them with versatile improvement tools to make their meetings and teamwork efficient, involving, and productive. Communicate your expectation of accountability, that is, that every department manager is responsible for proactive problem solving in his or her own realm of influence.

A myriad of quality improvement tools are available to help individuals and teams analyze and improve processes. Figure 7-12 summarizes the tools helpful at each step in our model. A solid bullet means "often used," a hollow bullet means "used less often," and an *x* means "rarely used at this step."[14]

Consider Suggestion Programs

Another approach to problem solving and process improvement involves creating incentives that encourage employee suggestions. Most suggestion programs are focused on cutting costs, and because of this fact many use financial incentives to spark a high volume of high-quality suggestions.

We recommend suggestion programs that improve customer satisfaction (if they also cut costs, great!). If there is no funding for satisfaction enhancements, a ground rule for a service-oriented suggestion program can be "It can't cost anything," while still keeping the focus on customer satisfaction.

Suggestion programs have proved to be productive at such health care organizations as EPIC Healthcare in Dallas, Texas; University of Michigan Medical Center in Ann Arbor; Presbyterian Health Services Corporation in Charlotte, North Carolina; and Kaiser Permanente Medical Center in San Francisco.

We don't see suggestion programs as essential to every service improvement strategy for the simple reason that improvement teams are a more immediate and effective fountain from which suggestions spring. If you want to institute a suggestion program to complement (not replace) process improvement teams, consider these caveats so that you can make it optimally effective:

- Suggestion programs require constant publicity or they fade away.
- Suggestion programs need to change periodically. When programs are focused on service, you can rotate the customer group that is the focus of suggestions. For example, the first quarter can encourage patient satisfaction suggestions; the second quarter can encourage physician satisfaction suggestions; the third quarter can encourage employee satisfaction suggestions; and the fourth quarter can encourage visitor (or payer) satisfaction suggestions. Otherwise, the programs get stale and suggestion volume drops off drastically.

Figure 7-12. Guide to Use of Tools

● = Often used
○ = Used less often
× = Used rarely

	Identify outputs, customers' expectations	Describe current process	Measure and analyze	Focus on an improvement opportunity	Identify root causes	Generate and choose solutions	Map out a trial run	Implement a trial run	Evaluate the results	Draw conclusions	Standardize the change	Monitor; hold the gains
Focus groups	●	●		×		●	○		●	●	○	○
Surveys			●		○	○			●			●
Interviews	●	●		×	○	○	○		○	○	○	×
Check sheets			●					●	○			●
Logs			●					●	○			○
Histograms			●		○			×	○			×
Pareto charts				●	●					●		
Trend charts			●					●	●			●
Flowcharts				●	●	○	●				●	
Control charts			●					●	●			●
Brainstorming				●	●	●	○				●	
Affinity charts					○	×	○				○	
Relationship diagrams					●	○	○					
Cause-and-effect diagrams					●							
Force-field analyses					●		●		○		●	
Multivoting					×							
Decision matrices				○		●			○			
Action planning							●				●	
Tree diagrams			○		○	●	●				●	

- Ideally, a steering team guides the program. This team should consist of managers and frontline people, because both are key to publicizing the effort, developing fair ground rules, refreshing the focus, and making it credible by taking an active role in idea implementation.
- When employees submit what appears to them to be a bright idea but one they have not thought through, you run the risk of creating disaffection if the idea is not accepted. It's helpful to require the idea to be fleshed out in the original submission, including a measuring device for establishing the success of the suggestion.
- A good system ensures response to all signed suggestions. Lack of follow-up means certain and sudden death. Most organizations use a computer to track the status

of suggestions and trigger follow-up in a timely fashion. A response gives the message that "someone listened to me," and this has more power than financial incentives.

- Recognition is essential whereas financial reward is not. The research on suggestion programs indicates that financial rewards for suggestions might undermine your broader goal of building employees' stake in the organization and your message that continuous service improvement is inherent in everyone's job. For that reason, the most successful suggestion programs use symbolic incentives (for example, ceremonies or tokens of appreciation). For example, Alliant Health System in Louisville created a company store in which employees could exchange points earned (by team participation and documented improvements) for Alliant memorabilia. This incentive fostered loyalty as well as team spirit.

Some organizations encourage, train, and reward teams (including cross-functional teams) for making implementable suggestions, thus encouraging both teamwork and the quality of the suggestions made. Other organizations require those who made the suggestions to become involved in their implementation, even if the suggestion applies to an area of the organization outside the suggester's purview. This encourages employees to broaden their perspectives, take a break from their everyday routines, and gain the kind of valuable tactical skills that are key to implementing innovations and improvements.

Suggestion programs may appear to be simple to run, but they require extensive commitment and labor. If your goal is suggestions and innovations, consider the alternative of quarterly employee focus groups that consist of intensive group brainstorming. These can be very exciting and surprisingly efficient; follow up by appointing a committee that sorts the ideas and reports back to everyone the yield of promising ideas.

Engage in Benchmarking

To speed up process improvement and innovation, to bring more minds to bear on the problem, and to force process owners to look beyond the familiar, many organizations have incorporated the strategy of benchmarking. Benchmarking entails identifying the "best-in-class" or "best-of-the-best" practices of other institutions and making process improvements that strive for those highest standards. According to the Healthcare Advisory Board Report, IBM calls benchmarking a "management tool to raise the bar."[15] Milliken defines it as "stealing shamelessly."[16] Benchmarking frees improvement teams from the boundaries of their own thinking and from their organization's current practices.

The following five-step benchmarking process is recommended by the Healthcare Advisory Board:[17]

1. Develop interview guides for the process in question (that is, figure out what you want to know). A questionnaire should probe for:
   - Full description of process (including how process gets around problem areas a hospital has identified).
   - Reasons why process works (for example: What really makes this process run so smoothly? Is there anything unique to your institution that might prohibit our organization from achieving the same results?).
   - Evidence that process is successful at achieving a hospital objective (for example: How is the process measured? What are its inputs? What have the trends been in these over time?).
   - Recommendations on what (if anything) they would recommend changing in their process, and why.
2. Once you know precisely what the hospital is looking for, begin a search for "best-practice" companies. Possible sources for benchmarking candidates include consultants, library data bases, professional associations, industry publications, annual reports, industry analysts, and university professors.

3. If possible, narrow list; then conduct phone interviews.
4. Select companies for site visits.
5. Prepare interview team and conduct site visits.

Wherever possible, obtain details on the process under study through literature searches, by phone or by mail; site visits are optimal. Because site visits are potentially expensive and time-consuming, however, they may not be necessary. For a more comprehensive discussion of benchmarking, see Gerald Balm's *Benchmarking: A Practitioner's Guide for Becoming and Staying Best of the Best.*[18] Other excellent resources on benchmarking are available from the International Benchmarking Clearinghouse (713/685-4609), a service of the American Productivity and Quality Center, and from the Healthcare Forum (415/421-2411).

Institute Structures and Special Supports for *Team* Improvement Initiatives
Because most service processes involve many people and many departments, *team* initiatives are needed to tackle significant problems and achieve significant improvements. By creating ongoing structures and support systems, you ensure that improvement efforts are easy to initiate and continuous—with parameters and expectations made clear in advance. For example, it would be helpful for your administrative council or service strategy steering team to address planning questions such as those shown in figure 7-13. Such an exercise would result in clear-cut parameters for a team.

Alternative structures and supports range from highly organized and enduring service improvement teams to the focused problem-solving task force that comes together to attack a single, finite problem. The point is that you need a deliberate plan that weaves service improvement processes into everyday life. Such a plan would support those who are motivated to make improvements and eliminate many of the hurdles that might be encountered in trying to get an improvement initiative up and running.

Consider training a squad of skilled facilitators to help build and facilitate a network of service improvement teams. Select a group of employees to receive special training

Figure 7-13. Sample Planning Questions

- As you see it, what do you want the teams to accomplish? What will satisfy you in terms of results? What is the role of each team?
- Who should identify the focus of the team's problem-solving efforts? (e.g., systematic look at customer requirements up front? Group's own perceptions of key problems/opportunities? Administrative suggestions? Can each group decide this? Other?)
- Are teams recommenders? Decision makers? Action planners? Implementers? Under what conditions? What latitude does each team have to act, spend money, etc.?
  —If they are recommenders, to whom do they recommend their proposals? In what detail? How, by whom, and by when will they get a response? How can "no response" be prevented?
  —When decisions made to implement solutions/innovations involve people outside the team, who communicates new expectations? Who runs interface? Who "sells" the change?
- What is the role of each administrator and the administrative team in relation to Service Improvement Teams?
- What is expected of each team facilitator?
- Everybody's busy. Is the frequency of meetings up to the team?
- What is expected of the boss of each team member? (e.g., number of meetings, degree of priority?) How can they be held accountable?
- What is expected of each team member's supervisor? How can they be told this? How will they be held accountable?
- What is the role of the advisor to the team? How can advisors be held accountable?
- What is the relationship between the team chain of command and the usual chain of command?
- How is each team supposed to communicate with its advisor? With other teams? With the administrative team? With departments or individuals needed in implementing team decisions? With the managers whose departments are affected by their proposals/decisions? With team members' bosses? With all employees?
- How can employees/physicians have input into teams?
- How are physicians/all employees involved in teams?

and consequently to serve as facilitators of improvement teams. Train them in process improvement, problem solving, and group process management. Once they are trained, assign the facilitators to teams engaged in tackling processes that need improvement.

Along with skilled facilitators, a simple process chartering improvement teams should be in place. Determine whether you want to control or approve the establishment of improvement teams and the priorities they decide to address. For example, can any interested manager initiate a team? Is there a system for starting cross-functional improvement teams? Do you want the administrative council to consider proposals for team start-up and decide whether to charter the team? Or would you rather clarify parameters for team start-up and let managers start the teams at will?

Also, do you want to structure or encourage departmental teams, cross-functional teams, interdepartmental "liaison" teams, or a combination of those? For problems that go beyond "turf lines," consider structures that engage people from a variety of departments in solving problems that affect all of them. Following are some options:

- *Interdepartmental liaison teams:* For two departments that interface a lot and need to have effective service partnerships, liaison teams bring people from the two departments together to solve problems. This option improves the flow of people, papers, supplies, and services across turf lines.

  Interdepartmental process improvement can be a challenging experience, because most processes involve many departments. Whereas it is ideal that all departments involved in a particular process should work on its improvement, there is an alternative: Liaison teams involve *only two* departments. Their task is to smooth out the processes and relationships between them that affect service performance toward key customers. One hospital, for example, set up a series of two-department teams, including nursing–pharmacy, utilization review–social services, nursing–laboratories, admissions–nursing, and dietary–nursing.

  By singling out only two departments, you help the team focus on a range of issues narrower and more manageable than the host of problems that emerge in multidepartmental teams. These teams work best when they consist of a mix of department manager (director or assistant director), supervisors, and staff. Typical team size is four to eight people with equal representation from each of the two departments.

  Skilled facilitators can help the teams function effectively; however, team managers can share the facilitator role if they are trained in group facilitation and process improvement skills. By singling out only two departments, both departments and their managers develop a shoulder-to-shoulder partnership in approaching the problems that might otherwise fall between the cracks.

- *Cross-functional service improvement teams:* Because many problems involve several departments and because most important processes are cross-functional, some improvement efforts need to include key players from several interlocking departments. Some examples of cross-functional processes are discharge planning, bed facilitation, results turnaround, and clinic flow. These teams typically adopt a step-by-step model of process improvement and follow it—drawing on the multiple perspectives represented on the team to untangle and rebuild a problematic process.

- *Customer-centered teams:* In establishing ongoing teams that focus on specific customer groups, each team becomes an advocate for its assigned customer group and takes steps with appropriate people to smooth out the kinks in service delivery that affect that group. For example, you might develop a Patient Satisfaction Team, a Visitor Satisfaction Team, a Physician Satisfaction Team, a Managed Care Buyer Satisfaction Team, and an Employee Satisfaction Team. The agenda for each team would be to translate the organization's service mission into reality for their assigned customer group and to handle problems that the Service Improvement Clearinghouse channels to them. Specifically, these teams solve problems that interfere with their customers' satisfaction and generate service enhancements that make service to them distinctive.

For each customer group, identify the constellation of departments most central to and most influential with regard to that customer group's satisfaction. Form an interdepartmental team of representatives of each of those key departments. For example, your service improvement team charged with enhancing "Group-Buyer" satisfaction might include representatives from billing, nursing, medical records, utilization, and administration.

- *Persons on sabbatical as internal consultants:* Interested, respected managers are replaced for two years so that they can fulfill a two-year term of office with one priority: to focus all their attention on helping other people tackle process improvements with the variety of resources available to the organization. These people need a clear mandate from the administration as well as the "four Ts"—training, tools, time, and teams—to help them. Some organizations invite managers to compete for this opportunity.
- *Peer consultation among managers:* Create arenas that encourage managers to generate mutual helping relationships among peers. For instance, hold weekly sandwich seminars in which managers voluntarily join with peers to seek and give help on service improvement. One 1-hour meeting format involves dividing managers into trios in which each manager gets 20 minutes of free consultation with two partners. Thus, three people get a turn in each trio's 1-hour meeting. In time, managers get the hang of it and, valuing the help other managers can give them, cross turf lines to ask for the help they need—without the necessity of a structured meeting.

Whichever option(s) you choose, the quality improvement literature abounds in resources helpful to team start-up and facilitation.[19-25]

☐ Final Suggestions

Once you gather information about customer satisfaction and complaints, funnel this input into clear mechanisms to figure out what to do. Depending on what's needed, these mechanisms invariably involve top management, middle managers, supervisors, all employees, and a dedicated squad of patient representatives. To the extent that you harness this people power to prevent problems and handle complaints effectively, your organization will cultivate a loyal following that praises you for your responsiveness to their concerns and your concern for their comfort and well-being.

Ask yourself the following questions:

- What am I already doing to solve problems, handle complaints, and improve service processes?
- In what ways are my current systems working or not working?
- What alternatives can I consider that would strengthen these systems?
- What priorities have to be identified if needed change is to occur?

In examining your problem-solving, complaint-management, and operational systems, consider the following:

- *Create formal problem-solving systems:* Many administrators claim that they listen to complaints, review findings from customer and employee surveys, and keep the findings in mind as they set their priorities. Those methods alone don't solve problems. You must have formal systems for problem solving and complaint resolution so that problems and complaints are *systematically* reviewed and processed. Again, they must not be permitted to fall through cracks.

- *Make sure the systems for problem solving are simple:* For example, once a week five people sit around a table, read through the complaints of the week, and then assign follow-through responsibilities. At the next meeting, they review what happened since the last meeting.
- *Concentrate on results:* Some people think that a problem has to be processed by committees and more committees, teams and more teams. The result is that the problem is processed ad infinitum, with no solutions on the horizon. Many problems can be solved by one person if the culture permits this and trusts its members to make a move without layers of bureaucratic review.
- *Provide a climate for risk taking:* To fuel the problem-solving mentality in your organization, allow more responsibility (and more mistakes). Traditionally, hospital cultures have discouraged decision making among their managers because making decisions involves risk taking. Consequently, no decision making—or decision by default—has become the norm. Do people in your organization fear that if they try a solution and it proves unworkable, they will be belittled or punished? If so, why should they bother? If you really want to promote innovation, you have to be willing to accept autonomy of action and occasional mistakes on the part of people who seek to improve the system.
- *Involve employees in complaint management and in process improvement:* Not only are employees closest to the problem, they understand the root causes and may have viable solutions. You spark their investment in implementing solutions and build greater job satisfaction.
- *Avoid problem-solving processes that focus on Band-Aid solutions:* Look instead for root causes so that your time is well spent.
- *Don't make your work impossible by picking unrealistic processes or problems:* Select breakthrough objectives and then recognize, value, and take delight in achieving incremental improvements. If you try to tackle an elephant-sized problem, you run the risk of debilitating frustration. Trust that fixing each link in a chain of service delivery will help you strengthen the whole chain or, if necessary, redesign it.
- *Invest time and energy in training facilitators:* So often, problem-solving meetings regress into gripe sessions unless someone in the group can move the group to a constructive and responsible attack on the problems and the underlying processes that turn well-intentioned employees into victims of dysfunctional processes. Group process as well as process improvement facilitation skills help teams succeed.
- *Once you install solutions, monitor implementation and results:* When you see positive effects, celebrate. When you identify problems, go back to the drawing board.

Remember, if you do not channel the information gathered from your customer groups about their perceptions of your services into an aggressive and determined problem-solving process, then don't bother with gathering the information in the first place. The hospitals that survive in the challenging years ahead will be those that can unstick themselves from past methods and create systems that serve every one of the organization's customers.

References

1. Joint Commission on Accreditation of Healthcare Organizations. *Accreditation Manual for Hospitals.* Oakbrook Terrace, IL: JCAHO, 1992.

2. Goodman, J. Closing the service gap III. Presented at the Lakewood Conferences, Memphis, TN, October 29–30, 1990.

3. TARP Technical Assistance Research Programs. Membership services as a revenue center: cost justification and marketing impact of an aggressive service program. Working paper. Washington, DC: TARP, Feb. 1986.

4. Newbold, P. A., and Stover, D. S. Patient satisfaction pilot reveals gains and limits. *Healthcare Forum Journal* 34(6):51, Nov.–Dec. 1991.

5. Kalafat, J. A systemic health care quality service program. *Hospital and Health Services Administration* 36(4):571, 1991.

6. Labovitz, G. Presentation at ODI sales presentation, Philadelphia, PA, Jan. 1988.

7. Labovitz.

8. Healthcare Advisory Board. *TQM: 14 Tactics for Improving the Quality Process.* Washington, DC: Healthcare Advisory Board, 1992, p. 24.

9. Healthcare Advisory Board, p. 25.

10. King, B. *Hoshin Planning.* Methuen, MA: GOAL/QPC, 1990.

11. Leebov, W., and Ersoz, C. J. *The Health Care Manager's Guide to Continuous Quality Improvement.* Chicago: American Hospital Publishing, 1991.

12. Leebov and Ersoz.

13. Leebov and Ersoz.

14. Leebov and Ersoz.

15. Leebov and Ersoz.

16. Leebov and Ersoz.

17. Leebov and Ersoz.

18. Balm, G. *Benchmarking: A Practitioner's Guide for Becoming and Staying Best of the Best.* Schaumburg, IL: Quality and Productivity Management Association, 1992.

19. Aubrey, C., and Felkins, P. *Teamwork: Involving People in Quality and Productivity Improvement.* Milwaukee: Quality Press, 1988.

20. Scholtes, P. *The Team Handbook.* Madison, WI: Joiner Associates, 1988.

21. Leebov and Ersoz.

22. Brassard, M. *Memory Jogger.* Methuen, MA: GOAL/QPC, 1988.

23. Brassard, M. *Memory Jogger Plus.* Methuen, MA: GOAL/QPC, 1989.

24. Johnson, D., and Johnson, F. *Joining Together: Group Theory and Group Skills.* Englewood Cliffs, NJ: Prentice-Hall, 1975.

25. Goodmeasure Inc. *Solving Quality and Productivity Problems.* Milwaukee: Quality Press and the American Society for Quality Control, 1988.

Chapter 8
Communication

Employees will be invested in and committed to service quality improvement only if management keeps them informed about organizational performance, challenges, and improvements. To advance service quality, overcommunication is the guideline. People at every level of your organization, including customers, rely on you to give and receive information about your organization's activities and priorities overall and about the activities, current thinking, and progress related to your service priority in particular.

You need communication loops that are both horizontal (from person to person at the same level) and vertical (between levels). No part of the organization and none of your customers should feel left out of this process.

Before reading further, take the self-test in figure 8-1. "True" answers show that you're on the right track. "False" answers suggest possible directions for revamping communication so that it supports and advances your service commitment. If your score is high, you have systems in place that keep people informed and engaged. If your score is low, you need to build new systems or strengthen existing ones for sharing information with customers and employees, maintain open communication, and build the quality of interpersonal relationships that are key to ongoing problem solving and teamwork.

This chapter will describe communication strategies that advance the big picture, allow for listening and responding to employees, and facilitate sharing of feedback and progress. In discussions of what and how to communicate, employee updates, the grapevine, and storyboards (among other techniques) will be examined.

□ Communication Strategies

You will need a mix of strategies to accomplish four key communication objectives. These objectives are to enable everyone throughout the hospital to see the big picture; to listen and respond to employees and physicians; to reinforce your service commitment through written devices; and to share feedback and progress. The remainder of this chapter is devoted to each objective and the techniques needed to advance it.

Figure 8-1. Self-Test

Communication. *Circle the appropriate answers. The more "true" answers, the better. "False" answers indicate areas that need improvement.*

1. Our employees at all levels are regularly informed about our organization's performance, including our financial situation and what we're doing to fulfill our mission. — True False

2. Our service record (summaries of customer surveys, phone interviews, compliments) is shared with employees regularly. — True False

3. Decisions made by top management and the reasons for those decisions are shared openly with employees. — True False

4. When we make a service improvement here or solve a service problem, employees are told about it. — True False

5. We regularly use a variety of methods of communicating with staff (for example, memos, meetings, newsletters, "town meetings," and informal visits). — True False

6. In our organization, people are encouraged to give each other feedback in order to enhance performance and teamwork. — True False

7. Our middle managers are actively encouraged to convey information to their staff on behalf of top management. — True False

8. Most employees feel relatively well informed about the organization's plans and programs. — True False

9. We use visible methods to publicize service performance and progress in making improvements (for example, trend charts, storyboards). — True False

10. The quality of communication in our relationships with one another is a priority here, and breakdowns receive constructive attention. — True False

11. In our organization's "image" materials (for example, annual report and employee and patient handbook), our high priority on customer satisfaction is stated and restated to reinforce its importance in our culture. — True False

12. Our house publications carry features on customer relations issues, events, and accomplishments. — True False

Total: ___ ___

Enable Everyone Hospitalwide to See the Big Picture

In an information vacuum, employees feel alienated and resentful of an administration that expects employees to get on the service excellence bandwagon and do all they can for the organization but fails to "let them in" on its objectives, challenges, and plights. Frequent employee laments are:

- "They think we're too dumb to understand."
- "Everyone knows but me."
- "Nobody ever tells me anything."
- "What are those people doing up there anyway?"
- "Who cares. They think we're nobodies."

These unfortunate sentiments are frequently the result of inadequate communication from administration, department heads, supervisors, the governing board, and indeed every layer perceived as having power over and a monopoly on dissemination of information. If administrators claim "This is your [employees'] hospital, and you are this hospital," then they should keep employees informed even on routine news. Communication about "the big picture" is essential for three reasons:

1. It builds commitment, investment, and ownership.
2. It gives people information on which to base their decisions and actions.
3. It shows caring and respect for employees and their commitment to the facility.

Communication Fallacies

Organizations can suffer from "infosclerosis," hardening of the communication arteries. This organizational affliction can occur in the health care setting whenever higher-ups fall victim to six fallacies:

- *Fallacy 1: No news means no need to communicate.* No news *is* news. If management fails to communicate about inactions or tabled problems, employees become paranoid, believing either that something has happened and everyone knows but them or that nothing has happened because management has not even *heard* the problem.
- *Fallacy 2: A problem must be 100 percent solved before it becomes news.* What problem in a hospital is ever 100 percent solved? Even slight improvements are news. You should inform employees when the process of exploring possible solutions to a problem has begun, and you should urge managers to inform each other when they initiate problem-solving or process improvement efforts—no matter how remote a solution may appear to be. Employees and physicians can better tolerate waiting for improvements if they know that improvement processes are under way.
- *Fallacy 3: News has to be big.* Even the repair of the cafeteria's ice machine deserve air time. If you communicate all the little things, employees are more tolerant of the difficulties involved in solving the big problems.
- *Fallacy 4: Employees should hear only good news.* Employees resent administrators and managers who act like overprotective parents.
- *Fallacy 5: Middle management is assumed to be an effective funnel.* Alas, department heads don't always hear what top management says, absorb it, and convey it to staff. A system of checks on middle management communication methods is necessary.
- *Fallacy 6: Only communicate news that makes you look good.* You'll be well served by being honest, even in conveying bad news.

Communication needs to be liquid, flowing through systematic, recurring, and habitual channels. Managers and supervisors at each level need to stay in touch with the information needs and concerns of their staff, to aggressively seek the information that responds to these needs and concerns, and then to provide information responsibly and responsively. This includes relevant information that may not have been requested.

What to Communicate

In the past, employees were rarely informed about their organization's financial health because it was taken for granted. However, in view of today's more competitive health care environment, employees are entitled to be kept up-to-date in this area if they are to expected to help their facility compete successfully. Figure 8-2 shows a reinforcing letter that one administrator sent to all employees to convey her vision about service excellence and also to put the vision into a larger economic context.

Specifically, employees want to know:

- Where the organization is going
- What vision its leaders have
- What values drive the leaders (and consequently the employees)
- How the organization is doing (areas of excellence, problem areas and consequences, and what improvement efforts are under way)
- What is expected of employees

Employees want to feel ownership in their organization, and that people at the top know it. Furthermore, they want to feel a sense of "we're in this together; if we don't hang together, we'll all hang separately." In simple terms, employees want to feel heard, cared about, respected, relied on, and appreciated by higher-ups.

Figure 8-2. Example of Reinforcing Letter to Employees

Dear Fellow Employees:

In an environment of increased competition, our division is undergoing change. Although these are challenging times, there is a danger. With so much on our minds and with not enough time to do what we need to do *yesterday*, there is a risk of neglecting the all-important human element—personal touch.

I am concerned that we do not forget the real reason for our hospital's existence—providing quality care to our patients. Unlike us, patients are not thinking about prospective payment or preferred provider organizations or hospital marketing. They only know that they are hurting or that they are scared. Although we are familiar with the hospital environment, most patients are not. We must strive to be aware that they may be seized with fright when faced with cold machines and cold voices.

As a hospital, we have much at stake. Hospital care is turning into a "buyer's market." Patients are, and for good reason, choosy about which hospitals they use. The advantage lies with the hospital whose employees are seen as friendly, sensitive, understanding, generous with time, compassionate, and attentive. I want our hospital to pursue that advantage.

In the last two years, we have made terrific gains in the *hospital*ity we extend to our patients and visitors. Although the pressures on us are greater than ever, I know that together we will meet the challenge, become distinguished for our *hospital*ity, and strengthen the quality of care and service we extend to our friends and neighbors. I believe we are special, and I want to get the word out.

During the last few months, you were asked to participate in several programs to reinforce and advance our *hospital*ity effort. I am enthusiastic about these programs and hope you found them stimulating and worthwhile to attend.

Thank you for your active cooperation and for giving our hospital your best.

A. Susan Bernini
Vice-President and General Director
Albert Einstein Medical Center

Reprinted, with permission, from Albert Einstein Healthcare Foundation, Philadelphia, Pennsylvania.

Employee Updates

Many hospitals, especially those with active strategies for service excellence, communicate by means of *employee updates* in the form of *live* presentations (for example, slide shows, speeches, and discussions). Ideally, discussions should be held by administrators for all employees. These strategies are designed to keep employees apprised of the organization's health and the challenges before it. Updates are a kind of progress report that helps keep the big picture in view. Updates also help leaders ensure that all staff are hearing the same information and message. The following subsections describe a few other ways to update employees.

Regular Leadership "Advances"

According to General Motors President Roger Smith: "You can't push people to do what we're trying to do. If they don't want to do something—and if they aren't dedicated to doing it—the human being, and particularly the American human being, has a marvelous capacity for screwing things up. And he (she) feels justified in doing it too. He (she) just says, 'I don't believe in it. I'm not going to do it.' "[1]

To give management the knowledge, respect, and opportunity to become committed, many organizations hold quarterly or semiannual leadership "advances." In these events, senior management restates the organization's mission, values, and priorities and helps managers seize the reins to lead the organization forward.

Variations on this theme include Management Grand Rounds, which are shorter, more frequent gatherings at which leaders describe goals, activities, and plans regarding specific facets of the organization. Some examples are "Emergency Department Update," "Our Growth Strategy for the Next Five Years," and "Top Priority Process Improvement Efforts."

Barry Brown, chief executive officer of the West Jersey Health System in New Jersey, created the *Corporate Open Forum* to help his people stay in the know. Here's how it works:

- All corporate officers meet as a group with the entire management staff of each of their four hospitals, one hospital at a time.
- The CEO presents a brief update on major initiatives in the system.
- All corporate officers then form a panel and field questions and complaints about anything and everything managers voice.
- Afterward, a social hour encourages further open exchange and team building.

Fireside Chats and Fishbowls

In periodic discussions, top-level executives talk with managers and physician leaders as a group, addressing questions and concerns in an intimate "fireside chat" atmosphere where all are encouraged to speak openly. Many find it helpful to hold a focus group with managers and physician leaders so as to solicit questions ahead of time. This ensures that the tough questions surface at the discussion meeting and that the executive team has a chance to prepare a full response.

In a variation on this approach, called the executive "fishbowl," executives sit in a circle in the center of the room. They talk with each other about tough subjects while managers and physician leaders listen in a theater-in-the-round arrangement. The circle includes two empty chairs, and listeners are invited to enter the fishbowl and sit in these chairs if they have a question or comment. In this environment, managers can learn important things while witnessing executive teamwork as executives grapple with tough questions and discuss their complexity, disagree constructively, and listen to each other. Executive teams who want to be role models of teamwork and healthy communication welcome the opportunity inherent in this approach.

Question-and-Answer and Round-the-Clock Briefings

At the University of Missouri-Columbia Hospital and Clinics in Columbia, Missouri, the hospital administration conducts updates at least twice a year using a question-and-answer format. Because everyone cannot attend the updates, the administration circulates to all staff a written communication sharing all the questions raised, along with their answers.

Some hospitals conduct round-the-clock annual briefings that are more structured and mandatory for all staff. Each employee is scheduled into a 90-minute session with an administrator–facilitator. A session presented in figure 8-3 includes eight steps as well as a sample agenda.

Videos, Speakers Bureaus, and Other Update Vehicles

Other hospitals use video methods to keep their employees informed. For example, every three months, Rockdale Hospital in Conyers, Georgia, produces a 5- to 10-minute *video* news magazine called "Communilink" and makes it available to all staff through the hospital library, at department meetings, for home use, and for lunchtime viewings. Content of videos typically includes the following items:

- Winners of employee recognition awards and contests
- Introduction to new services
- New programs offered to the community
- Acquisitions of new and/or innovative technology
- Updates on buildings or renovations
- Meetings with people from behind-the-scenes programs that deserve attention
- Motivating words from the hospital director

Another approach to employee updates involves developing an internal speakers bureau. With administrators and managers as speakers, each quarter several topics are

Figure 8-3. Round-the-Clock Briefing Agenda

Statement of Goals

- To increase employee understanding of our organization's strengths, accomplishments, and plans
- To provide employees with a structured way to ask questions of the administration
- To heighten employees' awareness of their power to shape our organization's reputation by word-of-mouth

90-Minute Session Agenda

1. Welcome, introduction, and overview of objectives.
2. Employees form small groups and generate a list of questions they'd like answered by administration, questions that, if answered, would help employees feel "in the know."
3. Every employee question is recorded on a flipchart.
4. The administrator presents (preferably using slides) an update on "What's New at the Hospital." This includes:
   - The challenges we face as a medical center
   - How we're doing (satisfaction results, competitive position, quality indicators)
   - What we're doing to succeed
   - Our accomplishments and strengths
   - Our priority problems to solve and processes to improve
   - How all staff and physicians can help
5. Administrator returns to the employees' questions and, with their help, scratches out the questions that have been answered. A few additional questions are answered and the administrator promises that any remaining questions will be answered within a fixed time period in the employee newsletter.
6. Employees turn to a partner and discuss recent positive (+) events and accomplishments in the hospital—
   - + about our people
   - + about our services
   - + about the work here
   - + about improvements made
7. Partners are invited to share their lists with the larger group. Administrator makes the point that employees are crucial to the future of the hospital because of what they do and what they say about the hospital.
8. The administrator closes the session by thanking employees for their participation and encouraging them to share with their families, friends, and community what they've learned about the organization's strengths and plans.

---

listed and promoted. Departments sign up for speakers who come to department meetings as news ambassadors. Topics include new program initiatives, expansion plans, service changes, and also process improvement stories told by people who have served on improvement teams.

Following are more vehicles for getting the word out:

- If your organization is going through construction, renovation, or a move, publish a *facilities update*.
- Place *tent cards* on cafeteria tables announcing updates.
- Have your administrator convene an *Opinion Leader Committee* and give the committee regular updates. In their everyday interactions, opinion leaders (people widely respected by peers) spread the word informally through your organization's grapevine.
- Set up a *speakeasy* in which 10 employees have breakfast or lunch with the CEO and discuss current events.
- Establish a *direct-line phone information service*.
- Put a *Daily Slice of Life* (a news brief) on your hospital's TV system, if you have one.
- Post *bulletin boards* along waiting lines in the cafeteria.
- Post *key indicators* (for example, number of admissions and average length of stay) daily for all to see.

The point, in short, is better communication by every possible means. The result is improved morale; a work force that has information, not hearsay, guiding their actions; and a work force more likely to climb aboard your service excellence bandwagon.

Listen and Respond to Employees

Updates, grand rounds, and the like expedite the flow of communication from leaders to staff. You also need to foster communication from staff to leaders, providing for interchange and discussion. The following subsections describe three examples of methods to make this happen: the employee "sound-off" meeting; the grapevine; and employee hotlines.

The Employee Sound-Off Meeting

Employee sound-off meetings structure exchanges between employees and their administrators, department directors, or employee relations specialists. Here's how a meeting works:

1. The convener (manager) introduces the meeting's purpose—to create an opportunity for employees to take stock of how things are going so that communication is open and problems can be addressed.

2. The convener divides people into trios and gives each trio a worksheet for use in guiding their discussion. Each group is asked to select a recorder, who writes down every idea expressed (not just those that people agree on), so that the feedback can be shared with the whole group and collected later for follow-up. A general sound-off worksheet might have the following sections (with space after each for writing in the group's ideas):
   —How have you been feeling at work lately?
   —What's going right? What have we accomplished? What have we appreciated?
   —What's been frustrating lately about work? What barriers have made it difficult to serve our customers? What problems have made it difficult to work with coworkers cooperatively?
   If something in particular is going on that needs employee feedback, the worksheet questions can be more specific. For instance, if you've been focusing on service improvement for several months, these questions might be asked:
   —How has service improved for patients?
   —How has service improved toward internal customers?
   —How has service improved toward physicians?
   —What remain as priority service problems to solve for patients?
   —What remain as priority service problems to solve for internal customers?
   —What remain as priority service problems to solve for physicians?

3. After small groups brainstorm responses, the convener reconvenes the large group and invites small groups to report on each question in turn. The convener writes down key words on a flipchart and then, before moving to the next question, asks if people see any themes or patterns.

4. The convener asks people to break again into small groups and reach agreement on two things they wish management would take responsibility for improving/addressing and two things they think employees should take responsibility for improving/addressing.

5. These desires are then shared in the larger group, which discusses them and decides how best to follow up (whether teams are needed, or a deadline for reporting back).

6. The convener thanks participants and reinforces the importance of keeping communication lines open in an effort to improve service and achieve a quality of work life that serves everyone.

After the meeting, follow-up is essential in accordance with promises made.

The Grapevine

At Children's Hospital of Michigan, The Grapevine has been designated to create employee access to information and to dispel rumors. Fliers were distributed to all employees explaining The Grapevine, how to fill out its question-and-answer form, and that employees can request that their questions remain confidential. The flier also explained that human resources would track response time so that each question submitted is answered within 15 working days. A mailbox was placed outside the cafeteria to collect forms, which were picked up once a day and returned to human resources.

The Grapevine forms include space for a code number, so that when a question and its answer are published, the person who submitted the question remains anonymous. The name is required only if an answer is to be returned personally to the questioner.

Questions are submitted to training/development personnel and are then routed to the appropriate administrator or department head. The answers are returned to training/development where they are reviewed and forwarded to The Grapevine. All signed questions are answered, but names are kept confidential; very few questions are submitted without a name. The Grapevine publishes a wide variety of questions and answers, on an average of twice monthly, in the widely read employee newsletter. This tactic serves as a reminder to use the system.

Employee Hotlines

According to Jean Altman, public relations director, El Camino Hospital in Mountain View, California, CEO Dick Pettingill has two phones on his desk: one for typical business calls, the other an employee hotline. From anywhere in the hospital, employees can dial 7777 and reach Pettingill with complaints, suggestions, or concerns. Clearly, El Camino leaders think of employees as assets, not overhead.[2]

While many management teams make a common practice of inviting employee and physician complaints and suggestions, few have installed regular systems for *responding* to what they hear. The glow from participation only lasts if management *responds*. Avoid the communication vacuum that develops when you invite employees to submit ideas and then communicate nothing further. Follow these guidelines:

- *Respond in writing:* You can't depend on a small group of people (for example, department heads and other managers) to communicate accurately to *all* employees. Messages get lost and mixed up.
- *Respond in a timely fashion:* Employees need *responses,* not necessarily *solutions,* and they need them quickly so they don't think you've forgotten about them or ignored their ideas.
- *Respond to all suggestions:* Employees need to know that their input is important and that what may be small suggestions to improve daily work life are just as important to the organization as larger ones. Respond, even if you don't adopt the ideas.

Of course, when you ask for employee input, you often get a lot more than you want or need. Here's a method for categorizing an onslaught of ideas and complaints from employees so you can respond in a systematic fashion:

- *Step 1. Categorize all of the ideas and complaints:* For example, are they environmental or technical in nature? Do they relate to problems with systems, people skills, amenities, or programs or services?
- *Step 2. Pick one category and classify each item in that category using the following scheme:*
  - "We've already done something about that." (Perhaps you've already solved that problem or fixed the broken item but never told anybody. Communicate that information now.)
  - "We know that's a problem, and here's our plan for addressing it." (For instance, "We're chartering a process improvement team to work on this" or "We have the director of engineering looking into this").
  - "We didn't know that was a concern. Now that we do, here's our plan for looking into it."

— "We know that's a problem, but we can't do anything about it now. Here's why."
- *Step 3. Write a memo and distribute it to all staff:* Use paycheck stuffers, a column in your in-house newsletter, or any other method to reach *all* employees. Don't rely only on verbal communication to small groups of employees. Your responses won't reach everyone.

Frequent and honest response to employees about their complaints and ideas keeps them involved, motivated, and thinking on your organization's behalf. *Ask, listen, and respond.* Figures 8-4 and 8-5 show a sample report from an administrator in response to suggestions and a sample form letter in response to an unsolvable problem, respectively.

Reinforce Your Service Commitment through Written Devices

Your organization already produces a mixture of written devices to communicate about matters of importance. You need to align these written devices with your service strategy and use them to reinforce and advance your strategy in yet another way. To start, consider using your existing newsletters and other house publications to highlight important service issues, results, and events.

Some organizations develop a newsletter dedicated exclusively to service excellence. It includes patient interviews, visitor interviews, patient survey results, a "doctor's corner," skill-building features, puzzles, cartoons, and announcements about forthcoming service/quality related events. Figure 8-6 (p. 149) shows excerpts from MetroHealth Medical Center's "People First" newsletter designed to update employees on what people have accomplished in their service improvement efforts. Also consider letters from leaders reinforcing their service priority and sharing anecdotes, information about your service strategy, people's reactions, and results.

Figure 8-4. Administration's Response to Suggestions

Report from Administration

In response to your steady stream of suggestions, we're continuing to improve our service toward patients. Here's a nutshell summary of recent improvements:

- **Signs** (at last!): The maintenance department designed and installed a whole series of directional signs. Hopefully, these make it easier for patients and visitors to find their way and relieve the burden you've carried of answering so many questions and handling so many lost people.
- **Newspapers:** You asked that newspaper boxes be moved inside. We can't because of lobby clutter. But we have arranged for the gift shop and coffee shop to sell newspapers.
- **Free and Available Radio and TV:** In February, we installed two TV channels and two radio stations on every patient TV. One TV channel carries regularly scheduled patient education films. The other will show a clock, advertise hospital services and events, and offer special programs. (Patients still have to pay for access to other TV channels.)
- **Employee Nametags:** Soon, we will be providing you with bold, new nametags that can be read from a distance.
- **Employee Lounges:** You will have lounges. The new buildings and Levy (after renovations) will contain employee lounges on every patient floor and in the OR and lab areas.

If you've submitted a concern or suggestion and haven't heard any response, give me a call at Ext. 6010. We'll do our best to follow up with you if you leave your name and number.

I see steady gains in the quality of service we extend to our patients and their families and want to thank you for all you're doing to help.

Sincerely,

CEO

Figure 8-5. Form Letter for Responding to Unsolvable, but Plaguing, Problems

---

Dear Friends,

I want to get back to you on a problem raised by many employees during our recent workshops on service excellence. People complained about _____, a very complex problem. I agree that this problem has difficult consequences for us, like _____ and _____. With the help of _____ and _____, we've researched possible solutions. Frankly, every possibility that might help the problem seems to lead to several other problems, for instance, _____.

Until we can figure out a way to tackle this problem that doesn't create more problems than it solves, we are not going to take action.

I am asking for your understanding and patience. I am also inviting you to contact _____ to discuss any ideas or approaches you would like us to consider.

Meanwhile, I assure you that we are not forgetting about this problem. It's important, and we know it. I'll keep you informed about any new angles we might decide to pursue.

Sincerely,

CEO

Stories and articles highlighting the importance of customer satisfaction and ongoing service improvement should appear in your annual report and in your physicians bulletin. Use any printed tool produced by your organization and take advantage of every opportunity to keep people informed and alert to the organization's issues and priorities.

As you move forward implementing piece after piece of your strategy for service excellence, communicate with employees about each step of the implementation process, as well as their reactions to that step, and the plans that emerge from the reactions. This communication helps keep service excellence in the forefront of peoples' consciousness.

If you invite employees to sound off about your organization's service strengths and weaknesses, publish these comments and administration's responses to keep the communication ongoing. In your employee publication, include a service feature on such topics as:

- Evaluation results that include employee, physician, and patient perceptions of employee behavior
- A feature on administrators' findings regarding improvement of service processes
- A thank-you from the CEO to everyone for the strain the staff endured and the cooperation they offered one another in order to make attendance at the service refresher programs possible
- The major issues raised during employee sound-offs (what's been done, what's being done, what will be done, what can't be done, how interested people can get involved in solutions)
- The status of service-focused process improvement teams
- Service recovery stories in which staff used a customer complaint as a second chance to make things right and found creative ways to win back customer satisfaction and loyalty

Service Excellence Bulletin Boards

Some hospitals also create one or more bulletin boards with changing displays that highlight service improvement efforts of departments, feature thank-you letters from satisfied customers, and recognize people deserving recognition for outstanding service. You can also post storyboards that describe process improvements achieved by teams. Figure 8-7 illustrates a possible format for such a bulletin board.

Figure 8-6. MetroHealth Medical Center's *People First* Newsletter (Excerpts)

****

Performance Standards: Are You in Compliance?

A major goal of the **People First** Steering Committee this year is to increase compliance with the **People First** performance standards. Projects aimed at reaching this goal are in progress.

A **People First** subcommittee is developing a plan to increase employee awareness of performance standards and compliance in following them. They are also looking at incorporating the performance standards into job descriptions.

Under consideration is incorporating bargaining unit employees' performance standards in their annual evaluation. The Employee Reward and Recognition Service Enhancement Team is considering a proposal in which "mystery shoppers" (individuals posing as customers) will reward employees "caught" being in compliance.

This year, every department at MetroHealth Medical Center must have at least two **People First** performance indicators in its goals. Help will be offered to set these indicators, using the performance standards as the basis.

****

What Does **People First** Mean to You?

"I mainly see **People First** as an attempt of the hospital to put in a very obvious, straightforward way the philosophy it's had all along. And that is dedication to serving the people who come here—the patients. They are not new ideas, but through **People First** they are being focused on to try and make people remember them every day." Linda Headrick, M.D. Medicine

Dr. Headrick, an attending physician with MetroHealth Medical Association, is a long-term supporter of **People First,** having served on the committee which recommended that the MetroHealth System adopt a strong customer service strategy—now named **People First.**

****

Which Way Do We Go? Contest Winners Know!

What are the correct names of the buildings located in the new Outpatient Plaza? Just ask Linda Simons, Faculty Business Office; Margaret Jones, Admitting; Blanche Valancy, Social Work; Bill Downer, Jr., Management Engineering; Scott Marella, MetroHealth Referral Service; Rich Moriarty, Facilities Engineering; Tom Tuckerman, Information Systems; and Terri Jaruscak, Cardian Catheterization Lab. They were the winners drawn from all the correct responses in the first two versions of the "Which Way Do We Go?" Wayfinding Contest. The contest was sponsored by the **People First** Hospitality Service Enhancement Team.

"We want employees to use consistent terminology when giving directions to our customers," said Terry Podrapovec, R.N., unit manager on 7B, and member of the Hospitality SET. This helps eliminate confusion and uncertainty for those unfamiliar with the MetroHealth Medical Center campus.

The contest is part of an effort to acquaint employees with the correct names of buildings, streets, and other areas. "While employees learn the names, they'll have fun at the same time and remember to use this information when giving someone directions," said Sue Sammons, R.N., PM&R Nursing. Sammons co-chairs the hospitality SET with Becky Moldaver, Community Affairs.

All the correct responses from each game were pooled together and names were drawn from the pool. Prizes were donated by Employee Services, the Hair Care Center, and the Art Studio.

Reprinted, with permission, from MetroHealth Medical Center, Cleveland, Ohio.

Figure 8-7. Service Excellence Bulletin Board

Letter from Administrator	Upcoming Events	Service Improvements
Department of the Month	Steering Committee	Notes/Updates

The printed word, although inadequate by itself, is a must-do vehicle for keeping employees informed. If you circulate substantive information, and not just image-making hype, your readership will steadily increase because people hunger for information that matters.

Share Feedback and Progress

There's no benefit in measuring service performance unless you consider the results and use them to celebrate success and guide decisions about improvement. *Communicating the results systematically* (not sporadically) to the people with the power to act on them makes your measurement efforts pay off. Routine memos and charts posted on walls are important because they display results visually. But you also need to devote meeting time to the examination and discussion of results to decide what to do to follow up on them appropriately.

The Routine Memo

Once you've identified your performance indicators, you can create report formats to share performance feedback with staff. This report or memo would be distributed with results for each measurement period (weekly, monthly, or quarterly, depending on your monitoring schedule). Regular or routine distribution using a previously designed format is important, otherwise production of this kind of feedback report becomes an afterthought and a burden. An effective memo or report includes the following:

- Charts that display performance over time, because pictures speak a thousand words
- Prose summaries of what the charts show, because some staff are more verbal than visual and find it difficult to see what charts say (for example, "We managed to increase our response speed by an average of 10 minutes per patient this month.")
- Implications of the data (for example: "That means we can congratulate ourselves for a substantial improvement over last month" or "Because this score is substantially below our standard, I want us to see if we can get to the bottom of it. I'd like whoever thinks they have some insight about what happened to join me in a discussion about this.")

Because progress plotting is a powerful device, plotting performance data on charts and posting them on walls or bulletin boards visible to all staff is another way to communicate feedback. User-friendly computer software can help you produce eye-catching bar and line graphs and charts.

Feedback Meetings

Supplement visual and written performance-related communication with regular meetings in which appropriate managers or work teams examine and discuss the feedback. This builds understanding of important service criteria (those important enough to measure), focuses staff on these criteria as performance objectives, and gives work teams the chance to identify improvement opportunities. An example of a meeting format for this purpose follows:

- Ask people to guess how they think the department or organization performed on each indicator during the recent period. (This builds interest in the results.)
- Show the results in a trend chart. Give people a chance to digest them. Answer questions to make sure people understand what they see.
- Invite people to share their conclusions: "What do you see happening here? How do you interpret what you see?"

- Discuss actions that need to be taken:
  - When the results are disturbing, talk about short-term measures for improving performance and, if the performance problem has lingered over time or gotten worse, decide how to investigate the underlying causes and remedy them (for example, charter a team or brainstorm possible solutions then and there).
  - When the results are great, decide how to celebrate and gloat.
- Summarize the findings and the actions the group has decided to take with time lines for follow-up.

Figure out regular vehicles for sharing qualitative feedback about service performance. Some hospitals have an ongoing "Complaints and Compliments" column in their house organ. Consider the excerpt from the "Letters" column in MetroHealth Medical Center's *People First* newsletter (figure 8-8).

Others have a well-planned clearinghouse and routing system for compliment and complaint letters. For instance, all compliment letters are sent to the patient representative. The patient representative sees to it that the editor of the house publication, key executives, the supervisor of the staff involved, and the employees mentioned all receive a copy of the compliments letter along with a thank-you letter and customized margin note from the CEO.

Storyboards

If your organization has improvement teams working to improve service processes, you also need to ensure communication about their processes, experiments, and results. Storyboards are a wonderful vehicle for this communication. A storyboard is a visual portrayal of the steps a team goes through to improve a process. It shows the tools used to measure performance, identify root causes, select a key cause, develop changes, do a trial run, monitor results, and so forth. By visually portraying the "story" of their work together, people learn not only about what they achieved but about the process of improvement and teamwork.

Storyboards can be displayed on bulletin boards, circulated in an employee "Teams on the Move" magazine, and transferred to slides for live team presentations at management meetings, team leader meetings, and department staff meetings.

The vicarious learning that occurs from storytelling using storyboards is phenomenal. Also, your staff develop respect for each others' energy and work toward improvement and optimism that staff can collaborate successfully to make systems more friendly, efficient, convenient, and effective for internal and external customers.

Renovating Your Meetings

Some people estimate that 30 percent of the personnel time in a health care organization is consumed in meetings. Yet if you ask the people who go to meeting after meeting about the productivity of these meetings, the response is often depressing. We're wasting resources when we fail to use meetings as essential and powerful communication

Figure 8-8. Letter in *People First* Newsletter

Just a note to let you know about my experience with Radiology.

When I went for my mammogram, the receptionist was very pleasant and helpful. Your technician was so very nice and really had a calming way about her. I was very apprehensive after my previous mammogram, but her professional and efficient manner made this experience 100 percent better.

In my opinion, you have two very good employees.

Del P.

Reprinted, with permission, from MetroHealth System, Cleveland, Ohio, 1989.

tools to convey results, to address barriers to service delivery, to refresh service consciousness, and to share ideas, priorities, and plans.

Try evaluating your standing meetings with the following questions:

- Does this meeting in any way help us serve our customers better?
- Does the process used in this meeting better equip individuals to serve their customers better?
- If a visitor listened in, would our commitment to service quality and customer satisfaction be clear to him or her?
- Are we spending our time tackling issues that affect customer satisfaction?
- Is our process reflective of the value we place on humane and respectful treatment of people in this organization?

☐ Final Suggestions

Convene a group of influential, informed people to consider together your existing communication practices, their effects, and possibilities for improvement. Then make decisions and implement them.

The following is a possible process to use with your key people:

- Find out what formal and informal methods you already use to ensure a vertical and horizontal flow of communication.
- Examine how each existing vehicle is working. Don't guess, ask employees.
- Identify gaps and needs.
- Generate alternatives. What else might be done?
- Check out the doable options with your target groups.
- Identify changes you want to make.
- Make the changes. Specify a trial period.
- Evaluate the changes after your trial period.
- Refine the changes based on what you learned during the trial period.

When considering your systems for communication, keep the following in mind:

- *Mix your methods:* People learn in many different ways: Some need to hear it, others need to see it, and still others need to experience it. Because of this, it's important to use many methods and say the important things over and over. Most administrators say that key information eventually filters to employees; but according to employees, the filter is often opaque. You will ensure that communication is indeed reaching people if you have a healthy mix of methods for communicating down, up, and across your organization.
- *People pay more attention to things that interest them:* When building your communication strategy, keep checking back with your target audience to find out what *they* want to know. If you "listen" to surveys, focus groups, interviews, and questions people ask, you'll be better able to keep your information interesting and valued by your customers and employees.
- *Watch out for one-way communication:* Ensure that communication flows in both directions, from the bottom up and from the top down. Communication is a two-way street.
- *The medium is the message:* Consider carefully the style of both oral and written communications. The style is at least as important as the content. Be frank, empathetic, and humane.
- *Better late than never, but better early than late:* Get information to people quickly. You can be sure employees and physicians will fume if they read about their

organization in the newspaper or hear about it from friends before anyone on the inside spills the beans.

- *Not just employees, not just physicians:* Some organizations do a great job of communicating to the physicians but insult employees by communicating inadequately to them. In other places, the opposite happens. The point is to install timely, regular, forthright communication vehicles that reach both groups.
- *Occasionally, check out the absorption rate of what you're communicating:* Don't rely on "I said it. Why didn't they hear it?" Keep evaluating whether your vehicles for downward communication are *reaching* the right ears.
- *Be careful of communication overkill:* Whether communication overkill exists is debatable, but nevertheless, remember to hit the main points in manageable segments. Your communication vehicles have to be carefully honed to help people see the forest through the trees. To check that you've presented the essence, be sure to answer these three questions:
  - —What? (the news)
  - —So what? (Why am I telling you this?)
  - —Now what? (Here's what I'm going to do; here's what I want you to do.)
- *"What will the neighbors think?"* Adopting the mind-set of your target group is vital when preparing your communication. How will what you have to say look to the public? Don't become gun-shy and clam up because of possible public perceptions. *Consciously* fashion the optimal way to get your message across.
- *Communication with the pen is not enough:* Communication from person to person cannot be replaced by mass media vehicles. Dedicate attention to building the *teams* and *relationships* you need to make informal, everyday communication happen productively and in ways that foster trust, initiative, and openness to ways of doing things.

The idea is to communicate by many possible means and to design your communication strategies to align with and advance your priority of ongoing service improvement.

References

1. Smith, R. Roger Smith takes on GM's critics. *Fortune* 114(4):26, Aug. 18, 1986.
2. Altman, J. Personal telephone communication. April 6, 1993.

Chapter 9

Staff Development and Training

For years, health care organizations have focused the lion's share of their training dollar on technical and clinical training, as if that's all that counted. Now, as we realize increasingly that patient satisfaction is a function of service quality even more than clinical quality, this allocation of resources needs to shift to include training on service skills.

Twenty of the top-rated applicants for the 1988 and 1989 Malcolm Baldrige National Quality Award escalated their focus on customer satisfaction. They shifted to a philosophy that acknowledges the customers' definition of quality and they strive to achieve quality on the customers' terms as stated in a study released by the General Accounting Office and reported by Craig Steinburg in the *Training and Development Journal*.[1] What's more, the study shows that these companies are reaping tangible benefits, including a 2.5 percent annual average increase in customer satisfaction and an 11.6 percent drop in customer complaints.

Learning International investigated further to find that companies esteemed for service excellence dedicate substantial resources to training. They believe that service representatives are professionals who merit continuous training to enhance their service skills.[2]

The companies in Learning International's study allocate between $750 and $10,000 to the training of *each* employee in the first year of employment alone. Employees are typically trained in problem solving, listening, communication, and stress management. The study pinpointed the following competencies as key to excellent service performance, competencies you can use to audit and improve the substance of training provided by your organization:

- Building customer loyalty and confidence
- Communicating effectively
- Empathizing
- Handling stress
- Listening actively
- Demonstrating mental alertness
- Working well as part of a team
- Demonstrating reliability and loyalty
- Solving problems

- Maintaining a professional image
- Understanding the organization and the industry
- Maintaining high energy levels
- Applying technical knowledge and skills
- Organizing work activities

An ambitious overall training agenda? Absolutely. But then your organization can't expect skillful service from employees unless you invest seriously in their development. Says James Barksdale, executive vice-president of Federal Express:

If you train people well enough, you can get out of their way and let them do the job.

A human resource executive magazine survey suggests that in the 1990s the following trends will continue to be emphasized in training:[3]

- Tailored rather than generic training programs will be important. Firms will train personnel in skills directly related to company goals and objectives.
- More training will be offered to help managers work with ethnic and racial minorities.
- More training will be provided to middle managers and secretaries as each one increases in importance because of reduced layers of management.
- Senior managers will demonstrate more interest in people development, especially as related to organizational strategy.
- Business will pay closer attention to hiring the right employees the first time. Emphasis will be placed on people who seem capable of making on-the-job decisions.

These trends apply to service organizations in particular. People at all levels need to become learners in order to apply the concept of continuous improvement to themselves.

Executives need to demonstrate fervor for service quality and appropriate behaviors that reflect personal alignment with service excellence. They need to skillfully coach managers in service management, recognize their progress, and hold them accountable. They also need to be effective in their interactions with customers, installing customer-listening systems, handling complaints effectively, and playing a leadership role in making process improvements. To accomplish this ambitious agenda, executives need training.

Middle managers also have a far-reaching role to play in service quality improvement; many organizations make the mistake of devoting too little attention and development to this role. Managers need to establish expectations for themselves, implement effective service management practices, and involve staff in continuous improvement. They also need to be personally aligned with service excellence, reflecting the behaviors that model personal effectiveness.

Employees need training opportunities to help them execute your plans, service performance expectations, and service processes at the front line and do so with excellence and confidence.

This chapter will discuss various approaches to training in today's health care environment. Emphasis will be on building skills for all levels—including administrators, middle managers, and supervisors. Strategies will be presented for handling difficult people and situations, telephone protocol, and coworker relationships. The chapter will close with thoughts on what to do when training is *not* the answer.

☐ Learning Opportunities Extend beyond "Training"

Organizations have discovered the importance of becoming "learning organizations" as indicated by the far-reaching effect of Peter Senge's book *The Fifth Discipline: The Art and*

Practice of the Learning Organization.[4] This orientation involves measuring processes and outcomes, listening to customers and using feedback to identify improvement opportunities, hypothesizing about ways to improve processes, and applying the experimenter mind-set to testing these and learning from them. Being a learning organization also involves equipping staff with the skills they need to contribute fully to service delivery and continuous learning and improvement.

Some service strategies have placed a great emphasis on offering training opportunities for all levels of staff, but few have provided this training in the context of a learning process that results in concrete change and demonstration of new behavior on the job. It is more powerful to think in terms of creating "learning" opportunities than "training" opportunities. Too often, "training" implies an instructor and a classroom, when in fact this kind of learning neither is the only option nor tends to be the most effective. Following are some shifts in training approaches (summarized in figure 9-1):

- In the past, most training occurred in classrooms. Current thinking is that, although training usually was limited to the classroom, learning was not. Training should not be equated with learning. You need to consider alternative approaches to fostering staff development, such as learning labs.
- There is a shift in popularity and effectiveness from intensive up-front coursework to training programs offered "just in time" for implementation of skills.
- Instructors are no longer exclusively training professionals. Now managers are learning to train their staff, and peers with expertise are being called on to mentor, coach, and support skill building.
- Learning of concepts is giving way to a strong emphasis on on-the-job application. Conceptual learning has no teeth without observable changed behavior on the job.
- Multiple methods are replacing one approach for all staff and the normal curve of results. Most learn adequately, people on the high end of the curve learn wonderfully, and people at the low end learn little. Now multiple learning approaches bring everyone up to a level of mastery, because mastery by all is the only way to meet service standards consistently.
- It used to be that regular attendance or "completion of training" was used as the organization's success indicator. Now changed practices are the essential accountability indicator.

This chapter describes the skills that staff at all levels need to develop in order to enhance service quality. But beyond that, learning systems are presented that go beyond classroom training and favor on-the-job skill use and experimentation.

☐ Skill Building for All Levels

In service strategies, the skills that constitute excellent performance and foster contributions to making service better are instinctive. Staff development and training help

Figure 9-1. Recent Shifts in Approaches to Training

From	To
Classrooms	Learning labs
Intensive up-front coursework	Just-in-time training
Expert instructors	Peer mentoring, coaching, and mutual support
Intellectual learning	On-the-job applications
The same approach for all with normal curve results	Alternative learning processes with everyone expected to achieve mastery
Accountability for attendance	Accountability for changed practices

managers, staff, and physicians sharpen skills such as listening, problem solving, explaining, handling complaints, designing process improvement, and sensitive handling of upset people. As a result of such training, people build their sense of professional identity and increase their effectiveness. Training is necessary because some people don't know how to act in an *excellent* manner toward customers. Most know how to be inoffensive or even good, but excellence requires the seizing of opportunities.

Training helps people recognize opportunities for excellence and develop the skills needed to capitalize on them. And it does more. It helps people to identify less than wonderful behavior. If you don't train your people in the skills you really value, you'll never know whether they have the capacity or willingness to do what you require. When training opportunities are provided, you can make this determination. Training is also important because people need time to polish their skills and build their sense of professional identity.

Before going on with this chapter, take the self-test in figure 9-2 to evaluate your organization in terms of its employee training systems. The more "true" answers, the better. "False" answers indicate areas that need follow-up if your service strategy is going to succeed.

□ Training—When and Where

Do not begin training until after you've laid the foundation for the successful application of skills learned to the job. People shouldn't be trained to be great until the systems, management style, and job expectations in your organization support greatness. If you don't wait, you'll see a quick fading of the effects of training and conclude that the training didn't work. The training worked, but the environment didn't support it. Training too soon hurts morale and frustrates eager-to-excel employees, thus creating attitude problems that really are justified. This is why staff development and training were not discussed earlier in this book.

Figure 9-2.   Self-Test

Staff Development and Training. *Circle the appropriate answer. The more "true" answers, the better. "False" answers indicate areas that need improvement.*

1. Our employees demonstrate excellent service skills.	True	False
2. Effective learning opportunities are available to help managers and supervisors sharpen their service management skills and apply them to the job.	True	False
3. We provide the support needed so employees can and do attend training programs designed to strengthen their service skills.	True	False
4. People here are trained in the tools of process improvement.	True	False
5. Problems or frictions within groups and between groups are addressed through strategies to enhance intergroup cooperation and teamwork.	True	False
6. Learning opportunities are available to help frontline employees sharpen their service skills.	True	False
7. Supervisors know the difference between adequate and excellent service skills and coach their staff to demonstrate excellence.	True	False
8. This organization's staff development and training efforts attend to both the technical aspects of people's jobs and service aspects.	True	False
9. In this organization, there are substantial resources devoted to developing staff.	True	False
10. We emphasize and support application of learning to the job, not attendance at training sessions.	True	False
	Total:	___ ___

Training too soon also consumes resources. These resources typically include time, use of room, refreshments, costs of instructor, planning time, and participant time. The cost of a typical day's training may break down as follows:

- 20 participants × 7 hours × average pay of $11 per hour = $1,140
- Food for 20 at $5 = $100
- Instructor salary or consulting fee = $200 to $3,000
- Space use = $150
- Materials for 20 people at average of $10 per person = $200 plus

In addition, other costs such as time spent scheduling, developing materials, prepublicity, registration, short staffing or replacement hassles in the participants' departments, raised expectations, and much more contribute substantially to the cost. Training is not cheap. The time and money is well spent only if you first create the optimal conditions for successful training and for the successful transfer of training from the learning setting to the job *beforehand*.

As already observed, not all training should occur in a classroom, where training can seem ethereal, unrealistic, and too disconnected from the job to take hold. The most intense training occurs directly on the job, one-on-one, with the novice "shadowing" the expert who coaches, provides feedback, and engages in instant replays of a situation. Ideally, each department head or supervisor should have a list of standard operating procedures (SOPs) for each job (just like the ones hotel people have). Job instruction then focuses on implementing these SOPs skillfully.

The pool manager at the Marriott, for example, goes down a list of 14 steps when opening the pool every morning. This list was developed after study and discussion with the employees who actually do the job and therefore could help determine the best way to open the pool. A similar process of SOPs should guide customer relations coaching on how to use a telephone effectively, how to ease long waits, and how to handle patient complaints.

☐ An Orientation Kickoff

If you're just starting an explicit organizationwide service strategy, consider a systematic, awareness-raising *kickoff* that orients every person in your organization to your service priority and your plans to achieve service excellence. Do this before you start skill building. If you've already started skill building, then use this kickoff as a refresher to reinforce your commitment to service excellence.

Employees should be oriented to your service strategy through a widely publicized session at which attendance is mandatory. The session should be repeated for all shifts. Consider having at least one top administrator present at every session to show the importance of this effort and to demonstrate a commitment that encourages employees to take the service excellence effort seriously. The session should launch (or relaunch) the service excellence mandate, introduce or review relevant policies, and, through careful program design, enlist employees' energy and cooperation.

To be effective, the session must use state-of-the-art adult education and motivation principles. You're at an advantage if you have in-house people who can design the program; otherwise, numerous outside consultants can help. If you do use an outside consultant, make sure the program is customized to your specific setting, culture, and issues.

Here are the basics of a successful kickoff:

- Tell employees the truth about why your organization is launching a full-scale focus on service quality and continuous service improvement. Are you motivated by image problems, an economic downturn, fierce competition, or internal conflict resulting from staff insecurity and change? Tell it like it is. If survival is an issue, then explain that if the organization does not survive financially, employees will lose their jobs.

- Describe what your organization is doing to compete successfully in an increasingly competitive health care environment and indicate that through your strategy for service excellence, you're asking every employee to play a role in helping your organization not only to survive but to thrive.
- Acknowledge the positive role employees have always played in providing high-quality care, but emphasize that in these competitive times, everyone can do even more. Everyone must do what they can to distinguish your organization's quality of service provision so as to improve its competitive status.
- Emphasize that although employees certainly are not responsible for the economic climate, they can help solve or prevent problems that result from it.
- Have employees evaluate your organization's service from their own viewpoints (use the self-test in figure 9-2). Give people a chance to vent their frustrations about the obstacles to service excellence in their particular workplace. Allow problems to be confronted openly, acknowledge them, and reassure employees that their views will be channeled to people with the power to act.
- Present concrete performance expectations ("House Rules") that define what you mean by excellent service. Make these rules clear, unequivocal, mandatory, and applicable to all.
- Present relevant policies and personnel practices that put teeth in your new standards; for example, through job descriptions, supervisory practices, performance appraisal, and commendation systems.
- Announce your plan for aligning the organization with your service mission and securing their full participation.

The kickoff session for *all employees* usually runs 2½ to 3 hours. From then on, training should be targeted to specific groups so that you use their time optimally by focusing not on generic skills but on job-specific skills. In many organizations, employee "opinion leaders," rather than professional trainers, conduct this session, using a train-the-facilitator approach.

☐ Targeted Training

Generic programs, such as a kickoff, can build a customer-oriented mind-set and raise behavior awareness. They can also engage employees in activities that sharpen needed skills. However, to move people to *excellence* in service and not just to eliminate blatant rudeness or other offensive behavior, staff need help in *identifying and capitalizing on previously missed opportunities in their specific jobs*. For example, an admissions clerk greeting an incoming patient with "Good morning, may I help you?" is acceptable behavior but not excellent behavior. More impressive would be: "Good morning. My name is Sue Martin. Welcome to Community Hospital! May I help you?"

The distance between giving good service and great service lies in thousands of "moments of truth" that happen between customer and staff. Consistent excellence and missed opportunities in these moments of truth are two areas to focus on in staff training. Targeted training involves job-specific skill building with selected groups whose performance suggests a need for further development. Or they may merit special attention because of their disproportionate influence on the first and last impression customers form at your facility's doorstep.

For example, the quality of nursing care has an obvious impact on patient evaluations of a facility. Nurses, then, stand to gain from the program's emphasis on caring, courtesy, and cooperation. However, nurses face challenges that few other hospital employees face.

How can they meet, even surpass, the demands for empathy required by their intimate contact with patients, shift after shift, hour after hour, patient after patient? How can they best cope with the difficult patient and the difficult physician? Every other specialized role, particularly those involving patient contact, has its own unique set of problems and opportunities, and each respective role needs to be examined individually.

Of course, you can't tackle the specifics of every special group simultaneously. The number of relevant groups and the need to go beyond the superficial preclude treating them all at one time. The question then becomes: Which groups require specific action first? It depends—each organization has different needs. One way to establish priorities is to let patient survey data guide you. Maybe the data at one facility are positive toward the nursing staff but indicate dissatisfaction with the transport and tray delivery personnel. If so, you start there.

What skills are needed to improve the job-specific performance of special groups? Again, the answer depends on the groups in question. To use the example of transporters, ask them to give one another fast stretcher rides so they can experience for themselves the difference between their job done poorly and done well. Create dexterity impairment exercises for tray delivery staff, for instance, eating with splints on their fingers or with gloves on, so that they become sensitized to how an arthritic patient eats a meal. By examining the nitty-gritty aspects of specific roles, you identify the problems in each job and treat them as opportunities to exceed patient expectations with spectacular behavior.

You can assess needs by using focus groups, think tanks, interviews, observations, complaint analyses, and patient survey results. You should have an adequate patient feedback system that points you toward the groups that need the most help. If you don't have such a system, focus on the areas with the most public contact and start there: admissions, billing, outpatient services, emergency department, and housekeeping.

The following sections provide ideas on training for specific groups and in specific subject areas. These suggestions are just a smattering of staff development and training needs and possibilities. You must first find out who needs skill building, morale boosts, and attention. Then develop appropriate programs that translate your stated service priority into an actual investment for your staff. These descriptions may expand your own image of the possibilities and in some cases even strike a chord of "Oh yes, we need that." If you have in-house training resources, you can perhaps develop your own training agenda; if not, seek out knowledgeable consultants. However you do it, again the key is to match the program to your organization's needs.

Development Opportunities for Administrators

Skill-building opportunities for administrators help them examine the special roles they need to play to assert their leadership, inspire cooperation throughout the organization, and prevent problems that may impede progress. Administrators need to be able to identify and concretely tackle obstacles to service delivery, be role models for *all* expectations of managers, develop skills in mentoring and coaching that will help them help their staff, and acquire facilitation skills for running team meetings designed to improve service processes.

Many administrative teams also need training in communication skills, especially constructive feedback and confrontation; nondefensive listening; positive assertiveness; giving effective presentations; and straightforward writing, to name a few. All of these skills are key to communicating effectively with staff and customers. Administrative teams frequently need team-building interventions that promote unified commitment to their service mission, mutual support, and resolve in serving as coaches and cheerleaders as they roll out their service strategy.

Development Opportunities for Middle Managers and Supervisors

The middle-management layer is your organization's internal accountability mechanism for ensuring that employees meet the standards for service excellence. Special attention to the role of middle management and supervisors is a necessity because middle management is often the weakest link in your strategy.

Managers need to identify their customers and how these customers define excellent service. Managers need skills and systems for staying in close and regular communication with customers, which entails managing not by instinct or intuition alone, but by systematically gathering meaningful information and using high-quality tools to make good decisions. Managers also need to engage in effective communication across lines, with staff, customers, and suppliers, reflecting an organizational (not territorial) perspective and partnership attitude.

Three Models for Management Development

Three approaches to service management development have been found to be effective in advancing service quality. One approach, *Service Management Essentials*, applies to organizations that want to train all managers with the methods of customer-driven management and the steps in the departmental alignment process described in chapter 16. The second approach uses *just-in-time* training with a pilot group of managers. This approach may be for organizations that have conducted management development programs in the past but saw no concrete benefits (the organization might prefer to focus more on the implementation process and less on the training process). A third exciting and innovative approach called *Quality Merit Badge* was developed at Baptist Memorial Hospital in Memphis, Tennessee. These three approaches are described in the following subsections.

Model 1: Service Management Essentials

The first model for organizations that want to train *all* managers in service management begins with "Service Management Essentials"—a series of skill-building modules. This approach helps managers to:

- Mobilize employees to focus on satisfying their internal and external customers
- Raise their standards of service performance so that patients, families, physicians, and coworkers all receive courteous, compassionate, timely, and responsive service
- Embrace continuous service improvement as their primary everyday priority
- Implement the departmental alignment process described in detail in chapter 16

The approach includes two phases—groundwork with leaders and workshops on the essentials of service management (as shown in figure 9-3). The modules in phase 1 include needs assessment, setting expectations for managers, and systems to support skill implementation.

Needs assessment devices, including interviews with executives; focus groups with managers, supervisors, and staff; and surveys, are used to identify particular training needs. These crystallize the previous history of management development, the perceptions of priorities from multiple perspectives, and the managers' current levels of proficiency.

Setting expectations for managers occurs after surveying the results of the needs assessment. Executives decide on the actions they expect of managers as a result of the training and the components of the training plan. They also decide on supporting management training through role modeling, coaching, follow-up discussions, and reinforcement. They then establish measures for monitoring management performance and effectiveness.

Executives then identify *systems to support implementation*, that is, what system they want to use to ensure that skills learned in the classroom setting are applied to the job. They set up a system for providing interim, on-the-job support as managers apply what they've learned to their everyday realities. A select group of managers then receives training in how to facilitate peer support groups using simple formats that help peers share experiences, experiment with new ways, and build unbeatable teamwork.

In phase 2, six management development modules are offered in the nuts and bolts of service management. Training is reinforced with interim "homework," implementation guides, a system of peer support groups, and executive coaching. Modules considered to be "staples" include the following:

Module 1: The Service Management Mind-Set

This module provides an overview of the manager's role in service excellence and builds the customer-oriented mind-set that is prerequisite to proactive service improvement. This module accomplishes six objectives in building a customer-focus mind-set:

- Strengthens management commitment to pursuing service improvement
- Briefs managers on what's happening in health care to advance service quality and customer satisfaction and builds a common language
- Explores and helps managers embrace role shifts essential to proactive service management (see figure 9-4)
- Helps the team identify and commit to achieving specific group norms that will support these pivotal role shifts

Figure 9-3. Skill-Building Modules

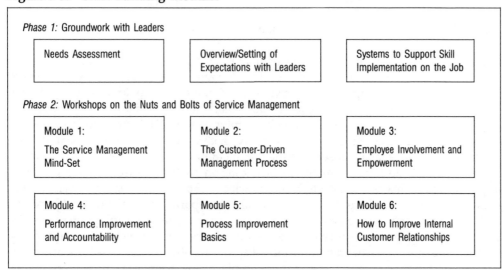

Phase 1: Groundwork with Leaders

| Needs Assessment | Overview/Setting of Expectations with Leaders | Systems to Support Skill Implementation on the Job |

Phase 2: Workshops on the Nuts and Bolts of Service Management

| Module 1:
The Service Management Mind-Set | Module 2:
The Customer-Driven Management Process | Module 3:
Employee Involvement and Empowerment |
| Module 4:
Performance Improvement and Accountability | Module 5:
Process Improvement Basics | Module 6:
How to Improve Internal Customer Relationships |

Figure 9-4. Role Shifts Essential to Proactive Service Management

From	To
Provider orientation	Customer orientation
Tolerance	Continuous improvement
Directing	Empowering
Employee as expendable entity	Employee as customer
Reactive	Proactive
Tradition and safety	Experimentation and risk taking
"Busy-ness"	Results
Turf protection	Teamwork across lines
"We-they" thinking	Organizational perspective
Cynicism	Optimism

- Develops a group-generated action plan for making these norm shifts happen in practice
- Crystallizes the manager's role in service quality improvement

Module 2: The Customer-Driven Management Process

Who are a department's internal and external customers? How do they define excellent service? Which processes and performances are needed to meet their expectations? How can managers monitor performance and satisfaction levels so that they can use the results to guide service improvement?

Every manager needs to base his or her departmental routines on the answers to these questions, thereby instituting and sustaining a cyclical service management process that ensures customer satisfaction. This module, enhanced by a simulation exercise that requires customer-driven goal setting and planning, helps managers build the skills they need to start up and sustain the Customer-Driven Management Process outlined in chapter 16. For managers to sharpen their skills they need to do five things:

- Clarify their key internal and external customers
- Effectively consult these customers to identify their key, reasonable expectations
- Translate customer expectations into operational or process requirements
- Establish and install measures for monitoring service processes and customer satisfaction
- Engage staff in using data to identify improvement priorities

Module 3: Employee Involvement and Empowerment

Employee involvement and empowerment are key to achieving far-reaching service improvements and retaining talented staff. Involvement is real when employees embrace the organization's challenges as their own and contribute actively to improving service. Empowerment is real when employee responsibility and authority are in balance. This occurs when employees are entrusted with the information, skills, and autonomy needed to meet diverse customer needs in ways that serve both the customer and the organization.

In this module, managers examine the tough emotional and practical aspects of effective involvement and empowerment—from holding on to letting go, from directing to trusting, and from manager as expert to team knowledge. Specifically, managers will be able to educate employees about the organizational and departmental mission and priorities and thus confidently shift responsibility and autonomy to employees; sharpen their skills at substantive delegation; build trust in employees' judgment by skill building and coaching to ensure that employees can think and act appropriately in tough situations; and facilitate simple staff meeting formats and other employee involvement techniques to trigger participation and to reap the benefits of employees' special knowledge and ideas.

Module 4: Performance Improvement and Accountability

To effectively raise the standards of service performance, the quality of performance must have consequences. Managers and supervisors who communicate high expectations, who give employees frequent behavioral feedback, and who coach employees help stretch the standards upward. This module helps managers sharpen their use of the tools of accountability so they can help employees perform well consistently. Managers learn six skills:

- Modeling high performance in their own interactions with customers and employees
- Clarifying and communicating job-specific expectations to staff

- Giving employees frequent constructive behavioral feedback
- Coaching employees to improve their performance
- Describing and confronting unacceptable behavior effectively
- Recognizing and rewarding exemplary behavior

Module 5: Process Improvement Basics

As quality expert Joseph Juran has emphasized since the early 1950s, more than 80 percent of the enduring problems in an organization are the fault of systems controlled by managers. Not even 15 percent of the problems stem from employee performance. To better equip managers to improve work processes, this module builds skills in process improvement. It demonstrates the power of process improvement and enables managers to facilitate departmental meetings and work teams using user-friendly process improvement tools. Specifically, managers learn to follow a scientific approach reflected in the 12-Step PDCA Model for Process Improvement shown in figure 7-12, p. 131. They also learn to make their meetings and teamwork efficient and productive with the help of the versatile tools shown along the outside of that model. As a result, managers will be able to do five things:

- Analyze work as a process, identifying suppliers, inputs, the process itself, outputs, and customers
- Follow a rational and thorough approach to improving service processes
- Use the powerful tool of flowcharting to make rapid and far-reaching improvements—to clarify current reality, plan purposeful measurement, and design and visualize improvements
- Supplement their common sense with user-friendly tools for collecting, displaying, and reporting data; solving problems at their root; and designing and sustaining effective improvements
- Facilitate "improvement meetings" with staff in ways that foster energetic and widespread participation as well as persistence in achieving results

Module 6: How to Improve Internal Customer Relationships

Relationships and the flow of people, paper, supplies, and information across department lines need to be managed efficiently and effectively. This module examines tactics for strengthening these relationships to create "seamless" service processes that serve customers and staff alike. Managers learn to identify their internal customers, negotiate and crystallize effective service partnerships across turf lines, monitor performance, and keep communication lines open—all with an eye to building even better relationships over time. Managers sharpen their ability to target key internal customers and consult them to verify their main service requirements; negotiate and ratify service partnerships across turf lines, using a variety of techniques including user groups, service contracts, and liaison teams; use constructive negotiation and confrontation skills with other managers to strengthen teamwork across departmental lines.

As a result of Model 1, *Service Management Essentials*, managers can:

- Pursue service improvement with focus, determination, optimism, and stamina
- Express to staff a sincere commitment to customers and continuous service improvement, making that commitment contagious
- Act as role models and coaches to help employees behave in exemplary ways toward their customers
- Install a regular system for obtaining customer feedback and using this feedback with staff to guide service improvement

- Create a culture and quality of work life in which everyone feels valued, demonstrates teamwork, and contributes actively to service improvement
- Scientifically study and constantly improve the processes by which service is delivered
- Cross turf lines to solve problems; streamline the flow of patients, paper, supplies, and communication, creating a "seamless" organization
- Build the confidence and optimism vital to tackling long-lived inefficiencies and service snags with a probing mind, spirit of experimentation, and old-fashioned persistence

Model 2: Just-in-Time Training

The second management development model engages a pilot group of managers, in a just-in-time training and coaching process designed to help them work their way through the departmental alignment process described in chapter 16. This approach is particularly suited to an organization in which the following conditions exits:

- Your current service strategy focuses on individual performance only, and you now want to make the transition to quality management.
- Your efforts to build a customer orientation among your employees have been largely successful, but your middle managers haven't changed their everyday practices all that much. They still don't run their departments like customer-driven service businesses and they don't involve their employees in service improvement.
- You have instituted a service excellence or quality management strategy but have not attained the middle management buy-in or the degree of implementation needed to see results.
- You want to institute quality management but lack the time and/or widespread commitment to advance a hospitalwide strategy.
- You want to follow up on your past tactics to improve service, but not simply with awareness-raising refreshers. You want to achieve new depths by using a systemic approach that adds structure to service management in every department.
- You wish you had a core group of really strong, solid middle managers who could help their peers become "believers" in systematic service management and upgrade their departmental management habits, before working to engage all managers hospitalwide.

This approach involves a six-month process that gets a small group of managers up and running with a sound departmental system for customer-driven management, employee involvement, and continuous process improvement. Between 10 and 20 *interested* managers and administrators participate. These can be "volunteers"; managers encouraged to join in because they manage pivotal projects, service lines, or departments; and/or managers who are likely to succeed and be effective later as resources to their peers.

This training process involves periodic meetings in which the managers are provided just-in-time coaching on key skills (such as identifying customers, developing customer surveys, running a focus group with internal customers, and running a staff meeting in which customer requirements are prioritized and translated into target objectives). By the end of the first six months, the organization has a core group of managers who have thoroughly and successfully integrated customer-driven management into their departmental routines. Participating managers and their staff should achieve measurable improvements in the satisfaction levels of their departments' internal and external customers. Also, their departments should be making data-driven improvements.

Once this core squad of managers is confident that the process works, they share both process and results with other managers. They help in recruiting additional "waves" for new groups that are forming and then act as informal mentors to other managers who are learning and applying the process to their respective departments. With the just-in-time model, quality management unfolds steadily and at a manageable pace—without the organization committing itself to a more extensive (and perhaps exhausting) hospitalwide approach. As a result of just-in-time training, managers will be able to:

- Express to staff a sincere commitment to customers and continuous service improvement, making that commitment contagious
- Use facilitation and team-building techniques that build a cohesive staff team with shared commitment and healthy communication
- Assess their department's culture and modify it to better support customer focus, employee involvement, and continuous improvement
- Target their key internal and external customers and consult with them to pinpoint their expectations
- Translate customer expectations into operational or process requirements
- Install a regular system for monitoring customer satisfaction and operational processes, so that staff can use data and feedback to identify improvement priorities
- Engage staff in making process improvements by:
  - Analyzing work as a process, identifying suppliers, inputs, the process itself, outputs, and customers
  - Using user-friendly tools for collecting, displaying, and reporting data, solving problems at their root, and designing and sustaining improvements
  - Facilitating "improvement meetings" with staff—fostering energetic, widespread participation as well as persistence in achieving results
  - Pursuing process improvements with the help of a rational step-by-step plan
- Create a culture and quality of work life in which employees feel valued, demonstrate teamwork, and contribute actively to service improvement

This technique also yields beneficial by-products, including more trusting and mutually supportive peer relationships, less focus on turfdom, a network for idea exchange and support, and managerial role models for higher standards—managers who experiment, engage in an active learning process, and promote change.

A variation on this approach for organizations that emphasize *peer* coaching involves these activities:

- Managers attend a course to develop an overview of the skills, steps, and actions key to service management.
- Managers are divided into teams and assigned a coach who is equipped with tools and short training modules that address steps in departmental alignment with the service strategy. If and when the team needs "training," the coach can provide just-in-time training.
- Teams members (peers) are responsible for getting each other through installation of a systematic approach to continuous service improvement (for example, using the Customer-Driven Management Process as a model) in whatever way they wish; that is, through a buddy system, periodic meetings with homework in between, or some other method.
- Department head meetings include team reports and storyboarding that describes what the teams are doing and shows examples of individual steps and results along the path to departmental service management.
- Recognition events celebrate milestones in the team's achievement of key objectives.

Model 3: Quality Merit Badge Approach
Baptist Memorial Hospital in Memphis, Tennessee, developed an innovative approach that moves management development from training to "habit building." Their Quality Merit Badge system, developed by Marcia Boyd and Claude Haraway, has these goals:

- To build new *habits* that reflect service management by integrating a system of learning and doing that supports managers through the departmental alignment process
- To get managers focused more on learning and doing what they need to do with their work groups and less on how they look to their bosses
- To provide a structure that encourages managers to experiment and recognizes managers who take initiative to improve their practices in pursuit of service improvement

Managers can pursue three merit badges. They earn a badge after they have completed *all* of the requisite actions for that particular badge. Figure 9-5 shows the key actions required for each badge in a comparable Champion Program that is in the planning stages at the Albert Einstein Medical Center in Philadelphia.

The Albert Einstein Medical Center approach rewards interested managers for *following through* on key actions instituted in their department/program alignment process. This reinforcement helps managers to repeatedly try actions that are key to *continuous* customer-driven management until these actions become habitual. When a manager completes certain actions, he or she achieves "model" status (column 1 of figure 9-5, the first achievement level). Upon completing the additional key actions (column 2), "mentor" status is achieved. And when the key actions listed in column 3 are completed, the manager earns "champion" status. By that time, the discomfort of implementing new management actions that align with the values should have worn off, with managers now reaping the benefits that result from these management actions.

The program is voluntary; managers *choose* to pursue the achievement levels. Every manager is eligible (up to and including the president). A manager who chooses to pursue an achievement level is assigned a coach (another manager who is at least one step

Figure 9-5. Possible Actions to Earn Each Achievement Level of the Champion Program

Model Level	Mentor Level	Champion Level
Hold two staff meetings that explicitly advance service	Hold two additional staff meetings that explicitly advance service	Four more staff meetings that explicitly advance service
Consult and survey your customers on their expectations	Consult and survey your customers on their expectations	Consult and survey your customers on their expectations
Review customer feedback with staff and set improvement priorities	Review customer feedback with staff and set improvement priorities	Review customer feedback with staff and set improvement priorities
Make measurable progress on improvement objective	Make measurable progress on improvement objective	Made measurable progress on departmental alignment objective
Meet with two interrelated departments to monitor conformance to previous service agreements and identify improvement needs	Meet with two interrelated departments to monitor conformance to previous service agreements and identify improvement needs	Meet with interrelated departments to monitor conformance to previous service agreement with an additional internal customer
Recognize staff using at least one of several alternative methods	Recognize staff using at least two methods	Recognize staff using at least three methods
Pursue one individual learning need that helps you align with the values and show evidence of accomplishment	Pursue one additional learning need that helps you align with the values and show evidence of accomplishment	Pursue one additional learning need that helps you align with the values and show evidence of accomplishment

- Complete every action in the first column to earn a "Model" award.
- Complete every action in the second column to earn a "Mentor" award.
- Complete every action in the third column to become "Champion."
- By the time managers achieve Champion Status, they will have become more comfortable with the action and continue it because they know it works.

ahead). The coach assists the manager throughout the process and checks his or her results along the way. Recognition ceremonies and symbolic rewards mark successful attainment of levels.

Applied to service management, this approach begins with an overview course on service management and continuous improvement. A second phase helps managers *apply* the concepts and processes described in the course. Individual managers set their own learning goals and pursue them by opting to work toward earning merit badges in service management.

Development Opportunities for First-Line Supervisors

This is the most often neglected area for training and development within the context of service strategies. Many organizations offer substantial training to department directors, but do little if anything for the first-line supervisors who work day in and day out with frontline people.

Supervisors need basic supervisory development. *Most* supervisors were promoted to supervisory positions because of excellence in the technical skills they used in their previous positions. Few have had any orientation to the dramatically different responsibility and role they take on in a supervisory position.

To equip supervisors with skills specific to service management, some organizations institute basic supervisory development programs in which service issues are used as case examples and integrated into every component of their basic training approach. Other organizations train supervisors in two phases. Phase 1 offers "Basic Supervision" that defines the role of supervisor and builds skills in performance management, team building, motivation, safety management, and the like—the staples of any management job. Once supervisors learn these basic skills, phase 2 focuses on "Service-Oriented Supervision." In this more advanced level, supervisors build skills in setting job-specific expectations, developing service protocols that reflect excellence, coaching employees to handle complaints effectively, running service improvement team meetings, coaching and counseling employees on what appear to be elusive behavioral or attitudinal problems, monitoring frontline service effectiveness, and recognizing staff for service excellence.

Both approaches can work. The key is to value the role of supervisors enough to provide training opportunities in the context of an effective training delivery system (with clear up-front role expectations, peer support during implementation, coaching by the supervisor's manager, and accountability for effective application of skills learned to the job). It is not sufficient to just train department directors; they have too little contact with frontline staff to make a difference on that level.

Development Opportunities for Frontline Employees

All nonsupervisory employees need skill development opportunities (workshops, programs, seminars, for example) that heighten their motivation with regard to service and boost their development of sophisticated service skills. Following are descriptions of a smorgasbord of workshops and programs that can help accomplish these objectives.

Developing Frontline Communication Skills

A few employee groups repeatedly generate first and lasting impressions of your organization—for example, personnel at the information desk, transporters, tray deliverers, security guards, and housekeepers. These public contact personnel are your frontline people. Inherent in these positions are special problems and special opportunities. The continued effectiveness of your strategy for service excellence depends on reinforcing employees' views of themselves as public contact professionals and strengthening the attitude and skills that optimize your organization's image. Highlights of this workshop may include:

- Understanding the vital role of frontline people in customer relations
- Identifying key moments of truth in their contacts with your organization's customers
- Creating powerfully positive first impressions
- Developing the verbal and nonverbal behaviors essential to customer satisfaction
- Using initiatives to ease long waits
- Practicing techniques for handling irate customers and other difficult situations
- Understanding the basics of customer-conscious and sales-minded telephone communication

You can use a program similar to the above to cultivate positive relationships between your facility and the staff in physicians' offices. This program can also strengthen the customer relations skills and awareness of physician staffs.

Handling Difficult People and Situations

Even those individuals with the best skills and attitudes encounter patients, physicians, and other customers who test their coping abilities to the limit. This workshop builds the skills necessary for handling a wide range of difficult people and situations while maintaining personal emotional health and a professional demeanor. Workshop highlights may include:

- Personal prejudices and preconceptions that sabotage encounters
- Control through action, not reaction
- Active listening to uncover hidden meanings
- Step-by-step process for handling an irate person
- Assertive communication of your message
- Nondefensive complaint management
- Strategies to use when you're at your wit's end
- Dissatisfied customers as opportunities to win loyal customers

Building Effective Coworker Relationships

Most health care jobs are stressful enough without having additional stress imposed by problematic relationships with coworkers. Turning a problem relationship into a relationship that works for everyone involved leads to both successful and satisfying work. This workshop builds skills and problem-solving techniques that improve those all-powerful, day-to-day relationships with coworkers. Workshop highlights may include:

- Getting what you need from your coworkers
- Communicating to get results
- Resolving conflicts productively
- Negotiating terms in the worst of situations
- Expanding your skills repertoire to enhance your own on-the-job comfort

Practicing Telephone Tact and Tactics

Because they feel shielded by anonymity, employees typically lower their expectations of their telephone performance, which can result in a tarnished organizational image. If a health care organization wants to project a professional image and build goodwill, its public contact personnel need to develop skill and sensitivity in telephone communications. These professionals, such as receptionists, secretaries, medical clerks, and telephone operators, need to understand, and be understood, while at the same time making callers feel cared for and respected by the organization.

This workshop is concerned with how they answer the telephone, how they put people on hold, and how they handle the angry or impatient caller. Workshop highlights may include:

- Making the connection between telephone communication, customer satisfaction, and the organization's image
- Responding with care and tact to the obvious and hidden aspects of a conversation
- Presenting yourself, your boss, and your organization in the most favorable light possible
- Building people's confidence in the organization through impeccable competence and courtesy
- Practicing specific telephone protocols for handling typical daily challenges

Making the Most of a Minute

Some employees resist customer relations standards because they don't have time. This workshop is for staff (such as tray delivery workers, housekeepers, and maintenance workers) who have, or think they have, only fleeting contact with patients. Workshop highlights may include:

- The impact moments of truth have on patients
- Verbal and nonverbal skills that help staff make the most of even brief contact with patients, for example, how to greet patients warmly and how to make the most positive impression in two or three sentences
- A repertoire of impressive customer relations behavior that enables the employee to establish contact with patients without interfering with the employee's work, for example, wearing a pleasant facial expression when entering the patient's room and using a few standard sentences to acknowledge the patient's presence and importance

Learning Service Skills as a Professional Asset

Consider providing employees with a set of service skill-building courses that enable them to earn certification in service excellence. For instance, you can offer a basic program of required modules, electives, and a supervised "internship." When employees successfully complete the required combination of program components, they become certified in service excellence. You can hold certification ceremonies so that other employees, family members, and friends can witness the granting of the certificates.

This kind of program can be a powerful motivator, especially for the nonprofessional people who have fewer chances to become "credentialed" than do nurses and managers. A certification program enhances the message that service excellence is substantive and takes work. Also it leads to recognition (at the very least), to increased self-esteem, to the employee's enhanced marketability, and—better yet—to salary increases, promotions, higher grade jobs, or other perks. A certification program is one way to inspire perseverance in developing service skills of the depth that pushes people beyond less-than-acceptable, or even acceptable, performance to service excellence.

Development Opportunities for Nurses

Many nursing staffs have come under the budgetary scalpel. Nurses who have survived layoffs are expected to do more with less: work more shifts, attend more patients, perform a broader range of duties. With the heightened emphasis on service excellence, they're also expected to do their job with greater sensitivity, patience, and empathy.

In this environment, many nurses and their nurse managers vigorously resist their hospital's strategies for service excellence because they view pressure to pamper the customer as cosmetic, superficial, and commercial. Special workshops and programs, some of which are described in the following subsections, are needed to build nurse manager support for service excellence and to approach the special needs of the staff nurse in appropriate ways.

Promoting Service Excellence for the Nurse Manager

Resistance to customer relations strategies on the part of nurse managers may stem in large part from the fact that many nurse managers have not been sufficiently involved in the design or scope of their hospital's approach to service excellence and customer relations. Tailored training prevents or overcomes their resistance, replacing it with active, enlightened support.

This workshop shows the big picture of service excellence to give the concept depth and meaning. It then examines the nurse manager's vision of service excellence in tough, everyday situations and provides suggestions for educating nursing staffs to fulfill this vision. Highlights of the workshop may include:

- Defining service excellence in nursing
- Discussing conflicts in nursing that lead to a breakdown in service (for example, the multiple demands on nurses and the emotional drain of working with sick people)
- Managing for service excellence, including suggestions for increasing empathy and handling difficult patients and demanding family members

Enhancing Professional Renewal for Nurses

Many organizations acknowledge that nurses need substantive help in coping with the emotional challenges and frustrations of their new environment and the demands placed on them. Because of the evolution of nursing in relation to physicians, many nurses hear "servitude" when you talk of "service." Many need help in feeling more positive about themselves, more in control, and more equipped to avoid negativity and disabling stress. In short, to strengthen your service effort, nurses need a philosophy and tool kit for working happy.

The Einstein Consulting Group, as exemplified in its program "Harmony: Professional Renewal for Nurses," recommends the following guidelines for training nurses to cope with their hyperstressful environment:

- Identify patterns of thinking and action that drain energy and undermine a nurse's ability to sustain a positive outlook.
- Redirect the interactions between nurses and patients and other staff so that they enhance pride, emotional availability, and sense of accomplishment.
- Build skills for gaining a greater sense of control while handling multiple demands.
- Examine strategies for working smarter, not harder.
- Rekindle the satisfaction inherent in working with and for patients.
- Explore healthy ways to handle stress.

Assertiveness training for nurses, including how to handle the difficult physician, and an advanced program stressing more sophisticated customer relations skills is also time well spent to engage nurses in building a repertoire of interpersonal skills that make a difference to customers. Possible items to include in such programs include:

- How to give intense personal attention so that patients and visitors feel special
- How to respond empathically
- How to turn complaints into opportunities to heighten customer satisfaction
- How to deal with the difficult patient and the difficult physician

The options are many. The important thing is *to do something special for nurses* who, whether justified or not, perceive their situation as unique and therefore need special understanding and an especially sensitive approach.

Hospitalwide Training

Other attitudes and skills are needed by everyone, regardless of their position. Many hospitals (for example, Grady Memorial Hospital in Atlanta) are providing extensive *training in diversity.* Because their work force is diverse, their customers are diverse, and interactions are powerfully (and often negatively) affected by differences—in race, gender, religion, sexual preference, nationality, age, and so forth. These forward-looking hospitals want to cleanse interactions of discriminatory practices and prejudicial assumptions that interfere with effective communication and healthy service attitudes.

Every employee at every level hears complaints, whether these complaints are by internal or external customers. Handling complaints effectively has dramatic and lasting consequences for the quality of the employees' and the organization's *future* relationship with customers, which is why *service recovery training* is essential. First, it can help staff view complaints as a precious second chance to make things right for the customer. Second, staff can be reminded of the importance of empathy in confronting customer frustrations and can develop a step-by-step approach to making quick, resourceful responses to patient, visitor, and physician complaints. Service recovery training emphasizes what employees can do to minimize the number of patients and physicians who go away mad or just go away.

All employees also need to be educated about the importance of *work processes* and the tools of process improvement so that they can make improvements in their daily work and can participate effectively on improvement teams. Just-in-time training on the occasion when teams are launched is an effective way to accomplish this.

☐ Beyond Training: Other Learning Approaches

In addition to variations on training in which someone serves as instructor and groups convene to learn from the person or from his or her coordinated learning approaches, other methods can help staff develop their service skills. Some of these methods are job aids, mentor relationships, assessment devices, and instructional literature.

Job aids are usually written methods of instructing employees about how to handle situations; for example, service protocols or procedures on index cards or manuals in the format of "What to do or say if the customer does this or that." Too often, organizations—and managers in particular—neglect to put in writing instructions for handling specific service situations. Consequently, serious inconsistencies arise in handling service situations because there are no instructions to serve as the protocol. Well-intentioned employees are left in the lurch.

A job aid can be as simple as taping the word "opportunity" to every telephone to remind employees of the importance of making a good first impression and presenting themselves in a positive way. Or, consider a "who-to-call" list for various problems or a laminated pocket-size reference card that includes key steps to a particular procedure. Consider this job aid on constructive, customer-oriented language:

Make Your Customers "Thankful"

Thank you for going to the trouble to call about this.
Thank you for expressing your concern.
Thank you for giving us a chance to correct this situation.
Thank you for getting all the facts together.
Thank you for understanding.
Thank you for your cooperation and help.

Figure 9-6 shows an example of a job aid for transporters that, according to people at MetroHealth System in Cleveland, circumvents the need for extensive classroom training or performance counseling.

Mentor relationships, or "each one teach one," programs are another "training method" that hotels, for instance, use with new personnel. Each new staff member is assigned a coworker experienced in the same job to serve as a mentor to the new employee, showing him or her the ropes and acclimating the new hire to a very high standard. An example is the Management Mentor Program at the Albert Einstein Healthcare Foundation in Philadelphia. Its objectives are to:

- Help new department managers learn about key organizational practices right after their arrival, including information about the culture, key people, and how to get things done
- Give people a personal, warm welcome into their new jobs and prevent feelings of loneliness and floundering common to new managers
- Acknowledge and recognize excellent managers by appointing them as mentors of new managers

Managers eligible to be assigned to a mentor include those hired from the outside and those who are promoted internally into department manager positions. The duration of

Figure 9-6. Sample Job Aid: Transporter Performance Standards (Excerpt)

Purpose: Transportation personnel/volunteers are a key link in the health care team, interacting with nursing units, various departments, patients, and the general public every day. You provide a unique opportunity to make a major contribution to a warm and friendly environment for patients, their families, and staff members.

Initial patient contact

7. Knock on the door before entering, if you need to enter patient's room.
8. Establish eye contact with patient, introduce yourself in a friendly manner, and state the purpose of the transport.
9. Use the patient's name and check the wristband for positive identification. Address the patient as Mr., Mrs., or Miss unless the patient prefers to be called by the first name. (If the patient does not have an ID bracelet, notify the unit personnel.)
10. Greet the patient's family/visitors and inform them of the approximate length of time the patient will be gone. Check with the staff regarding this time.
11. Communicate only nonmedical information to family/visitors.
12. Assist patient in preparation for transport according to departmental guidelines. Use proper draping to ensure patient comfort and privacy.
13. If needed, patient's chart will accompany patient in pocket of wheelchair or at foot of stretcher.

On route to department with patient

14. Answer questions tactfully; take care not to divulge confidential information.
15. When encountering visitors in the hall who need assistance, supply needed information if asked or refer them to the appropriate person or department.
16. Consider the patient's dignity and condition at all times.
17. Use patient elevator, when available, for patient transport.
    - Carts should be placed head first in elevator.
    - Wheelchairs should be backed in so that the patient is facing the elevator doors.
18. Assure that the patient and any equipment (IVs, tubes, oxygen tanks, etc.) are positioned properly.
19. Be aware of patient's needs during transport.
    - Stand where patient can see you and maintain eye contact if possible;
    - Reassure and talk directly with patient;
    - Adjust transport speed to the comfort level of the patient;
    - Note changes in patient's condition and report these to the appropriate individuals;
    - Ensure that the patient is covered at all times;
    - Ensure that proper patient positioning is maintained.
20. Follow infection control procedures as indicated.

General Information

27. Do not have private, social conversations with other employees during transport.
    - Avoid patients overhearing personal or work-related problems.
    - If delays occur, apologize and briefly explain what is happening.
28. Do not sit on wheelchairs or on stretchers.
29. Limit the transport of un-self-propelled wheelchair users to no more than two patients. (Refer any questions regarding this to your supervisor.)

the formal relationship between mentor and new manager usually is three months. Each new manager receives *two* mentors: a generic mentor and a specialist mentor.

A *generic mentor* is a department manager from a different department who is expected to:

- Greet the new manager personally on his or her first day and be a lunch partner during the first week. The generic mentor also may provide a special welcoming note, make a welcoming stop-in visit, and leave flowers on the new manager's desk
- Devote four hours to the new manager the first week (for such things as tour of key locations, introductions to others over lunch, and other methods of paving the way—a "walk-through" the manager's manual and organizational chart
- Join the new manager for lunch at least once a week for the first month and expect to spend two hours with him or her weekly for that first month
- Devote an hour a week during the second month
- Devote time as needed during the third month
- Provide phone number and easy access
- Anticipate and address questions and concerns

The *specialist mentor* has duties very similar to those of the new manager and therefore can provide very job-specific help. For example, a new administrator of a clinical department may be assigned an administrator of another clinical department; both deal with revenue and accounts receivable, for example. Likewise, a new director of one service department will be matched with a director of another service department, nurse managers with nurse managers, and so forth. These specialist mentors are expected to:

- Have lunch with the new manager during first week
- Urge the new manager to call the mentor whenever necessary
- Schedule dedicated time with the new manager to lay out common elements of the job (for example, billing, payroll, staff scheduling, revenue reports) and what the new manager needs to know related to these tasks
- Take the new manager under wing and hold a series of proactive meetings to help him or her handle responsibilities effectively and without undue frustration
- Lay the groundwork for networking by helping to structure meetings with people the new manager needs to know

The mentor pool at Einstein was developed by the following methods:

- Department heads were invited to volunteer for mentor service.
- Administrative staff were invited to nominate possible mentors.
- Members of the Mentor Committee invited specific managers to participate.

Another method of skill building capitalizes on the power of feedback. *Self-assessment devices* help employees tune into important features of service by assessing themselves in relation to a particular standard. In addition to self-assessment devices, coworkers and customers can complete *written questionnaires* about a particular employee (or many employees can complete forms about each other). Used confidentially as skill builders, feedback helps individuals improve by calling the employee's attention to important behaviors that reflect service skills.

Instructional literature, such as pamphlets or booklets, can also be helpful, especially if key skills are reviewed, discussed, and experimented with in staff or team meetings. For example, American Hospital Publishing, Inc., publishes a series of booklets on customer relations skills. These booklets include assessment devices and formats for skill building at staff meetings. Receptive employees learn from such educational and "refresher" materials.[5-10]

☐ When Training Is Not the Answer

Training efforts fail for many reasons, but two appear to stand out: lack of skills was not the problem in the first place; and skills are learned in a vacuum.

In situations where lack of skills was not the problem in the first place, training efforts are misplaced. Sometimes unwillingness is mistaken for inability, and skills "training" is imposed on people who already have them. The problem is that people are not inspired to *use* their best skills on the job. Usually the reasons have to do with the quality of teamwork, supervision, or communication. Often low morale permeates interactions with customers, and dysfunctional behavior toward customers and coworkers is attributed to lack of skills when in fact it is due to dysfunctional dynamics within the work group. When morale dips, service slips. When groups fail to work as teams, the customer knows it.

Although process improvement efforts often address these problems, many organizations have found it necessary to provide team-building facilitation in which coworkers address their own dynamics and, as a group, set norms and build skills key to working together as a more effective service team. Organizational development professionals are particularly helpful toward this end.

As for the second reason, skills learned in a vacuum, the classroom does not necessarily reflect the employee's real world, as mentioned earlier in the chapter. Training is a waste of valuable resources unless it is provided as one step in the following sequence of events:

1. The supervisor communicates clear performance expectations to the employee, making the skill important to develop.
2. Using a needs assessment process, the supervisor determines whether the employee has the skill already.
3. The supervisor communicates the reasons for providing the employee with the training experience and clarifies how he or she will follow up on what has been learned.
4. Upon returning from training, the employee is asked by the supervisor to describe and demonstrate what was learned. The supervisor gives feedback and incorporates the new skills as standards.
5. The supervisor provides frequent feedback to the employee about performance and uses answerable skills to hold the employee accountable for use of the newly tuned skills on the job.

In other words, it is not enough to send people to training. Follow-up makes training stick. Lack of it makes training fade.

☐ Final Suggestions

Opportunities for promoting learning abound. Because training and development can be expensive in terms of time and energy (among other resources), consider these tips so that you can see definite results from your training investment:

- *Don't train before you install service excellence as an organization priority:* First-chosen training candidates are bound to ask, "Why us? Are we so bad?" If a systemwide orientation has been effected, they'll understand why you're singling them out.
- *Root training in expectations:* Decide up front what you expect of people in various positions. Next, figure out what skills they need to meet your expectations. Then focus your training on building these skills. This way, your training efforts will be clear routes toward success on the job.
- *Beware of Band-Aid skill training:* Training perceived as having failed may in fact not have failed but was undermined or was applied in a vacuum. To reap results,

a foundation should be in place that enforces and reinforces the skills learned. Strategy coordinators who promise behavioral improvements as a result of short-term training without adequate system supports at best treat only the symptom and offer no more than short-term (or Band-Aid) relief.

- *Don't be punitive; empower people:* People need to build and apply new skills in an atmosphere of acceptance and motivation. In a culture that supports learning, workers can experiment and be permitted to take risks. In an atmosphere of fear, this won't happen.

- *Don't set your standards too low:* Train for excellence, not merely for adequacy. Simply eliminating offensive behavior is not enough.

- *Don't leave desirable behavior to people's imagination:* In a recent program, 30 supervisors were divided into groups of three. Each trio was asked to spend 20 minutes preparing a demonstration of making the most of a brief time with a patient, such as delivering a patient tray, changing a light bulb, giving directions in the hallway, or checking the TV. Two of the 10 demonstrations were excellent; most were mediocre, although inoffensive; but two had offensive elements in them. The trainer had to devote substantial time to helping the groups polish their scenarios to eliminate offensive aspects and tap missed opportunities. A short exercise turned into an all-day activity, for good reason. If your managers don't know what excellence looks like in everyday situations, how can they move their people toward it? Excellence is not always obvious, and training programs need to direct the group's attention to defining it in concrete terms for each person's job.

- *Don't overuse scripting:* Some businesses teach a standard script and require every employee to use it with every customer, the so-called programmed robot approach. In a health care setting, this approach can be fraught with problems: lack of sincerity, lack of patient individuation, employee boredom, loss of spontaneity, to cite a few. On the other hand, scripts can be considered as *fallback positions* for those times employees cannot allow a negative mood to dictate behavior. Also, if all employees learn at least one "excellence script," they understand at least one definition of excellent behavior.

- *Use a mix of methods:* This way people with different learning styles all have a chance to build their unique degree of effectiveness.

- *Don't bypass managers and supervisors:* Because they set the pace, they need to have clear expectations for service leadership and the skills to meet them at a high standard of excellence.

According to R. H. Hayes and S. C. Wheelright, coauthors of *Restoring Our Competitive Edge: Competing through Manufacturing,* the Japanese recognize that well-trained employees can make or break a company. As a result, Japanese workers typically spend 25 percent of their first six years with a company in various training programs. Hitachi, an electronics giant, spends more than $80 million a year on employee training, an amount equal to about two-thirds of the company's advertising budget.[11] Furthermore, according to the authors, over the long haul, American managers would be wise to rethink their training strategies if they want to stay competitive. Hayes emphasizes the importance of up-front investments in training to instill the discipline, skills, and pride essential to providing the high-quality services that win consumer favor.[12]

References

1. Steinberg, C. In practice: buying into customer service. *Training and Development Journal* 45(9):11–12, Sept. 1991.

2. Learning International. *Lessons from Top Service Providers.* Stanford, CT: Learning International, 1991.

3. Survey: Training in the 90's. *Human Resource Executive,* Mar. 1988.

4. Senge, P. *The Fifth Discipline: The Art and Practice of the Learning Organization.* New York City: Doubleday, 1990.

5. Leebov, W. *Customer Service in Health Care.* Chicago: American Hospital Publishing, 1990.

6. Leebov, W. *Effective Complaint Handling in Health Care.* Chicago: American Hospital Publishing, 1990.

7. Leebov, W. *Job Satisfaction Strategies for Health Care Professionals.* Chicago: American Hospital Publishing, 1991.

8. Leebov, W. *Positive Co-Worker Relationships in Health Care.* Chicago: American Hospital Publishing, 1990.

9. Leebov, W. *Practical Assertiveness for Health Care Professionals.* Chicago: American Hospital Publishing, 1991.

10. Leebov, W. *Telephone Tactics for Health Care Professionals.* Chicago: American Hospital Publishing, 1990.

11. Hayes, R. H., and Wheelright, S. C. *Restoring Our Competitive Edge: Competing through Manufacturing.* New York City: John Wiley & Sons, 1984.

12. Hayes and Wheelright.

Chapter 10
Physician Involvement

One of the most complex challenges in achieving service excellence is mobilizing and involving the medical staff in ways that help the institution reach its service objectives while also benefiting the physician. The question "what to do about the doctors" is usually an agonizing one. Before continuing with this chapter, take the self-test in figure 10-1 to see how involved your physicians are in your *current* efforts to improve service. The more "true" answers, the greater their involvement. "False" answers reveal opportunities to expand your efforts to enlist physicians as stakeholders in service improvement.

Figure 10-1. Self-Test

Physician Involvement. *Circle the appropriate answer. The more "true" answers, the better. "False" answers indicate areas that need improvement.*		
1. Physicians help plan their own form of involvement in our service strategy.	True	False
2. Our physicians are aware of our organization's priority on service quality improvement.	True	False
3. Our physicians see themselves as an important part of our service quality improvement strategy, not just as people who will benefit from it.	True	False
4. Physicians are aware of the specific behaviors that constitute excellent service.	True	False
5. In their organization, problematic physician behavior toward nurses and other staff is confronted, not dismissed as unimportant.	True	False
6. Our employees know that physicians are customers whose reasonable expectations need to be met.	True	False
7. We take steps to strengthen the service relationship between our organization's staff and physician office staff.	True	False
8. We involve physicians in helping us solve service problems that affect care for their patients.	True	False
9. We actively involve physicians in helping us identify priorities for service improvement.	True	False
10. We have a clear system for responding to physician complaints and needs.	True	False
Total:	___	___

Excellent service on the part of physicians is obviously important. Physicians interact with and affect patient and staff satisfaction. Also, nonphysician staff resent double standards they perceive when they are expected to excel at service while physicians (their so-called partners in caring) are not. Benefits of physician involvement include the following:

- Your strategy will gain credibility when employees see that service excellence is for *all* caregivers, including physicians.
- By inviting physicians to join service improvement teams, you improve communication between hospital management and your medical staff while showing your interest in improving the satisfaction of physicians as internal customers.

Achieving physician involvement in your service strategy is easier when physicians are salaried employees and, like other employees, can be held accountable to service expectations. However, some doctors have admitting privileges at several institutions. These "voluntary staff" are customers of the hospital, so imposing service standards on them is a lot trickier.

Whether to treat physicians as customers, as accountable partners in care giving, or as both is an important decision. Many service strategies fall apart when standards that purportedly applied to *all* caregivers were lowered to avoid holding physicians accountable.

Before exploring alternative approaches, let's look at what physicians stand to gain from excellent service. After all, if you want your approach to work, it must address a compelling question that physicians invariably ask: "What's in it for me?"

This chapter will offer specific strategies for recruiting physician participation and commitment to your strategy options. The delicate task of improving physician behavior will be examined in detail, along with encouraging physicians to be partners in your service improvement endeavors.

☐ Benefits for Physicians

Before the health care economic climate changed, how many physicians really worried about attracting and retaining a steady flow of patients? How many even thought of patients as customers? With today's competitive atmosphere and changing health care utilization trends and technology, physicians who don't worry may find themselves managing a gradually eroding practice. Physicians who resist the fact that patients (and their families) are customers, with the power to make or break a physician's practice, may find themselves losing patients to the practice down the street.

Excellent service is key to this quest. If they want customer loyalty, they must satisfy the customer criteria used to judge health care quality, criteria that are service-focused. Also, in interactions with hospital personnel, physicians rely on the support, cooperation, and service of hospital employees and thus benefit from treating coworkers with respect, courtesy, and cooperation as well.

Here are 9 arguments to use when describing to physicians benefits of their participation in service improvement efforts:

- *Technological advantage:* Physicians in almost any specialty can assume that others in their specialties have similar training and access to state-of-the-art technology and clinical protocols. The consumer sees so many alternatives that look—and frequently are—clinically alike and, until proved wrong, assumes competence on the part of every provider. Therefore, the competitive edge for the physician, the way to be different and better, does not lie with technical skill but with service excellence from the patients' point of view.

- *New breed of consumer:* Physicians are also faced with a new breed of consumers who are increasingly more knowledgeable and discriminating in choosing a provider. Knowing that they pay dearly for health care, and expecting value for their money, consumers *shop* for physicians or managed care plans. According to *Healthcare Marketing Report,* Tom Moody, vice-president and general manager of the Marketing Prescription, reported that 58.6 percent of patients switch physicians because of unsatisfactory relationships.[1] Once viewed with awe and from a respectful distance, physicians are now more likely to fall under intense scrutiny by a discerning public that wants more than just medical expertise. After all, consumers are largely unable to evaluate medical competence. Market research firms (for example, the Harris research organization in a study commissioned by Pfizer in 1986) indicate that service factors, not technical competence, are cited as the major contributors to customer satisfaction. Consumers select and evaluate physicians on the basis of service criteria such as bedside manner, staff courtesy and attention, convenience of hours, and easy access.

- *The grapevine:* Scrutinizing physicians more intensely, consumers spread the word about what they see and experience. In that health care reportedly is one of the top three topics of conversation among friends, family, and coworkers, the grapevine is either a powerful referral source or a deterrent. Physicians who want their practices to thrive (not just survive) need that grapevine to work for, not against, them.

- *The negativity obsession:* The powerful grapevine gives more airtime to people's negative experiences than to their positive ones. Dwelling on the negative seems to be a human tendency. In 1985, the Technical Assistance Research Project (TARP) in Washington, D.C., conducted a massive study of consumer behavior in service industries and found that the average consumer tells five other people about positive experiences they've had with a service organization, including health care. On the other hand, they tell 20 people about an experience they perceived as negative.[2] Therefore, consumers speak to four times as many friends, relatives, and coworkers about negative experiences or dissatisfactions with a service provider than they do about positive experiences. The result is that the service provider has to satisfy four people for every one it disappoints just to stay even in terms of public image and reputation. This applies to physicians as well as hospitals.

- *Stereotype of the greedy, disinterested physician:* Many feel that the media have been unkind to physicians, having painted them as arrogant, greedy, and insensitive toward the vulnerable patient. The situation is aggravated by the fact that malpractice, medical treatment atrocities, fraud, and other physician offenses seem more newsworthy than does well-functioning and empathic physician care giving. Victimized by stereotypes, the physician who wants and deserves a positive image and reputation has to bend over backward to overcome widespread consumer suspicion and distrust. Their care giving must be so sensitive, humanistic, respectful, and *excellent* that it can topple negative stereotypes.

- *Liability and the predisposition to sue:* A wary public is quick to sue, so malpractice premiums climb. Physicians cannot afford malpractice suits either in terms of expense or reputation. A prime factor that determines whether people sue a physician for malpractice is their perception of that physician's attitude and manner toward them. Generally speaking, people don't like to sue a nice, well-intentioned physician, but given equal severity of medical outcomes, they are more likely to sue physicians perceived as cold or impersonal.

- *Dependence on hospital staff:* Physicians have a stake in harmonious working relationships with hospital staff, on whom they depend to meet the needs of their patients. The pharmacist who mixes and dispenses medication, the nurse who provides the bulk and continuity of care, and the medical secretary who maintains patient charts all affect the physician's care delivery. Physicians who demonstrate poor behavior and consequently have poor relationships with these coworkers tend to receive (some say deservedly) second-class treatment.

- *"I'll scratch your back if you'll scratch mine":* If a hospital's physicians can't satisfy consumer needs, consumers turn elsewhere for service. When this happens, physicians lose patients; so do their hospitals. Consequently, physicians look more and more toward their hospitals' resources to help deliver better service. Because of this interreliance, a hospital can justify asking physicians to be involved in its service quality strategy. Otherwise employees resent the unfairness of the double standard.
- *The user-friendly hospital:* The hospital intent on continuous service improvement cares about making it easy for physicians to practice—getting test results quickly, scheduling appointments and surgical procedures smoothly, and locating key equipment immediately. The physician who *helps* the hospital improve service processes ends up having a much easier time serving his or her own patients.

Physicians, then, can benefit from participating in service improvement efforts for humanistic, marketing, and financial reasons. Your challenge is to bring these benefits to the forefront in your efforts to engage physicians as part of your service team. The result is that the physician wins, the hospital wins, and—best of all—the patient wins.

☐ Approaches for Involving Physicians

If they approach physicians at all, most hospitals opt for a relatively low-risk, and consequently low-results, approach to physician involvement. They simply inform them about their efforts to improve employee behavior, and hope that the message rubs off, or they politely explain how physicians could help make the effort work, and hope for the best. Although either approach is far better than no approach at all, other approaches have proven to be more diplomatic and effective.

As you reach out to physicians, of course you have to consider the constraints on their time and (with some physicians) the reality of their alliances with multiple hospitals. Their participation in your strategy hinges on your timing and on how you sell them on the value of service excellence to their practices and to their ease of practice.

To figure out the best approach for your organization, first use your physicians to reach other physicians. That is, seek out physician mentors and opinion leaders to lead the way; get advice from them early on; then start small and test the waters. Don't give up easily if you meet with some resistance.

Meet with key physicians to plan your strategy. Through focus groups, physicians can pinpoint problems they have with employees and identify service issues that they themselves can and need to address. They can be led toward setting their own service objectives and offering suggestions on how to achieve them. Usually a small number of physicians express strong interest and, if supported, will spearhead a substantive effort.

In our experience with numerous hospitals nationwide, no two physician strategies have been the same. Many organizations have developed Physician Planning Committees to pinpoint the needs and expectations of their physicians; define the hospital's approach; install a system for monitoring results and providing ongoing corrective feedback; define physician standards; and build a system for implanting these standards into physician performance. Figure 10-2 identifies a series of questions you can use to guide your process for planning physician involvement strategy.

☐ Physician Involvement Strategy Options

It helps to plan for physician involvement by considering the three hats physicians typically wear in relation to your organization. These are (1) physician as customer,

Figure 10-2. Planning Physician Involvement Strategies

1. Several kinds of physician groups can be involved in the service strategy:
   - Clinical chiefs
   - Salaried physicians/faculty
   - Attending or voluntary staff
   - Residents
   - Students and interns

   Which categories are included in *our* medical staff?
2. Who has influence on or authority over each of the above groups? Who are the formal and informal leaders? And which physicians have a reputation for caring behavior toward patients and staff?
3. Which forums exist in which communication can happen with each physician group? How often? Who controls the agenda?
4. What should be expected of each group regarding involvement in our service strategy?
   - Do we need separate strategies for each group?
   - What should we do to make each group aware of our service strategy?
   - How do we want to help each group become more effective in their behavior toward patients?
   - How do we want to help each group be more effective in building their practices or careers?
   - What opportunities do we want to offer each group to be partners with us in identifying and addressing our service improvement priorities?
5. To what extent should we establish standards of service behavior that apply to each of these groups? How will we hold each group accountable? By which mechanisms?
   - How can we monitor?
   - What consequences should there be for nonconformance?
   - Whose job is it to hold them accountable?
6. Sequence
   - What should the sequence of events be? How should mini-strategies for each group be coordinated or integrated? Simultaneous involvement of the groups versus cascaded?
   - Suggested timelines
7. Which organizational resources are key to carrying out this plan?
   - People?
   - Material?

(2) physician as caregiver and member of your patient care team, and (3) physician as partner. The following strategy options will help physicians commit to active participation while wearing these important hats:

- Build up-front commitment.
- Help physicians enhance their own behavior.
- Use feedback to improve physician behavior.
- Help physicians build service-oriented practices.
- Engage physicians as partners.
- Hire physician liaisons to ease the physicians' way.
- Help staff relate to physicians effectively.

Build Up-Front Commitment

To educate physicians about your service strategy, start early by engaging them in briefings that invite their active involvement. Briefings, which ideally are presented by a respected physician and/or nurse, should emphasize the benefits described earlier. Usually, the briefing occurs during an existing meeting (for example, quarterly brunch, department meeting, or regularly scheduled grand rounds). The agenda can include the following elements:

- Reasons why your organization is pursuing service quality improvement (quality care, public scrutiny, pride and integrity, patient satisfaction criteria, liability, competition, and so on)
- Quick overview of your overall strategy

- Value of a service-driven medical practice
- Quick presentation of House Rules or behavioral guidelines that apply to physicians in their interactions with their own patients and with hospital and office staff
- Call for role modeling, cooperation, support, and involvement in service improvement initiatives
- Presentation of an easy method for analyzing service quality in a medical practice
- Emphasis on what physicians have to gain from the effort. Invitation to cooperate and become involved in the hospital's strategy as a full partner.

In these briefings, some organizations make an appeal for physician "leadership" in service improvement. As an example, consider the excerpt in figure 10-3, taken from a forceful speech given to physicians at a large teaching hospital on the West Coast, a hospital plagued by physician–administrator infighting. In that speech, physicians were asked to lead and take initiative to improve service. They were called to action, to help the organization reach a higher plane for the sake of patients and staff pride.

Help Physicians Enhance Their Own Behavior

Because employees resent double standards, at some point in your service strategy you need also to establish behavior standards for physicians—standards with implications for credentialing and preservation of privileges to practice in your organization. Many organizations ask physicians to abide by the generic behavior standards developed as part of the organization's service strategy; others develop a unique set of expectations specific to physicians. Behavior standards can best be developed in patient focus groups that solicit views of which behaviors count most. In teaching hospitals, these expectations can be communicated to residents and students during their orientation and monitored by staff physicians, residency directors, or clinical chiefs. Following is an example of such House Rules developed by The Einstein Consulting Group:

1. *Break the ice and the mystique:* Introduce yourself, address people by name, express words of concern.
2. *Listen and understand:* Patients turn away or sue physicians who don't. Encourage patients to tell their story; invite their questions. Digest the meaning of the illness from the patient's point of view.
3. *Inform and explain:* Information is power, and it promotes compliance. People are less anxious when they know what's happening and why.
4. *See the whole person:* See beyond the illness to the person. Manage the "case" to the benefit of the patient. Don't pass the buck.
5. *Share the responsibility:* Risk and uncertainty are facts of life in medical practice. Acknowledging risk factors builds trust. It also helps the patient face reality and share in decision making.
6. *Pay undivided attention:* Sit down, focus, reduce distractions and interruptions, maintain eye contact, and empathize.
7. *Secure confidentiality and privacy:* Watch what you say, where you say it, and to whom!
8. *Preserve dignity:* Treat the patient as though he or she could be your loved one. Respect modesty—close curtains, cover up, and knock before entering.
9. *Treat patients as adults:* Your words and tone should communicate respect, not condescension. Expect and encourage responsible choices and patient autonomy.
10. *Anticipate:* You'll often know what people need, want, or fear before they speak up. *Act!*
11. *Remember the family:* Families feel protective, anxious, frightened, and insecure. Extend yourself, reassure, inform, and act as advocate.
12. *Respond quickly:* Keep appointments. Return calls. Apologize for delays. Others' time is valuable too.

Figure 10-3.   Speech Calling for Physician Leadership in Service Improvement (Excerpt)

The Call for Physician Leadership in Service Improvement

What happens in most hospitals is that administrators and task forces sit in meetings and brood, "How do we get the doctors to work with us?" People expect resistance from physicians. Many people expect doctors to be too arrogant and self-centered to buy into the need to help the organization renew itself to meet the new demands of health care.

Perhaps the expectations and stereotypes are self-fulfilling. You're victimized by and subtly influenced by people's stereotypes about doctors as people uninterested in change for the sake of organization and the patient.

The scheming and brooding non-physicians do about how to engage physicians has got to stop. But the only way it will is if you share a leadership role in our service strategy.

It's time people stopped seeing you as resistant to important change—needing to be dragged kicking and screaming along in order to enable the organization to succeed. It's time you earned the reputation as change makers who use your power to move this organization forward and help our organization achieve a reputation for service and teamwork that's as positive as our reputation for quality medical care.

How?

How can you help this organization move forward? We need your leadership. Consider four leadership characteristics that, if demonstrated by you, would move this hospital forward in offering excellent service to our patients and a much healthier, more satisfying work environment for employees and physicians.

Leadership Quality #1. A powerful vision of service excellence

Many people—physicians and non-physicians—walk around this place saying, "There's no vision here." Everyone who wants to influence the place needs to become visionary and extend a powerful positive vision to others. Imagine positive visions coming from physicians! How good do you really want it to be here? What *could* it be like if everyone poured their talent and attention into making it better?

Leaders have a vision of possibilities. They see what health care can be and what they themselves can do to make a difference . . . and they want to make their vision a reality. When they make their vision contagious, they help to shape the reality they want—and they gain respect, because something inside us admires the person who stretches our own view of the possible.

Leadership Quality #2. Physician leaders MODEL constructive, cooperative work relationships.

Approaching a unit secretary, the physician thinks, "She doesn't treat me with the respect I deserve." The unit secretary thinks, "That doctor's a prima donna. Do I get the respect I deserve? Never! So why should I rush for that chart? That doctor can just wait!" The two are at a stalemate that is painful and paralyzing for both parties.

If you were to act like a leader, you would take the first step. You wouldn't let this relationship problem go on and on, interfering with people's job satisfaction, customer service *and* the cooperation *you get* that you sorely need to serve your patients efficiently and well. You could say hello to the unit secretary and counteract people's perception that you act aloof and superior. Experiment: Walk through the halls and say hello to everyone. People will ask, "What's happened around here?"

Leadership Quality #3. Physician leaders express a positive view of the organization.

You can see your work world and our service strategy through the lens of skeptic, cynic, or powerless critic. Or you can see it through rose-colored glasses. What you see depends on your point of view.

You've known two nurses on the same unit with the same boss, the same hours, the same responsibilities. Yet one always sees the glass as half full and the other always sees the glass as half empty. It's not the situation. It's the person and the lens he or she wears when looking at the world.

You have the power to help people focus *not* on what's *impossible*, but to dwell on what's possible . . . and to focus on achievements and strides forward, not only on all the work yet to be done, the problems yet to be solved.

You can make positive waves here if you dare to be positive in the face of others' negativity. Instead of joining the ranks of the complainers, become activists when you don't like what's happening. Confront the generalizations and "ain't it awfuls" that you think hold other people back. It's a matter of mind-set and you have a choice about the mind-set you apply to what's going on.

(Continued on next page)

Figure 10-3. (Continued)

Leadership Quality #4: Physician leaders exhibit personal involvement and initiative.

Now that this organization needs to change and change quickly in order to stay competitive, "It's not my job" thinking isn't helpful. We need your help.

- You already get feedback from patients. Take initiative to get helpful feedback from coworkers, nurses, front-desk people. Model an openness to feedback for the sake of improved coworker relationships. Set up a time with each person you work with and ask how they think your relationship is and how you might improve it.
- Join our process improvement teams. Together, we can be much more effective making our services physician- and patient-friendly.

In another hospital, physicians were frustrated with the slowness of solving systems problems, such as cumbersome scheduling practices, slow registration, incomplete and lost charts. The physicians formed a "skunkworks" effort that joined staff in tackling these systems problems. They made concrete recommendations. In short, they got involved in the solution and used their tremendous power in the organization to *move* the organization toward service excellence.

Closing

In health care today, it's not only survival of the fittest. To be among the winners, you need to be, not only FIT as a medical provider, but also a fully involved member of our care team. We need your active, tenacious help and support as change agents. We need your partnership.

The fact is, every one of you has the potential to demonstrate these leadership qualities. You don't have to be explicitly a chief or *designated* leader in order to do so.

Service excellence and continuous improvement are frankly impossible without your partnership. You're too pivotal here to be involved minimally. We need your leadership, your initiative, and your vision. You have a fine reputation as clinical professionals. I challenge you to become involved with us in our service strategy so that we can all benefit from a service reputation to match.

13. *Follow through:* Call or visit to show you haven't forgotten. Keep your promises.
14. *Think team:* Show respect for coworkers. They share your purpose. Recognize good work and effort. Collaborate. Speak well of staff. They reflect on you.

To make these standards worth more than the paper they're written on, consider a skill-building program for physician administrators. The program should be set up and mandated by your CEO for salaried chiefs and should engage the physician chiefs in an exploration of what they do to coach the physicians they supervise toward service excellence.

Four basic skills can be developed during such a program:

1. How to be a role model and culture builder
2. How to set and communicate clear service expectations to physicians, residents, and students
3. How to encourage input, suggestions, and involvement in service improvement initiatives from physicians with an eye to improving physician ease of practice in the organization
4. How to hold physicians accountable through feedback, coaching, confrontation, and the organization's credentialing and privileging practices

If your organization is a teaching institution, also consider special sessions for house staff. After all, house staff provide most of the firsthand patient care. As rovers without strong loyalty to the institution and as students who often feel oppressed and exhausted by an overdose of hours and responsibilities, they are the ones likely to generate serious service problems for both patients and staff. Special sessions, which ideally are run by chiefs as special luncheons or grand rounds, should:

- Provide an overview of your service mission and values
- Invite house staff to sound off on your organization's service strengths and weaknesses as they have perceived them

- Present behavioral service standards that you want residents and students to demonstrate with patients, families, and coworkers
- Confront the physician–employee dynamics that interfere with patient and employee satisfaction (involve nurses here)
- Examine how doctors stand to benefit now and in the future from commitment to and cooperation with standards of service performance that achieve patient satisfaction and loyalty

Use Feedback to Improve Physician Behavior

Beyond establishing standards, one of the most effective methods for improving physician behavior is through feedback. Medical schools and most residency programs emphasize clinical knowledge and skills and give short shrift to the nonclinical aspects of the physician–patient relationship. But once physicians are in practice, there is no ongoing vehicle for receiving frank, specific, constructive feedback about their behavior and its effects on patients. The result is limited opportunities for growth and improvement in the behaviors that constitute the art of medicine.

Consider helping your physicians strengthen their interactions with patients by developing (with their help) a brief patient feedback device that yields patient perceptions of the physicians' service behavior. For example, the strategy of instituting regular patient feedback to physicians has been tested successfully at two Kaiser Permanente Medical Centers in Northern California (at San Rafael by Paul Alpert, M.D., and Geraldine Alpert, Ph.D.; and at Santa Clara by Robert Pearl, M.D., and Joyce Reynolds, Ph.D.).[3] At both centers, each patient was asked (through the mail or in person) to complete a short questionnaire (see figure 10-4).

A feedback package was then given to each physician after the baseline testing and after each subsequent data collection. The goal was to provide the physician with as much information as possible about how he or she was rated and compared with other physicians in the department. Each physician received copies of all of his or her patients' questionnaires and comments. Each physician also was given his or her raw scores and the mean score for the department. With the exception of the physician's own scores, patient anonymity was maintained, and no one other than the investigators had access to individual physician data. At various points in the project, physicians were given explanatory letters along with the data, describing changes that were occurring, the implications of these changes, and the need for more response from those physicians showing inadequate improvement.

After repeated assessment and feedback to physicians, several changes occurred:[4]

- The patient satisfaction mean increased significantly.
- Of the physicians who were the lowest scorers initially, all moved well into the satisfactory range.
- The number of patients who gave their physicians low scores decreased by 55 percent.
- During 12 months in which no testing or feedback occurred, scores dropped somewhat but not to the original baseline levels. Most important, the physicians who were originally the lowest scorers were the ones who best maintained their levels of improvement.
- Most impressive of all was the remarkable increase in scores when physicians knew they were being evaluated.

The feedback system was enhanced further by providing brief skill-training programs for physicians that helped them to expand their skill repertoires. They were motivated to participate because they wanted higher ratings from their patients. A complete description of this study can be found in *Patient Satisfaction: A Guide to Practice Enhancement.*[5]

Figure 10-4. Physician Feedback Tool

(On outside of envelope)

Dear Patient:

We, the physicians of Kaiser Permanente Medical Center-Santa Clara, want to satisfy your health care needs. Please help us accomplish this by letting us know how well the physician you see today meets your needs and what else could or should have been done.

Each day, we are asking a small, randomly selected sample of patients to let us know how well we did. This envelope is provided to maintain the confidentiality and anonymity of your responses.

After your visit, please complete the enclosed card, put it in, and seal this envelope and return it as you leave to the receptionist or nurse who gave it to you.

Thank you for taking time to help us.

Sincerely,

Chris Chow, M.D.
Physician-in-Chief

(Side one of card)

Patient Care Survey
Kaiser Permanente Medical Center-Santa Clara

What is the name and department of the physician you saw today?

1. Physician's name _____

2. Department: _____

3. Is he or she your regular personal physician?

   [ ] yes   [ ] no   [ ] not sure

4. What is the main reason for your visit today? Please check one.

   [ ] 1. Urgent/Same Day

   [ ] 2. Return Visit/Continuing Care

   [ ] 3. Routine Exam (physical, check-up, etc.)

   [ ] 4. Consultation

   [ ] 5. Other: _____

5. When was your appointment? Please check one.

   [ ] Morning   [ ] Afternoon   [ ] Evening   [ ] Weekend

   How would you evaluate the physician that you saw today?

   Please circle one. A = Great   B = Good   C = Fair   D = Poor

6. Showed concern for your needs: A   B   C   D

7. Treated you with respect: A   B   C   D

8. Gave you clear information and explanations: A   B   C   D

9. Spent enough time with you: A   B   C   D

10. Was knowledgeable and competent: A   B   C   D

11. Your overall impression: A   B   C   D

12. When you return to our Medical Center in the future, would you want to see this same physician again?

    [ ] yes   [ ] no   [ ] not sure

13. Comments or suggestions about your physician based on above questions.

Also consider offering physicians the service of confidentially surveying patients in their practices to determine perceptions of physician performance and then feeding back the results. Dale Matthews, M.D., and Alvan Feinstein, M.D., asserting that patients are appropriate judges of physician performance and that their perceptions are one measure of physician quality, have developed a carefully researched questionnaire for soliciting patient perceptions of physician behavior and their degree of satisfaction with their physician. The researchers conducted in-depth interviews with 50 randomly selected medical inpatients to identify their favorable and unfavorable impressions and reactions to the personal aspects of care extended by their physicians. From these data, they developed a detailed taxonomy of desired physician attitudes and behaviors.

The measuring device, an excerpt from which is shown in figure 10-5, translates this taxonomy into a survey device for monitoring patients' perceptions of their physicians' performance.[6] Consider using it as an item pool for developing a shorter "physician report card" for your physicians.

Help Physicians Build Service-Oriented Practices

Physicians welcome assistance with enhancing their private practices. Fifty-eight percent say they would like help training office personnel on customer relations.[7] When physicians increase the service focus among their own staff, the raised consciousness to service factors will also have a beneficial impact on physicians' service focus in your hospital.

Your organization can sponsor team-building programs and training programs for physicians' office staffs. After an enlightening workshop on patient satisfaction and practice enhancement, office managers in particular tend to share their new insights and skills with the physicians. In other words, reach the physicians by reaching their office managers. Sometimes these workshops focus on such trendy topics as marketing physicians' practices or practice management for the physicians and office manager. These topics attract people, and once you've attracted them, include a substantive component on staff and physician behaviors that generate patient satisfaction and harmonious, cooperative coworker relationships.

The Bay State Medical Center in Springfield, Massachusetts, sponsors a very successful Breakfast Club for the medical office staff of its attending physicians. During a monthly breakfast, office staffers discuss their problems and needs with one another and with the no-longer-faceless people they interact with so often over the phone from the hospital's admitting and quality departments. The Breakfast Club has taken on a life of its own, serving the medical center's public relations and problem-solving objectives as well as providing a stimulating and supportive forum for networking among office staff. The medical center supplements the breakfasts by distributing their special newsletter, called *The Breakfast Club*, in each physician's office.

According to Marjorie Rittenhouse, assistant vice-president for operations support, the Lake Hospital System in Painesville, Ohio, uses its 15-member Physician Satisfaction Committee to identify needs and then design and promote physician/office staff educational programs to meet those needs, including programs on quality in customer service, communication, and collections. Some hospitals offer service enhancement workshops for staff from individual practices. Figure 10-6 shows a sample design for such a program developed by The Einstein Consulting Group.

Consider providing tools for your medical staff that help them evaluate and enhance their practices from a service point of view. The Ambience Audit in figure 10-7 and the books by Brown and Morley[8] and Leebov, Vergare, and Scott[9] are examples of such tools.

Engage Physicians as Partners

In the long run, the success of your efforts to involve physicians in service improvement will depend on your effort to engage them as partners. Two promising ways to do that

Figure 10-5. Questionnaire on Patient's Appraisal of Physician Performance (Excerpt)

Part One Directions: In this part, we would like you to think about your own doctor, Dr. _____, and only Dr. _____. We will list some things that doctors are known to do. Some of the things we will mention are good for all doctors to do, others are not so good for any doctor to do. Your own doctor, Dr. _____, may or may not do these things.

If your doctor, Dr. _____, usually or always does them, circle Y for "Yes." If Dr. _____ rarely or never does them, circle N for "No." If Dr. _____ sometimes does them and sometimes does not, circle S for "sometimes yes, sometimes no." It is possible that a certain item may not apply to you or to your doctor. For example, the item "gets my family involved in my care" will not apply to you if you do not have family members that are available to help you. For such items, circle D for "does not apply."

1.	Spends enough time with me	Y	S	N	D
2.	Uses words I don't understand	Y	S	N	D
3.	Makes me feel nervous	Y	S	N	D
4.	Asks me about my personal life, such as my interests and hobbies	Y	S	N	D
5.	Asks me to give my opinion about what type of treatment I would like to get	Y	S	N	D
6.	Avoids my questions	Y	S	N	D
7.	Calls me by the name I wish to be called	Y	S	N	D
8.	Hurts my feelings	Y	S	N	D
9.	Comforts me if I'm upset	Y	S	N	D
10.	Asks me to give my opinion about what's wrong with me	Y	S	N	D

-
-
-
-

51. Which three items from the above list items (1–50) best describe your doctor?
    Best description (Item number):   _____
    Second best description (Item number): _____
    Third best description (Item number):   _____

52. Which three items from the above list (items 1–50) are most important to you when you rate a doctor (any doctor) who is taking care of you?
    Most important (Item number):   _____
    Second most important (Item number):   _____
    Third most important (Item number):   _____

Part Two Directions: In this part, we would like you to think about your own doctor, Dr. _____, and only Dr. _____. We would like you to tell us how satisfied you are with the way Dr. _____ takes care of you. Choose one number from the group of numbers below (a number between 0 and 10) to describe how satisfied you are with Dr. _____ for each of the qualities listed. The higher the number you choose, the more satisfied you should be with your doctor for that quality. For example, for the first item on the list, if you choose 1 you are quite dissatisfied with your own doctor, if you choose 5, you are neither satisfied nor dissatisfied, if you choose 7 you are somewhat satisfied, and if you choose 9 or 10 you are very satisfied. Rate Dr. _____ on each item separately; you may use different numbers for different items, and you may also use the same number for more than one item on the list.

	Dissatisfied					Neutral				Satisfied	
1. Bedside manner	0	1	2	3	4	5	6	7	8	9	10
2. Common courtesy	0	1	2	3	4	5	6	7	8	9	10
3. Way s/he talks with me	0	1	2	3	4	5	6	7	8	9	10
4. Skill in treating my illness	0	1	2	3	4	5	6	7	8	9	10
5. Concern for me as an individual	0	1	2	3	4	5	6	7	8	9	10
6. Overall satisfaction	0	1	2	3	4	5	6	7	8	9	10

Figure 10-5. (Continued)

7. Which items from the above list (items 1–5) was the most important to you when you decided upon your overall level of satisfaction with this doctor?

Most important (item number): _____

Second most important (item number): _____

8. Are you going to do what this doctor has told you to do?   Yes   No

9. Have you seen this doctor before today?   Yes   No

10. Would you like to keep seeing this doctor?   Yes   No

11. Would you recommend this doctor for a friend or member of your family?   Yes   No

12. How long (in months) have you had the illness that brought you in to see the doctor today? _____

13. How many times have you been hospitalized in the past year? _____

14. How many times (outside the hospital) have you seen a doctor in the past year? _____

15. How sick do you consider yourself at the present time?
    (circle one)

    Not sick at all

    Somewhat sick

    Moderately sick

    Very sick

    Extremely sick

Reprinted, with permission, from Matthews, D. A., and Feinstein, A. R. A new instrument for patients' ratings of physician performance in the hospital setting. *Journal of General Internal Medicine* 4:14–22, 1989.

Figure 10-6. Service Enhancement Workshop for Practice Staff

Goals

- Increase awareness of the need for service excellence as an unbeatable competitive advantage
- Define standards for office staff behavior in interactions with patients and family
- Sample a few techniques for positive interactions
- Help people identify the service strengths and weaknesses in their practices
- Strengthen teamwork and cooperation

Outline of the Approach

1. Introduction, objectives, and agenda.
2. Warmup: Partners talk about themselves and their work.
3. "Think of a Place": People are asked to think of a place where the service is terrific and to identify the behaviors demonstrated by staff in such places. These are then shared in the large group.
4. Why Excel at Service?: Short lecture and group discussion on the need for service excellence, including such points as the effect of excellent service on quality of work life, patient comfort, satisfaction and retention, the financial viability of the practice, malpractice prevention, complaint prevention, quality care, and more. Draw attention to health care as a service industry and the practical reasons why medical practices need to excel at service.
5. "How are *you* doing?": Try a small group exercise that asks how well people are already providing excellent service. This is a chance for a pat on the back for strengths and discussion of improvement opportunities.
6. Service Goals: Explain the Service Matrix for medical practices and spark group discussion of the dimensions of service that this practice needs to target for improvement.
7. The Behaviors That Matter: Using anecdotes and demonstrations, present the behaviors key to customer satisfaction (for example, House Rules). Stress consistency, because most behaviors occur inconsistently.
8. Skill Modules: Focus in on a basic customer service skill (such as handling complaints, working with the angry patient, handling multiple demands when customers are watching, making people comfortable). Present a skill model, demonstrate, and ask people to practice in small groups.
9. Brainstorm: "What do we need more of here?"
10. Thank-yous and evaluation.

Figure 10-7. Ambience Audit

_____ Is the name of your building obvious and easy to read from several angles?

_____ Is parking clearly marked, close by, and well lighted?

_____ Are there special spots available close by for people with handicaps, casts, bad backs, or other conditions that warrant special convenience?

_____ Is it easy and safe for someone to drop off a patient?

_____ Is the drop-off location accessible to the front door?

_____ Are the drop-off area, the main entrance, and route to your office barrier-free?

_____ Are there taxis available nearby or a method for calling taxis as needed?

_____ Once people enter your building, is the way to your office clearly indicated?

_____ Is your office clearly marked in the hallway, so people know when they've arrived?

_____ Is your reception desk positioned so that your staff are quick to see people entering?

_____ Are work surfaces and equipment unrelated to registration invisible to people in your waiting area?

_____ Do you have non-glare lighting and non-glare coverings on counters and surfaces?

_____ Does your reception area have shelves, hooks, or closets for the personal items of patients and their companions?

_____ If possible, do you provide specially designed areas conducive to reading, child's play, and conversations?

_____ If you have a play area, do you have play materials that are durable, safe, and usable by more than one child at a time?

_____ Does the waiting area have windows to the outside and to the hallway?

_____ If you have a TV in the waiting area, is it positioned so that not everyone has to watch or hear it?

_____ Are chairs arranged so that people can sit alone or in comfortably closed groups, as they choose?

_____ Are your chairs comfortable for children, heavy people, tall people, pregnant women, older people, and weak people?

_____ Do your chairs provide support to people's backs and arms?

_____ Is the material used on your furniture comfortable, insofar as it does not stick to people or scratch them?

_____ Do you have chairs that are easy to get out of?

_____ Is there a phone available for use by patients and their companions?

_____ Do people find your waiting area to be comfortable during a long wait?

_____ Do you have soothing artwork in your waiting area?

_____ Do you have patient education materials easily accessible to people who are waiting?

_____ Do you have trash receptacles available in your waiting area?

_____ Do you have easy-to-read clocks in the waiting area and in exam rooms?

_____ When people check in, can they do this out of earshot of others in the waiting area?

_____ Are locations where staff interview patients conducive to communication and self-disclosure?

_____ Do furniture arrangements facilitate eye contact between people talking with one another without barriers?

_____ Do you have private offices, cubicles, or partitions that control noise and provide privacy?

_____ Do rooms where people undress have doors the patient can lock or ways the patient can indicate "Occupied" or "Do not disturb"?

_____ Do you have a convenient bathroom and water fountain for use by people in the waiting area _and_ patients who are gowned?

_____ Are exam and treatment rooms where people might be unclothed kept slightly warm?

_____ Do you have a mirror in rooms where people dress?

_____ Do you have a place for people to put their clothes and personal items when they undress, such as hooks, hangers, shelves, or hampers?

_____ Are exam and treatment room doors, exam tables, and curtains arranged to protect the patient from view from the hallway when someone opens the door?

_____ Do you have privacy curtains where appropriate, and do you insist that staff use them?

_____ Are examination and treatment rooms soundproof, so people can't hear what's happening from one room to another?

_____ Do you have an extra chair in exam rooms in case the patient brings a family member or companion?

_____ Are your exam and treatment rooms decorated in a way that is comfortable, colorful, and non-institutional?

_____ Do you have ways of protecting patients from contact with cold instruments and equipment?

involve (1) inviting their involvement in identifying and tackling process improvements, and (2) building teamwork with their care partners (for example, nurses). To illustrate this effort, figure 10-8 outlines a retreat conducted by The Einstein Consulting Group for hospital administrators and physicians. The purpose of the retreat was to help administrators involve physicians in identifying service improvement priorities and to engage their active help in finding remedies.

Many hospitals engaged in total quality management (TQM) involve physicians intensively in the development of clinical protocols or "critical pathways" that identify the optimal clinical and service sequence for patients with specific diagnoses. George Washington University Hospital in Washington, D.C., Alliant Health System in Louisville, and Intermountain Health Care in Salt Lake City are pioneers who have demonstrated the power of this kind of physician involvement for service improvement, improved clinical outcomes, and financial performance.

Beyond involving physicians in identifying key processes that need improvement and harnessing their energy in improving them, a few daring hospitals engage physicians in partnerships or team building with other key caregivers. In the June issue of *Nursing91,* the editors reported in "The nurse–doctor game" the results of their recent reader survey that solicited nurse perceptions of the nurse–physician relationship:[10]

- Fifty-six percent of nurses expressed dissatisfaction with their professional relationships with physicians. Nurses asked to react to this finding found it surprisingly low. According to one respondent, "For some of us, the disrespectful physicians loom large. It might be a small minority but they cause disproportionate aggravation."
- Fifty-seven percent of the nurses said that nurses are subordinate to physicians; only 29 percent say the relationships are collegial. This seems to be changing for the better, particularly in patient-centered care settings where the traditional hierarchies are being challenged.

Figure 10-8. Plan for a Physician Involvement Retreat

Objectives

- Identify top-priority physician requirements: Engage key admitters in identifying five key issues that physicians want the hospital to tackle over the next two years—issues that, if solved, would significantly increase physician satisfaction and loyalty.
- Go after these problems with a vengeance.
- Engage physicians in continuous service quality improvement.

Method

1. Convene key admitters in full-day session (or two half days).
2. Have them identify their frustrations in practicing at this hospital.
3. Use the Affinity Chart technique to cluster ease-of-practice issues, identify overlap, and see the patterns in physician perceptions. (This technique is explained in W. Leebov and C.J. Ersoz, *The Health Care Manager's Guide to Continuous Quality Improvement*; AHPI, 1991.)
4. Involve the group in generating criteria for narrowing down the possibilities in order to pick the Big Five.
5. Using the Decision Matrix technique, whittle down the list to the five big ones. (For an explanation of the technique, see Leebov and Ersoz, 1991.)
6. Engage physicians in writing the problem statement for each top priority and how the problem is currently affecting them and their practice.
7. Identify the influential factors and forces contributing to each problem.
8. Engage the group in generating possible solutions using brainstorming. Promise to provide these ideas as input to the team that will tackle each priority more thoroughly.
9. Identify roles and responsibilities:
   - "How many physicians here are willing to be process owners? consultants? customers only?"
   - Assign an executive to work with physicians on each of the Big Five. Also assign a clerical person to each to show degree of seriousness and support.
10. Identify measurement criteria and methods of tracking and displaying progress.

- Sixty-six percent of nurses think that doctors don't understand what nurses do. One nurse reacted by saying, "They would be shocked to see that we are so much more skilled technically than the handmaidens they think we are."
- Fifty-five percent said that physicians *occasionally* address them in an unprofessional manner; 11 percent said they *frequently* do; 33 percent say they rarely experience rude behavior from physicians. According to our nurse colleagues, a small minority are blatantly disrespectful, but most show unprofessional and disrespectful attitudes through such behaviors as acting too busy to listen to a suggestion; ignoring the nurse's notes (74 percent never read them); acting dismissive when the nurse says something substantive about the patient; using patronizing words like "Yes, dear"; using abrupt commands like "Get those people out of there" without adding "please"; and taking out their bad moods or stress on nurses by losing their tempers and occasionally throwing things.
- When asked "Do you feel that most doctors you work with respect your judgment?" 68 percent said *no.*
- When asked "Do doctors routinely consult you about care and treatment for your patients?" 51 percent said *no.*
- Seventy-two percent of the nurses surveyed said that physicians do *not* see nurses as partners. Asked if it's realistic to expect physicians to consider nurses as partners, 81 percent said *yes.*

Physicians and nurses need to work increasingly well as partners, and partnership requires mutual respect, understanding, and support. Many hospitals have launched initiatives designed to strengthen understanding and collaboration between the two. For example:

- Several hospitals (including Baptist Memorial Hospital in Memphis, Tennessee) have included physicians in their "Walk a Day in My Shoes" programs in which a physician "shadows" a nurse for four hours at a stretch to observe the minute-by-minute details involved in the nurse's daily work. Some of the more progressive residency programs require residents to work alongside a nurse for a day or two, so that they learn *early on in their careers* what a nurse does and the extraordinary demands involved in the job.
- Hospitals are teaming nurses and physicians in teams designed to use the tools of continuous quality improvement to make clinical process improvements.
- Hospitals (such as Montefiore Medical Center in the Bronx) engage nurses, physicians, and all staff in department-specific strategic planning and team building to align everyone *together* with the organization's vision.
- At the Medical College of Virginia, Tallahassee Memorial Regional Medical Center, and Upper Chesapeake Health System, hospital leaders have helped nurses develop their own skills in building collaborative relationships with physicians. The workshop called *Harmony,* available from The Einstein Consulting Group, helps nurses sharpen skills in assertiveness and self-talk that inspire more collegial, mutually respectful relationships with physicians.
- Many hospitals are presenting *entertaining* programs for physicians. The most powerful and effective example of this is the program by humorist Loretta LaRoche of the Humor Works in Plymouth, Massachusetts, who calls herself an MD ("mirth doctor"). She addressed in a raucously humorous fashion the destructive patterns of complaining, whining, finger pointing, and air of superiority demonstrated by physicians and other staff.

An example of a team-building intervention is provided by the radiology department at one medical center we observed. The center convened all physicians and employees to bridge gaps in understanding and develop mutual respect and a climate for open dialogue and problem solving. A summary of the design for that program is provided in figure 10-9.

Figure 10-9. Team Building for Radiology

A. Introduction

"To work well as a team, it helps to take the time to get to know each other better as people. Today's meeting is designed to help us do that. The better we communicate and work as a team, the more effective we will be in meeting patient needs, solving problems, and creating a high quality of work life for all of us."

B. "Boundary Breaking"

1. Have the group sit in a circle for the instructions. Everyone must be able to see every other member of the group.
2. Give the following instructions:
   "This is a quick team-building activity designed to help us get to know each other a bit better as people, since we have to work with one another well. Here's how it works. I will ask a question from my list. The person to my right will be the first person to answer the question and we will then go around the group until everyone has answered. When we complete this question, I will ask another and the second person to my right will begin. We will continue until all seven questions have been answered. If you draw a blank when it is your turn to answer, you may pass, but we will come back to you. Please focus on the person who is answering."
3. "Boundary Breaking" questions
   • What is one thing that makes your job easy to do?
   • What is one thing that makes your job hard to do?
   • What is the one most rewarding aspect of your work?
   • Name one big reason why you're good for our organization.
   • Name one big reason why our organization is good for you.
   • Identify one way you would like to grow in your job over the next year.
   • "Things could work a lot better around here if _____."
4. Notes to Leader
   • Maintain very focused eye contact and non-verbally acknowledge responses, giving empathy and support.
   • Use names when you begin a question.
   • Sometimes you will have to repeat the question as it goes around to refocus energy.
5. Solicit reactions to this activity. Ask:
   • What were your reactions to this activity?
   • Whose answers surprised you?
   • Who is most like you?
   • What have you learned about our team?

C. Share the objectives for the session
   • Clear the air.
   • Examine work norms.
   • Get to know one another better.
   • Identify ways we can work better with one another.

D. The Ideal versus the Real

1. Form groups by job, so that employees are together and physicians are together. Give each group a piece of flipchart paper and a marker. Allow each group five to ten minutes to brainstorm characteristics of the Ideal member of the *other* group. Help the groups feel comfortable creating their Ideal in a freewheeling fashion. It might help to draw a cartoon figure on the paper so the groups can draw as well as describe characteristics.
2. After 15 minutes, reconvene the groups to share their drawings or lists and explain their choices. Make these points:
   • Each group has expectations of the other. These expectations are based on many things. Yet it's impossible for any group to perfectly meet the other's expectations. Unfortunately, when expectations are not met, relationships are in jeopardy.
   • This is an opportunity to "clear the air" and allow groups to share, even if sharing what they would like from the others feels like "wishful thinking."
3. Now for Reality:
   • "Holding onto these ideal images can be damaging. We must put our standards of perfection aside and discuss what we really need and want from each other."
   • Small groups discuss:
     —What we really want from the other groups
     —Why we really need these behaviors/characteristics
     Give the small groups enough time to discuss what they really need from one another. Have these small groups then share in the large group.

(Continued on next page)

Figure 10-9. (Continued)

E. Work Norms

This discussion is designed to help people examine ways they are presently working together. Using a flipchart and markers, help the large group brainstorm positive and negative examples. These can be systems issues or behaviors, for example:

Positives	Negatives
• generally friendly atmosphere	• Radiologists aren't informed of changes
• all call each other by first names	• talking behind people's backs
• clear dress code	• hard to find radiologists during lunch time
• techs pitch in and help busy coworkers	• nonprofessional chit chat in public places
• high priority on patient care	

F. Where Do We Go from Here?

Option One: Group decides which problems need to be addressed and discusses possible solutions and options.

Option Two: Small groups could take two or three problems, generate options/solutions, and report back to large group at a subsequent meeting.

G. Wrap-Up

Thank participants for coming and let them know how much you valued their input and openness. Add a motivational pitch that reinforces teamwork and mutual respect.

Reprinted, with permission, from Albert Einstein Medical Center, Philadelphia, Pennsylvania.

If strained or nonsupportive relationships have existed between nurses and physicians in your organization, you don't have to *wait* for history to slowly take its course. You can act proactively and experimentally toward helping nurses and physicians *interact* their way into a more collaborative and empowering relationship that benefits patients, physicians, nurses, and onlookers. Convene nurses and physicians who are supposed to be working as care partners and build them as a team.

Hire Physician Liaisons to Ease the Physicians' Way

If you don't already have one, develop a physician relations function in which dedicated personnel serve as liaisons and ombudspeople with your physicians. Liaisons can arrange for special programs, expedite physician ease-of-practice problems, and serve as round-the-clock troubleshooters on physician concerns. Also identify department heads, nurse managers, and others whose jobs require that they interact with physicians. Develop them as an extended team of physician liaisons for the purpose of:

- Conveying the goals of your service strategy
- Soliciting complaints and suggestions from physicians
- Holding monthly one-on-one meetings with individual physicians to build strong relationships, invite and respond to their concerns, and communicate the hospital's priorities—including service excellence
- Aggressively pursuing systems changes and improvements by addressing two topics: how the hospital can improve the environment for the physicians, and how the hospital and its staff can better serve the physicians and their patients

Help Staff Relate to Physicians Effectively

Help employees influence individual physicians one by one so that they work better with the physicians. The following topics can do wonders for relationships, as staff can shape physician behavior through a concerted effort and with improved skills:

- Building positive relationships with difficult physicians
- Key skills in communicating with physicians
- Conflict resolution

☐ Final Suggestions

There are no panaceas here, but rest assured that hospitals have made headway with their physicians by involving them in strategy design and by experimenting with approaches that best fit their medical staff's culture and politics. As you proceed with physician involvement, consider these pointers:

- *Do something:* If you're afraid of physicians and allow your service strategy to suffer as a result, you alienate employees. Decide what you're going to do, tell your people, and do it. If it doesn't work, try something else.
- *No one has the secret formula:* If you wait for the perfect approach, you'll do nothing. However, doing something is vital. Experiment after consulting with the best advice givers you can find.
- *Create a mix of approaches:* Use approaches that engage physicians as members of your care team, some that treat physicians as valued customers, and some that consider physicians as open-minded learners who want to do right by patients.
- *Know your target groups and the politics of working with them:* If you're working with attending physicians, tailor your approach to them. If you're working with physician chiefs, consider their special problems. Generic programs miss these potential and specific targets.
- *Ask physicians how to reach physicians:* Even though you have experience with physicians, don't think you can read their minds or know what they need. Don't decide what's best for physicians without asking them.
- *Beware of stereotypes and generalizations:* Physicians are a varied lot. The numerous stereotypes about them—for example, "they blow in, blow up, and blow out"—may convey self-fulfilling expectations. Expect to find concerned physicians, and work with them. Don't assume people are too busy, disinterested, or "above it all."
- *Physicians deserve empathy too:* Many physicians are hurting; their roles are changing, and they're understandably unsettled and ill at ease. Their territories are being invaded by new competitors; they're frustrated with red tape and systems problems that interfere with their ability to serve their patients; and they're threatened by the specters of malpractice suits and the financial burden of malpractice insurance. Being a physician is no longer a piece of cake.

Getting active physician participation and partnership in your service strategy *from the start* is your best hope. Consider bringing in specialized consultants just for that reason. However, once physicians are actively involved, you'll see the effects reverberating throughout your organization and your market.

References

1. Fact-finder. *Healthcare Marketing Report* 5(3):4, Mar. 1987.

2. Membership services as a revenue center: cost justification and marketing impact of an aggressive service program. Technical Assistance Research Programs working paper, Washington, DC, Feb. 1986.

3. Alpert, P., and Alpert, G. Personal communication. Aug. 19, 1987.

4. Alpert.

5. Leebov, W., Vergare, M., and Scott, G. *Patient Satisfaction: A Guide to Practice Enhancement.* Oradell, NJ: Medical Economics Books, 1990.

6. Matthews, D., and Feinstein, A. A new instrument for patients' ratings of physician performance. *American Journal of Medical Sciences* 31(3):159-71, Mar. 1989.

7. Professional Research Consultants. *Marketing to Doctors* (Newsletter) [The Beckham Co., Omaha] 1(2), Dec. 1988.

8. Brown, S. W., and Morley, A. P. Jr. *Promoting Your Medical Practice.* Oradel, NJ: Medical Economics Books, 1989.

9. Leebov, W., Vergare, M., and Scott, G. *Patient Satisfaction: A Guide to Practice Enhancement.* Oradel, NJ: Medical Economics Books, 1990.

10. The nurse–doctor game. *Nursing91* 21(6):60–64, June 1991.

Chapter 11
Reward and Recognition

Once you've identified the behaviors that constitute service excellence and contributions to continuous improvement, you need to install reward and recognition systems to reinforce these behaviors and celebrate improvements in customer satisfaction and service delivery. You need to acknowledge and reward those who deserve recognition—individuals and groups who distinguish themselves by their exemplary energy, behavior, and contributions. Before proceeding with this chapter, take the self-test in figure 11-1.

Figure 11-1. Self-Test

Reward and Recognition. *Circle the appropriate answer. The more "true" answers, the better. "False" answers indicate areas that need improvement.*

1. Our organization routinely recognizes employees who are courteous, helpful, and responsive to customers. True False

2. Experimentation and initiative in making improvements are prized and recognized here. True False

3. Work groups, teams, and departments, not just individuals, are acknowledged when they provide excellent service or make service improvements. True False

4. In this organization, employees are quick to appreciate coworkers for their efforts on a customer's behalf. True False

5. Our department heads and supervisors give frequent pats on the back to their staff for positive service performance and contributions to service improvement. True False

6. Our compensation systems reflect and reinforce the value we place on excellent service. True False

7. We publicize staff contributions to service improvements. True False

8. We recognize physicians who excel in their interpersonal relationships with patients and staff. True False

9. When considering people for promotion, we take into account the quality of their service performance and their contributions to making improvements. True False

10. We celebrate service accomplishments in ways that revive and strengthen people's energy for and focus on service excellence. True False

Total: ___ ___

If you answered "true" to all 10 questions, you're certainly on course. If you have a low score on this pillar, reevaluate your systems for reinforcing service-oriented behaviors, skills, and activities valued throughout your organization.

Most caregivers thirst for recognition; they have a fundamental need to have their efforts on behalf of customers and the organization acknowledged and appreciated. Too many organizations, however, fail to link recognition to performance. Instead, they recognize employees merely for their presence, conveying the message that "it doesn't matter how you act and what you contribute, as long as you're *here!*"

Make your recognition practices advance your service mission and influence staff to go the extra mile for customers. To do this, recognize their excellent service behavior and contributions to service improvement.

Who should give rewards and recognition? Your organization's leadership, the employee's manager, peers, and customers. Who should receive rewards and recognition? Individuals on your staff, teams (improvement teams, departments, services, work groups), and managers.

For such a diverse pool of awarders and awardees, you clearly need a carefully designed mix of strategies. Most systems already in place—for example, "Employee of the Year" or "Employee of the Month"—don't recognize enough winners. Every minute of the day in the health care arena, someone is performing acts of compassion. Competitive recognition methods among providers need to be supplemented with methods that allow for infinite winners and the reinforcement of teamwork and collaboration in the service of customers.

This chapter will present a variety of methods selected to reflect the following beliefs:

- Individuals need to be rewarded for improvement, not just excellence. People just starting to refine their skills may take a while to smooth out the rough edges, even though they're working hard at it. You should be generous with encouragement.
- Teams need to be rewarded. Health care staff are necessarily interdependent. Service improvements happen when coworkers and departments cross turf lines and develop delivery improvements together, recognizing that each party is a link in an interlocking chain of steps that constitute service processes. By rewarding only individuals, you breed unhealthy competition and downplay the power of teams.
- Specific behaviors (not "global goodness") that contribute to your organization's service quality should be rewarded. Whatever method of recognition you choose (a feature article in your newsletter, a special display, a mention at a department meeting, a note from administration, a prize, or a commendation form, for example), you must make it clear that *service behaviors* are being rewarded.

☐ Key Strategies for Implementing Methods of Recognition

To recognize employees for excellent service behaviors, consider these strategies when designing the best mix of methods for your organization:

- Audit your current reward and recognition practices to identify the impact they have on people's energy to excel on service dimensions. Then create a long-term improvement plan.
- Align your compensation system with your service mission.
- Ensure that managers recognize staff efforts in everyday words and deeds.
- Recognize teams for satisfying customers and taking steps to improve service.
- Recognize managers who exemplify your service commitment.
- Create positive feedback loops from external customers (patients and physicians) to staff.
- Make it easy for coworkers and peers to recognize each other for excellent service.

- Use visual and written media to recognize service contributions.
- Use recognition campaigns to focus attention and improvement on specific service needs (for example, phone skills).
- Celebrate your service mission and service accomplishments with occasional hoopla.

Audit Your Current Mix of Practices

Does your organization's mix of reward and recognition methods advance your service mission? Practices in many health care organizations suffer these weaknesses:

- The objectives for certain practices are sometimes unclear or they change over time without a conscious decision to change them.
- Many administrative teams continue practices just because they started them, without evaluating whether they still have the desired effect on target beneficiaries.
- Organizations have instituted reward and recognition practices without analyzing whether those charged with implementing them have adequate time and energy to do so effectively. The result is an undue burden on uncommitted managers.
- Typically, insufficient input is solicited from those who will implement the system and from those targeted for rewards before a new practice is instituted. Consequently, reward ideas are neither tested sufficiently nor debugged, which can defeat the strategy.

An audit can signal which practices should be enhanced or streamlined, which ones should be suspended in order to support your service mission. Specifically, a recognition audit enables you to:

- Evaluate your current recognition and reward programs from the point of view of your staff (employees and physicians), and check the fit between actual and intended results of these practices. Employee perceptions of theoretically wonderful reward systems have shown that these systems, although well intended, often have effects that are the opposite of those desired.
- Provide a framework or process for future decisions about which strategies to retain, add, or eliminate so that you have an effective, comprehensive program that is perceived well by your staff and is consistent with your service mission.

A group or committee can conduct the audit of your current practices. Focus groups can help you get started. For example, you might convene a diverse group of 12 employees and physicians for four different reasons at four different times during your recognition and reward decision-making process:

- *Focus Group 1: Take stock.* This focus group should ask:
  - What does this organization do to recognize and reward positive service performance and service improvements?
  - What does the organization do to recognize individual employees, physicians, and departments?
  - What methods are currently in use, and how do you feel about each one?
  - Where are the flaws in the current recognition and reward systems?
  - Where are the strengths?
- *Focus Group 2: Generate new options.* This focus group should ask:
  - What behavior related to service quality should be rewarded?
  - What rewards would work? What do employees value?
  - What methods can we use that may be effective?
  After you refine what your committee gleans as the best of the ideas, submit your tentative decisions to focus group 3.

- *Focus Group 3: Solicit reactions to the favored approaches before you implement them.* The focus group should ask the following questions about each proposed strategy:
  - —What's your reaction to it?
  - —What do you like about it?
  - —What bothers you about it?
  - —How can we strengthen it?
  - —What does its success depend on?
  - —What might make it fail?
  - —What can we do to make it work?
  After you have tested each suggested strategy, incorporate the advice from the focus group and implement your strategies for a limited trial period. Then reconvene members of your focus group for focus group 4.
- *Focus Group 4: Obtain feedback after your trial period and decide about the future.* This focus group should ask the following questions:
  - —How aware have you been of the new strategy?
  - —What's your reaction to it?
  - —Do you like or dislike it? Why?
  - —How can it work better?
  - —What else can our hospital do to strengthen its reward systems?

To determine the success of reward and recognition strategies, you have to find out how your employees perceive them. Good ideas on paper can bomb in real-life application. Perceptions are what matter, because recognition strategies are meant to raise awareness and reinforce what people are supposed to be doing so that the rewarded behavior becomes contagious.

Align Your Compensation System with Your Service Mission

Compensation practices raise a dilemma. Each employee makes myriad decisions daily about how to behave with customers. Of course, we want employees to choose behaviors that meet or exceed customer needs. Because some people behave better toward customers than others, it makes sense to reward some more than others.

On the other hand, customer satisfaction and continuous improvement are results of people working together. It's essential to send the message that cooperation is all-important. If your compensation systems are competitive, they tell people just the opposite—that the way to get more is to compete with each other. The following three subsections explore pros and cons of different compensation systems.

Merit Pay

In theory, merit pay is a good way to reward excellent service behavior. It reinforces positive work and motivates employees to try to do their best. However, as the mainstay for service or performance excellence, it breaks down for the following reasons:

- Pay is rarely connected to specific acts of service excellence. Both manager and employee lose sight of the link between pay and specific performance because of time lapse between act and compensation.
- Typically, the employee's goals and objectives are unclear or unrealistic. So linking rewards to vague goals and objectives makes little sense.
- Managers often base merit pay on nonperformance factors that may be subjective in nature. That is, managers may use whatever flexibility they have in merit pay decisions to reward what they personally value or to right other wrongs as they perceive them. Sometimes, length of service is rewarded as merit pay. In some instances, managers may reward mediocre work performance by a person they think has untapped potential, thinking that being rewarded will spur the person

to new levels of achievement. Many managers "fix" perceived inequities by using merit pay to help employees who earn less than their coworkers. The result in each of these examples is that the fundamental relationship between performance and merit pay has fizzled.

- The secrecy surrounding pay produces a knee-jerk perception of inequity. When performance appraisals aren't linked to clear and precise objectives and standards, secrecy flourishes because managers worry that their salary decisions will raise doubt and anger. So they become "loudly quiet." In "Merit Pay: Fact or Fiction," Edward Lawler III points out that in an atmosphere of secrecy, employees over-estimate [not underestimate] the pay of their peers.[1] This perception hampers the potentially motivating effects of merit pay.
- The increase pool has a low ceiling, especially in health care. If hospitals had enough money, maybe merit pay would work. However, most health care organizations are hurting financially and don't have enough money in the pool for increases to include significant rewards for performance. Typically a department is allotted a fixed percentage increase in its salary budget. Thus pay is determined not by performance, but by the size of the year's salary pool. Most managers use performance ratings to justify the only raises they can afford. Pay increases are only motivating in the long run if they cause a significant change in a person's overall financial condition. For most people, a significant change means at least a 15 percent raise.
- Because the increase pool is limited, merit pay is essentially a competitive system. It's a zero-sum game in which employees compete with each other for their share of the merit pool. If one employee "wins big," then others have to compensate accordingly by smaller raises—not much incentive for employees to improve team-work. In fact, this game may lead employees to backbite, sabotage, and fine-tune their political skills rather than their service or performance skills.
- Merit pay is grounded in the importance of individual performance. Yet most quality experts assert that about 85 percent of all service problems are a function of faulty systems and processes, not faulty employee performance. And systems and processes are generally fixed best by *teams*, not individuals.

Alternatives to Merit Pay
Because merit pay is adequate as a means of rewarding employees for service skills, you have to replace or complement it with other means that are more immediate, potentially more generous, and more reinforcing of teamwork and cooperation rather than competition. Compensation trends are moving away from step systems, in which employees get automatic raises year after year, toward systems in which employees are paid according to the market value of their jobs and motivated by bonuses based on individual—especially team—performance *if* the organization has done well enough financially to create a bonus pool. Following are some examples of alternatives to merit pay:

- *Gain sharing:* If excellent service enhances your organization's revenue potential, then gain sharing makes sense as an option. With gain sharing, a formula dictates how you divide up a portion of the organization's margin.
- *Win sharing:* With win sharing, you can define specific goals and, if money is available, reward individuals and teams according to goal attainment. For instance, staff of nursing units that achieve a targeted customer satisfaction level receive a certain percentage of the available money pool. The wave of the future is to use customer ratings, not supervisor ratings, to drive reward systems.
- *Zero-based individual bonus systems:* Employees receive base pay according to the market value of their jobs. Bonuses are given (if money is available) based on whichever behavior you want to reinforce; for example, teamwork, customer satisfaction results, or excellent service performance as judged by peer ratings. Or you

203

can install a system in which every individual has performance objectives that align with your service goals and then reward them based on how well they attain their individual goals.

- *Team incentives:* Some organizations supplement base salaries only with incentives for teamwork; for example, team satisfaction scores and process improvements made by teams.
- *Individual incentives:* At an IBM plant in Austin, Texas, employees earn $50 every time they serve on an ad hoc improvement team (they are limited to eight teams per year). At the end of the year, the best projects are selected, and three teams receive $15,000 apiece to divide among their members. This is only one example of how individual incentives might work.
- *Hybrids:* Hybrid systems can be an amalgam of merit systems with gain sharing, team incentives, or skill-based bonuses. For example, Motorola's Government Electronics Group has a semitraditional merit system *and* gain sharing, and a recognition program that provides immediate rewards to individuals and teams, *and* a team-incentive program.

The key to aligning your compensation practices with your service mission is to observe the following recommendations:

- Make sure financial incentives or raises are linked to clear contributions to service quality and customer satisfaction. Otherwise, you feed into an all-too-prevalent entitlement mind-set in which employees think that, "Because I come to work every day, I *deserve* more money." (This is the other side of the presence mind-set mentioned at the beginning of this chapter.)
- Ensure that your methods fit your mission and values. Only then will people recognize their inherent rationality and accept them. Because your mission and values are unique to your organization, you need a system that's tailored to your organization's culture.
- Involve employees in the design. Their input is invaluable in determining what measurements you'll use. You'll also benefit from their reactions to proposed plans and changes. Use employee and manager focus groups to test proposed changes and implementation plans.

Recognition, Not Reward

It's ironic that, despite the emphasis on compensation (real money) as a reward, the most effective methods for reinforcing service excellence and contributions to continuous improvement involve not money but recognition and gestures of appreciation. Some of these include:

- Tangible or intangible thanks for a job well done
- Opportunities for personal growth and development
- Increased job autonomy
- Enhanced status in the eyes of others
- A better work environment

Because such gestures make the best rewards, don't worry about your inability to raise the salary of every employee who demonstrates excellent service. Instead, spend your energy ensuring that they get what they deserve from the multitude of other meaningful rewards possible.

Ensure That Managers Provide Recognition to Staff in Everyday Words and Deeds

Think of how you'd feel if your boss called you on the phone for no other reason than to say, "I just wanted you to know that I think you're doing a great job in getting your employees more service oriented. I've really seen a difference and I appreciate all you're doing." Imagine receiving a card that reads "Bravo, your department achieved a terrific level of patient satisfaction this month. Please spread the word about how much we appreciate everybody's hard work!"

Recognition by managers and supervisors is the number-one best strategy. They need to acknowledge the contribution their employees make to the organization's important mission. To illustrate the point, when you ask street sweepers at a Disney theme park how they like their job, they respond, "I'm not a street sweeper, I'm in show business." When you ask bricklayers how they like being bricklayers, they respond, "I'm not a bricklayer, I'm a cathedral builder." What these responses have in common is that they reflect workers whose managers probably have express appreciation for their contribution.

Managers and supervisors also need to be generous with thanks and positive feedback. In a survey of nearly 30 reward and recognition programs at a large university hospital, employees cited "pats on the back from my supervisor" as the single most powerful incentive. However, despite being told that employees crave recognition, supervisors aren't always comfortable giving it. Perhaps they fear employee complacency or dependence on praise. Other managers withhold recognition because they don't get any or they take good behavior for granted and intervene only when problems arise. Still others are just plain mean-spirited when it comes to giving out positives. This kind of emotional starvation is probably one of the biggest problems an organization can have and one with the direst consequences. Managers can be effective only if they fuel their staff's sense of self-worth.

Revive positive feedback skills among managers and supervisors. Offer training to refresh their skills so that they give active, frequent, and generous reinforcement to employees. You must keep reminding managers that this is part of their job. Those who fail in this regard should be relieved from their position. Four components of excellent positive feedback are behavior, consequence, empathy with and recognition of good intentions, and appreciation.

Following is an example of a format that uses these elements in giving positive feedback:

- *Behavior:* "I noticed you sitting with Mrs. Higgins instead of going to lunch."
- *Consequence:* "Doing so helped calm her about her diagnosis, and it also demonstrated the kind of compassion that helps you, our department, and our hospital maintain the positive image we need to attract patients."
- *Empathy and recognition:* "I realize you missed your lunch hour, which I know is a much-needed break."
- *Appreciation:* "Helen, I really appreciate it."

Commendation letters are a more formal kind of recognition than everyday feedback. They provide a permanent record of positive employee performance. Also, service consultant Gail Murphy suggests that managers and supervisors keep on hand a supply of postcards like that shown in figure 11-2 to make thank-yous quick and easy.

There are many powerful, nonmonetary ways to reward outstanding service and contributions, as shown in the checklists in figures 11-3 and 11-4 (by Goodmeasure, Inc.). Use these examples with managers and supervisors to audit their current practices and set goals to enhance them.

Recognize Teams for Satisfying Customers and Taking Steps to Improve Service

It is not enough to reward acts of individual excellence. Recognition strategies that focus only on individuals risk being perceived as popularity contests, promoting negative competitive feelings; others prompt questions about fairness ("Why Helen and not me?"). Some fail to give a fair chance to employees in less visible departments.

Figure 11-2. Postcard Showing Appreciation

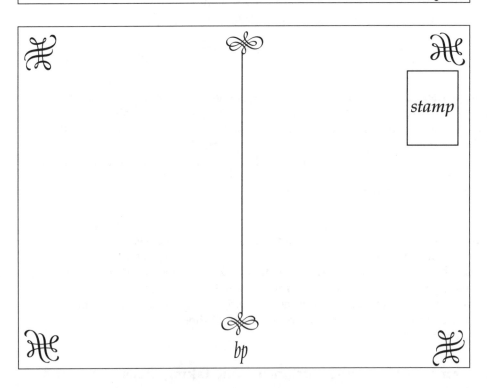

ap·pre·ci·ate (ə-prē'shē-āt')

1. To grasp the nature, worth, quality or significance of. 2. To value or admire highly. 3. To recognize with gratitude. 4. To hold in high esteem.

I appreciate you!

stamp

bp

Reprinted, with permission, from Gail Murphy, Philadelphia, Pennsylvania.

Figure 11-3. Checklist of Methods for Rewarding Outstanding Service

Actions	What I Do Now	What I Plan to Do
Greet employees when you pass by their desks or pass them in the hall.		
Have coffee or lunch with an employee or a group of employees.		
Thank your boss, peers, and employees when they have done something well or have done something to help you.		
Give credit where it's due when discussing an idea with other people, peers, or higher management.		
Involve employees in the discussion, analysis, and development or recommendations of issues they have shown interest in.		
Give special assignments to people who have shown initiative.		
Mention the outstanding work or idea brought to your attention by an employee at staff meetings.		
Mention the latest contributions of your employees and corrective action teams at meetings with your peers and management.		
Present "state-of-the-place" reports periodically to your employees and acknowledge their work.		
Ask your boss to attend a meeting with your employees in which you thank individuals and groups for their specific contributions.		
Ask individuals and groups to be part of or make presentations of their ideas and recommendations to higher management and to their own peers.		

Reprinted with permission from Rosabeth Moss Kanter and Barry A. Stein of Goodmeasure, Inc., One Memorial Drive, Cambridge, MA 02142, 617-621-3838. This material is from *Solving Quality and Productivity Problems: Goodmeasure's Guide to Corrective Action,* published by ASQC Press, Milwaukee, 1983, 414-272-8575.

Figure 11-4. Checklist of Ways Management Can Recognize Employee Contributions to Quality Improvement

Possible Actions	What I Plan to Do
• Send a letter to every problem-solving team member when they establish a team, thanking them for their involvement.	
• Briefly attend the first meeting of a problem-solving team and express your appreciation of their involvement.	
• Hold a luncheon meeting with every problem-solving team once they have interim findings. Express your appreciation and provide the lunch.	
• Hold a thank-you ceremony at the completion of a team's work. Provide breakfast, lunch, or refreshments. Invite their peers and higher management if possible.	
• Send a letter to problem-solving team members at the termination of their work thanking them for their contribution.	
• Establish a place to display information, posters, pictures, and so on thanking individual employees and problem-solving teams and describing their contributions.	

Reprinted with permission from Rosabeth Moss Kanter and Barry A. Stein of Goodmeasure, Inc., One Memorial Drive, Cambridge, MA 02142, 617-621-3838. This material is from *Solving Quality and Productivity Problems: Goodmeasure's Guide to Corrective Action,* published by ASQC Press, Milwaukee, 1983, 414-272-8575.

Another significant shortcoming is that team spirit, group pride and unity, and mutual cooperation for the sake of the group go unrewarded at a time when, more than ever, department staff need to see themselves as service givers to other department staff, pulling together as a team. Therefore, recognition strategies should include ways of commending *group* efforts that help the organization.

Some hospitals hold contests that reward a department or unit for initiating the best user-friendly improvements, improvements that enabled that department or unit to better serve its internal and external customers. Possible rewards might be to include in your publications and on bulletin boards pictures of the winning group with articles highlighting their achievements, augmented with a gift for the department or unit (for example, a microwave, new lounge chairs, $300 to spend as they please, a luncheon).

Consider also "Best Performance by a Department"–a method developed at Mother Frances Hospital in Tyler, Texas, as part of their Stars Program. The Stars committee invites individual departments to nominate a department (other than their own) by submitting their nomination on an Oscar Nomination Form that asks for the reasons why this department's performance is exceptional (see figure 11-5). The Stars Committee reviews all nominations and selects one department per quarter to receive the award based on established criteria. The winning department receives a gold Oscar inscribed, "Best Performance by a Department." The Oscar stays with the winning department until the next winner is announced. The winning department receives special recognition and is a member of the institution's Department Hall of Fame. Departments winning multiple times receive special recognition.

Internal customer satisfaction surveys can also be used to select the Department of the Month. Departments are asked to rate one another on key service dimensions (for example, responsiveness to phone calls, keeping service agreements, and customer orientation). You can then recognize the departments that score best and also the ones that show the most improvement.

Roanoke Memorial Hospital enhanced their Department of the Month program with a monthly sporting event in which the winning department challenged the last month's

Figure 11-5. Form to Nominate Best Performance by a Department

Best Performance by a Department

Is there a department or unit (other than your own) that you feel performs in an exceptional manner? Nominate them for the quarterly Oscar Award for Best Performance by a Department! The Stars Committee reviews all nominations and awards the Oscar to the winning department. The winners keep the Oscar during their reign and receive special recognition and entry into the Department Hall of Fame.

This is your chance to reward greatness!

I nominate _____ Department for the Oscar award for stellar performance!

These are ways this department consistently gives an outstanding performance:

_____

_____

_____

_____

_____

Name _____ Extension _____

Department _____

Send your nomination to the Guest Relations Department

winner in a well-publicized volleyball game that attracted throngs. The Big Game provided an excuse to call repeated attention to flagship departments. Everyone is invited to the Big Game, and at half-time people celebrate the new Department of the Month, which receives a banner that reads "We're the Department of the Month" to hang in their workspace.

The seven-facility Lake Hospital System in Ohio developed a team recognition system to reinforce the importance of interdepartmental teams and their accomplishments at Lake Hospital System. Here's how it works:

- A Team Recognition Day kicked off the strategy.
- Team Recognition bulletin boards were set up in all facilities.
- Team profiles and team pictures were requested from all departments.
- A rotation schedule was set up and the display was scheduled for at least one week at each facility.
- The 5 × 7 team picture was framed and returned to the departments for posting at the end of the rotation schedule.

Also consider "Milestone Recognition." In your quest for continuous improvement, you can spark employee commitment and energy by recognizing a department or work group when its service performance improves. Some managers identify specific milestones or benchmarks that they will celebrate with staff when these milestones are reached.

Picture the football team patting each other on the back after a great play and moving immediately into planning their next winning move. That's the spirit you want to capture with milestone recognition. You gather the team together, create a "Hurray for Us" atmosphere, and then engage the team in planning its next loftier goal and winning moves.

- Present the results on a banner. (For example, "We satisfied 5 percent more of our customers this month compared to last month!") Or post a big trend chart that shows this.
- Offer a toast to the group expressing your admiration.
- Invite team members to toast one another and the group, identifying people and actions that they believe contributed to this success.
- Eat together, provide a token of esteem (for example, a mug inscribed with "We're on the upswing") or have a subgroup of staff do a skit or do a mutual award ceremony in which pairs of people prepare awards for one another and then present them.

Another approach to team recognition needs to happen at the work-group level. Managers need to create opportunities for staff to recognize coworkers within the team. If people are helped to feel a sense of importance, not invisibility at the work-group level, they rely considerably less on recognition from higher-ups who don't see their work close up. Managers can make this kind of recognition happen during staff meetings. For example, they can facilitate short activities that recognize many staff members for their efforts. The "Proud Whip" is an example:

Proud Whip

- At the beginning or end of a staff meeting, announce, "We're going to take time out to recognize each other at a personal level by conducting an activity called "Proud Whip."
- Ask each employee to complete one of the following sentence starters. Then go around and ask each person to share their sentence with the larger group. "One service interaction I am most proud of this week is _____."

"One difficult situation I handled skillfully this week was _____."
"One way I'm proud to say I've grown or changed for the better on the job is _____."
"One way I've contributed to making things better here is _____."
"One thing I'm proud of about our department's services is _____."
. . . and other sentence starters you devise.

Following are some additional ways to recognize teams/departments:

- *Ring in success:* When positive monthly evaluation results come in, ring a bell and invite employees to convene for a quick announcement and popcorn or cookies.
- *Give the team resources for meeting service targets:* For each month that a department meets its service targets, put money into an employee fund to be used to enhance the department's quality of life (microwave, coffee machine).
- *Recognize one whole department or unit:* Each month, feature a department or unit in your organization's publication. Make sure you give extra attention to the behind-the-scenes departments that rarely get the attention they deserve. You might, for example, send pizza to an especially hardworking unit or present its staff with a surprise brunch or a thank-you visit from top management.

In today's stressful health care environment, team recognition needs to be stepped up. People need to pull together for a common purpose to satisfy your customers consistently and spiritedly.

Recognize Managers Who Exemplify Your Service Commitment

Manager recognition systems can acknowledge managers who have been able to instill a service excellence culture among employees and encourage the role modeling of desirable service behaviors and management styles. A manager can be selected by other managers using objective criteria such as his or her department's scores on an internal customer satisfaction survey, or a list of behaviors reflecting a service commitment on the part of the manager. This recognition usually includes a monetary award. The hospital also recognizes achievements by individual managers by sending a personalized letter of appreciation to the manager and including a copy in his or her personnel file.

The Arlington Hospital in Arlington, Virginia, instituted a Manager of the Quarter program. In a letter, managers and nonmanagers nominate a department head or supervisor for Manager of the Quarter, giving reasons for the nomination. At their quarterly supervisors meeting, the CEO announces the winner, who receives an engraved plaque, an escape weekend for two at a resort, and a free reserved parking space for three months.

Create Positive Feedback Loops from External Customers to Staff

Use positive feedback from customers to recognize employee service excellence. Chris Lee describes the ultimate reward of using customer ratings to determine a substantial portion of employee compensation.[2] Although difficult, customer satisfaction ratings can be designed into gain-sharing programs. But consider also using these ratings to trigger "thanks" and other incentives.

When patients report good behavior on the part of a caregiver, great lengths should be taken to ensure that the parties complimented know about it and that management does too. Many hospitals have carefully monitored and efficient processes for channeling all complimentary letters from patients to the people complimented, their supervisors, and their teams and for including with the letter a note of appreciation from the chief executive officer.

Good Samaritan Hospital in Cincinnati, Ohio, provides patients with a "Service First Gram" to make it easy for them to compliment staff (see figure 11-6). The UCLA Medical

Figure 11-6. "Service First Gram"

SERVICE FIRST
GRAM

Compassion, Care, and Respect

Employee: _____

Department: _____

Description of Service: _____

_____

_____

_____

_____

_____

_____

                           Signed: _____

                        Address: _____

                                   _____

                             Date: _____

------------------------------ Detach ------------------------------

SERVICE FIRST GRAM
Compassion, Care, and Respect

If you like the service one of our employees or departments has provided for you or a family member, we'd like to know about it. Please send us a Service First Gram today! Return it by mail or drop it off at either lobby information desk on your way out.

Reprinted, with permission, from Good Samaritan Hospital, Cincinnati, Ohio.

Center has a Humanistic Care Award Committee that recognizes employees who have received multiple compliments from patients by inviting them to a special luncheon and awards presentation. Patients are invited to compliment employees using the form in figure 11-7.

Here's how the Humanistic Care Award Program works:

Description: The Employee Humanistic Care Award is to be given each month to two employees, two employee groups, or to one nominee in each category who has been identified through patient feedback questionnaires as deserving special recognition. Each winner or group receives a check for $250, a special certificate, and a pin.

Eligibility: All Medical Center employees are eligible for the award, including outpatient areas, provided the employees are nominated by a patient. Finalists in one month are eligible for reconsideration in following months within that calendar year. Once selected as a winner, an employee is not eligible for the award until the following year. At the beginning of each calendar year, the selection process begins again with previous nominations and records being removed from consideration.

Figure 11-7. Form Inviting Patients to Compliment Employees

Please Let Us Know

Dear Patient:

We want you to feel that you are treated in a very special and caring way while you are a patient at UCLA Medical Center. We encourage our employees to offer that "personal touch" that will make a difference for you.

Because this is so important to us, we have a program here to recognize staff who show particular concern or caring to our patients. We want to identify those staff members, and we need your help to do this.

If an employee has given you exceptional service, would you please fill in his/her name on the attached card below.

You've probably met people here in the following classifications. You may want to consider these various people in making your choice.

Admissions Counselor	Patient Escorts
Cashiers	Patient Liaisons
Financial Counselor	Pharmacists
Floor Clerks	Physical/Occupational Therapists
Food Servers	Respiratory Therapists
Hospital Volunteers	Social Workers
Housekeepers	Telephone Operators
Information Desk Personnel	X-Ray Technicians
Medical Records Staff	Other Staff
Nurses	

Please fill out the lower part of this card, detach on perforated line, and mail.

....

Please print the name and title of your nominee on the appropriate lines below:

Name _____

Title _____

Can you tell us why you selected the person you did? What specifically did this employee do that impressed you?

_____

_____

_____

_____

_____

_____

_____

_____

Patient Name _____
(PLEASE PRINT)

Date of Admission _____/_____/_____

Room Number _____

May we have your permission to share your comments with the employee?   ☐ Yes   ☐ No

Reprinted, with permission, from UCLA Medical Center, Los Angeles, California.

Selection Process: A nomination form is submitted by a patient(s) nominating a particular employee for the Humanistic Care Award. The nomination and comments for each nominee are recorded in the department of human resources. At the end of each month, the cards are reviewed by human resources personnel and at least one other member of the committee, and the employee finalists for that month's awards are selected.

The supervisors of these finalists are interviewed individually. A final profile sheet for each finalist is then prepared from these interviews and submitted to the Employee Humanistic Care Award committee for final selection.

Selection Committee: The Employee Humanistic Care Award committee selects the two monthly winners. The committee is composed of six members, representing a cross-section of the hospital management group, and two human resource representatives. Committee members are selected through invitation, based on their management position within the hospital, their department, and their expressed interest in the award program. Committee members serve for one year and can remain longer by choice, provided their attendance and participation have been satisfactory.

Awards Announcement: There is a monthly presentation to award winners in the office of the director of the UCLA Medical Center. Recipients, their immediate supervisors, directors, and associate directors are invited to attend the ceremony. The director of human resources and the chairperson of the Employee Humanistic Care Award Committee are also present. In addition to the awards ceremony, the monthly *Medi-Scene* newsletter publishes an article on the winners and the human resources department posts their picture in the hospital lobby.

Selection Criteria: Finalists for the awards are evaluated by the committee based on a dozen criteria:

1. Number of nominations received
2. Quality of the nominations and comments received
3. Position within the Medical Center and job expectations regarding patient relations (humanistic behavior)
4. Supervisory comments
5. Overall job performance evaluation
6. Working relationship with coworkers
7. Other previous patient comments
8. Supervisory assessment of overall patient relationships
9. Years of employment
10. Other awards, recognition
11. Total number of employees within departments from which nominations are received
12. Departments represented by previous Humanistic Care Award winners

One way to discover what your patients value most, while at the same time rewarding outstanding performance among your nursing staff, is through a program called Report a Nurse. On randomly selected days, maybe twice a month, ask patients to report nurses who perform outstanding service. You can get patients involved by flashing an announcement on the patient television or by placing cards on meal trays. Patients are invited to make their reports by phoning a certain number. The person answering the phone must find out specifically what the nurse did that so impressed the caller. Volunteers can then deliver a rose or a lapel pin and a thank-you note commending the nurse.

The Report a Nurse program is an easy way to gain valuable data on what patients like. It is also a terrific morale booster among these too-often-unsung champions.

At Copley Memorial Hospital in Aurora, Illinois, a note on patient trays once a week asks patients to report staff who've made a positive difference for them. The staff person identified then receives the thank-you card shown in figure 11-8.

Figure 11-8. Thank-You Card: Copley Memorial Hospital

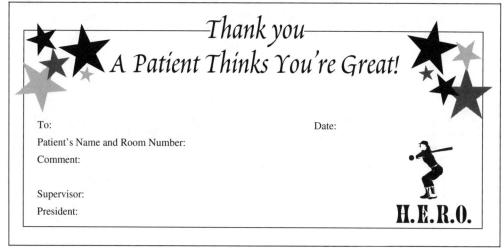

Also consider recognition triggered by survey questionnaires and letters from customers, since these at once link employees to their customers and remind employees of the power of customer feedback. The hospital distributes a customer satisfaction questionnaire to patients and/or family members, physicians, and visitors to obtain feedback on their satisfaction with services rendered. The questionnaire states that staff or departments mentioned as exemplary will be acknowledged through a letter to the employee or department. Figure 11-9 is an example of a letter of congratulations to a department with improved patient satisfaction ratings.

Make It Easy for Coworkers and Peers to Recognize Each Other for Excellent Service

The most popular approaches to peer recognition are variations of the Employee-of-the-Quarter program. Figure 11-10 describes the program at HCA Riveredge Hospital in suburb outside Chicago. Recognizing that programs like these inevitably have few "winners," many hospitals also have some variation of the Catcher program started at the Albert Einstein Medical Center in 1982. This program recognized a number of people daily for doing something wonderful. The objectives of the program were to:

- Reinforce excellent customer relations behavior, especially the extra efforts people make that are related to your behavioral expectations (for example, House Rules)
- Reinforce this behavior as soon as it occurs
- Reinforce this behavior in several people when they are "caught" doing something nice
- Encourage people to watch for and catch others doing something nice and compliment them for it

In the Catcher program, every month a squad of 20 employees and physicians were selected. Their job was to watch for instances of positive customer relations. "Catchers" who witnessed positive customer relations incidents were taught to approach the staff members who performed the acts, compliment them, find out their names and departments, and give them "hospital circle member" ribbons to attach to their ID badges, a coupon (figure 11-11), and an explanation of how to redeem the coupon. The "catcher" recorded the names of ribbon and coupon recipients and what they did to deserve them. The commendation was entered into the person's personnel file.

Coupon recipients could redeem them for a free drink in the cafeteria or coffee shop. On a quarterly basis, every person who received a coupon also became eligible for a drawing of prizes that have been donated to the hospital—for example, gift certificates, tickets to sports events and the theater, or dinner for two at a local restaurant.

"Catchers" were oriented to the program and given a packet containing the House Rules, ribbons, coupons, and commendation sheets. They were instructed not to award

Figure 11-9. Congratulations Letter

The 15 members of our Housekeeping Department, whose names are listed below, are being honored for their outstanding service this month. The department received seven letters of appreciation from patients as well as a big compliment from Drs. Wilson and Brown for excellent service before, during, and after their quarterly physician meeting.

In addition, the approval rating in our patient satisfaction survey is up from 79 percent to 84 percent and it's been noted that turnaround time for cleaning spills is down from 15 minutes to less than 10.

The hospital administration and the Service Excellence Committee salute our Housekeeping Department and its outstanding service-oriented members:

[list names, including management]

Figure 11-10. Hospital Employee-of-the-Quarter Program

It is the policy of HCA Riveredge Hospital to provide special recognition to those employees who demonstrate:

- A commitment to the mission of HCA Riveredge Hospital;
- Dedication to the goals and objectives of customer care as defined by Service Excellence:
  —Outstanding and extraordinary work performance
  —The qualities of QUEST (Quality through Understanding, Excellence, Service, and Teamwork)

Procedure

1) A nominating form will be available outside the Human Resources department or from PNAs/Dept. Directors.
2) Any employee can nominate any other employee (managerial staff excluded) whom he/she feels meets the criteria by completing the nomination form and returning it to Human Resources.
3) Human Resources will check the personnel file of all nominees to ensure there are no disciplinary actions or major problems with work performance.
4) Human Resources will give the completed forms to the committee chairperson for review. Employee names may be removed to ensure objectivity.
5) Committee members will meet, review all nominees, and vote for one by secret ballot. Each nominee will be considered on individual merit, not by the number of nominations received. If a tie occurs, the two nominations will be reviewed again, and a second vote taken.
6) The chairperson will count the votes and announce the "Employee of the Quarter" to the committee.
7) Administration, Human Resources, and the winner's department head will be notified of selection by the chairperson. A congratulatory letter will be drafted by Human Resources for the Executive Director's signature outlining the particulars. Administration will then arrange to personally present the selected individual with this letter.
8) Human Resources will make arrangements for refreshments through Dietary, will complete the check request, and send on to payroll for processing. HR will also arrange for the parking space through Plant Operations.
9) Administration will present awards to the selected employee at a special reception arranged at a mutually convenient time, usually 3 p.m., in the hospital cafeteria. In this photographed ceremony, the winner will receive $50, a reserved parking space near the hospital entrance, two meal tickets, and a day off with pay to be taken during the quarter.
10) Photographs and/or an announcement will be placed in the next issue of the employee newsletter. No employee can win more than once per year.
11) Each Employee of the Quarter will be automatically considered for the annual Employee of the Year award.

Q. U. E. S. T.

Employee of the Quarter Nominating Form

The Employee of the Quarter is the employee who not only exhibits a positive helpful attitude to those with whom he/she works, but also one who consistently exemplifies the qualities of Q.U.E.S.T. (Quality through Understanding, Excellence, Service, and Teamwork).

Person You Are Nominating:

Department in Which He/She Works:

Special Qualities That Demonstrate How This Person Exemplifies Our Q.U.E.S.T.:

Quality through:

Understanding _____

Excellence _____

Service _____

Teamwork _____

Additional Specific Reasons You Are Nominating This Person:

_____

_____

_____

Reprinted, with permission, from HCA Riveredge Hospital, Forest Park, Illinois.

Figure 11-11. "Catcher" Coupon

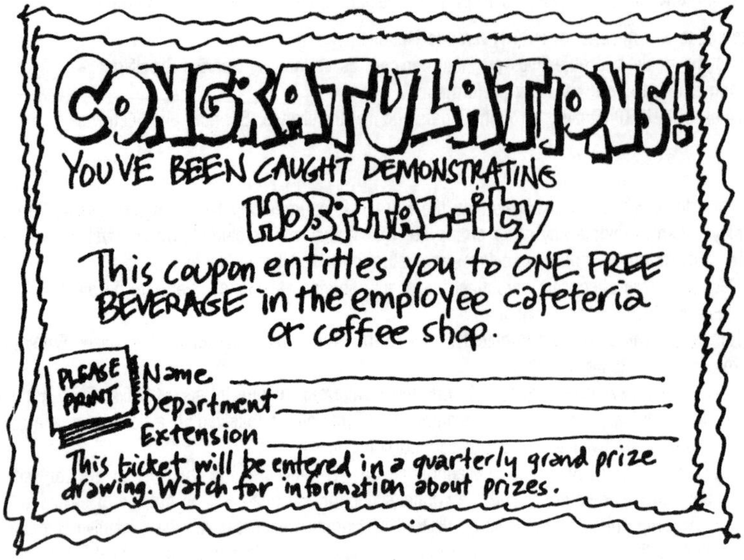

Reprinted, with permission, from Albert Einstein Healthcare Foundation, Philadelphia, Pennsylvania, 1983.

a ribbon to anyone in their own department. At the end of the month, a "catchers" wrap-up party was held so that "catchers" could share experiences, be thanked for their efforts, and receive a certificate of service signed by a top administrator.

Another approach to peer recognition involves creating a form and structure that prompt administrators, managers, or all employees to send "Appreciation Telegrams" recognizing a person for an act of cooperation, teamwork, going the extra step, or noticeable warmth and hospitality (see figure 11-12). Some hospitals set up "Appreciation Telegrams" as a project of the volunteer department. An employee, patient, or anyone else can call up and dictate a telegram, to be delivered by a volunteer. Some organizations charge 50 cents and use this tactic as a fund-raising project. At the University of Missouri-Columbia Hospital and Clinics, employees, physicians, visitors, patients, and, in fact, anyone can take a "You're Super" form from hallway racks if they want to express appreciation to anyone in the organization.

Peer recognition can extend to your facility's physicians too. Instead of complaining about physicians who don't uphold your strategy, recognize those who do. Develop service criteria for physicians to meet (for example, "Treat staff at all levels with dignity and respect; pitch in and help other staff serve the patient; be attentive, caring, and compassionate with patients"). Invite physicians and employees to nominate those who excel on these dimensions. Select winners by committee or vote. Present awards at a high-visibility event such as the annual physicians' dinner. As professional associations for physicians have discovered, peer approval is a powerful incentive for physicians.

Use Visual and Written Media to Recognize Service Contributions

Make provisions for individual contributors and teams to be lauded in available public media. For example:

- Verbatim comments from the Patient Delights Board at HCA West Paces Medical Center in Atlanta, Georgia, Caught Ya program are organized into categories (for example, Interpersonal Caring, Communication, Proactive Customer Service) and mounted on a storyboard display that rotates among departments.

- Take pictures of exemplary employees and teams on the job. Make slides and flash them on the wall of the cafeteria during lunch. After every 15 slides, insert one that reads "We Are the Hospital." You can spice up the program by adding a musical background. Or, consider a "Hall of Fame" where you display pictures of individual and team contributors to service success. Or, highlight one employee each week, including his or her writeup and picture in your facility's newsletter.
- Take pictures of staff who've been reported to provide excellent service. Make prints and tape them onto a permanent poster that you display prominently (see figure 11-13).
- Reprint complimentary letters from patients verbatim in your employee newsletter.

Use Recognition Campaigns to Focus Attention on Specific Improvement and Service Needs

You can target recognition campaigns to specific service areas and issues. For example, a Service Excellence Environment Award recognizes an entire department or unit for its teamwork in keeping its environment meticulous, thus raising the standards for other departments and teams.

The administrative team tours the facility quarterly to examine the environment in all areas. The department/unit they select to receive the Service Excellence Environment Award for that quarter is presented with the "traveling" plaque both at the department head meeting and in the department. The winning team is featured in the hospital newsletter.

Figure 11-12.   Appreciation Telegram

Telegram

To: Ann Jones, Nursing
From: Jane Smith, CEO

HEARD YOU MADE SALLY BROWN'S HIGH-RISK DELIVERY OF HER DAUGHTER A VERY POSITIVE EXPERIENCE. STOP. YOU PAID UNDIVIDED ATTENTION, SHOWED WARMTH AND CARING, STRONG SUPPORT DURING A VERY TRAUMATIC TIME. STOP. I REALLY APPRECIATE ALL YOU DO TO MAKE OUR HOSPITAL A SYMBOL OF HOSPITALITY. STOP. THANK YOU.

Figure 11-13.   "You're Making It Happen" Poster

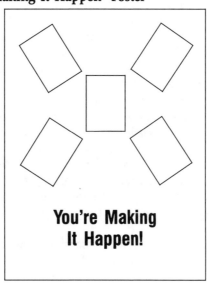

The recognition system built to reinforce telephone communication standards, designed by Elsie Miniscalco at Memorial Hospital in Hollywood, Florida, is meant to encourage and promote the use of telephone courtesy and excellent telephone tactics. Particular attention is given to answering the phone, filling the caller's needs, directing the call, and terminating the conversation so that every external and internal customer is left with a positive impression.

All departments were informed that random phone calls would be made to score them on criteria that reflect excellence in handling calls. Scores were tallied monthly or bimonthly. Memorial ran the program for six months, presenting six awards to winning departments.

Members of the Patient Relations Committee who served as the mystery callers rated the phone handlers on the following criteria:

- Was the phone answered in fewer than four rings?
- Was the unit identified?
- Did the person identify himself or herself?
- Was the tone of voice pleasant?
- Was the person helpful?
- Was the closing appropriate?

Callers telephoned departments they interacted with routinely but without identifying the purpose of the call. Each unit or department was called 10 different times. The department's score was the percentage of "yes" answers. The department with the highest percentage won each month and received the esteemed *Golden Phone* plaque (a small plastic toy phone spray-painted gold and placed on a decorated piece of wood). The plaque is passed from winner to winner and treasured by each department. A large poster-sized photo of the winning department's members was also displayed at the cafeteria entrance for a month, after which the winning department received it and hung it in their area for all to see.

Celebrate Your Service Mission and Service Accomplishments with Occasional Hoopla

Says Harvey Cox in *Feast of Fools*, "Preoccupied with producing and managing, people have lost touch with vast reaches of reality. Their beings have been borrowed and depleted. Therefore festivity is not just a luxury of life. It provides the occasion for people to establish their proper relation to time, history, and eternity."[3]

Celebrations are said to be high-touch events in a high-tech world, "festivals of the spirit," and opportunities to live the organization's vision. They can be used to honor individuals, teams, and your organization's progress in a festive, creative, and conscious manner. Celebrations give staff a chance to see and feel firsthand how your organization is transforming; they nourish people's spirit and help your organization run on high octane; and they cause employees to talk about your organization in the first-person plural.

What distinguishes celebrations from more routine recognition events? A strong values base, the use of symbols, ritual, storytelling, and a strong role for the organization's leadership are key features.

Similar to American Express's "Great Performers" event, the Kaiser Permanente Medical Center in San Rafael, California, holds a smashing annual Academy Awards banquet to show appreciation for employees' star service performance. Complete with glitter, tuxedos, gowns, champagne, excitement, and suspense, the evening generates rave reviews among attendees.

Another terrific example of a celebration of service improvement is the Service Olympics at Santa Clara Valley Medical Center (VMC) in San Jose, California. The process worked as follows:

1. A paycheck stuffer announced "The Games Are Coming!"– with VMC's Service Excellence logo.
2. An article in their in-house newsletter explained the rules and summarized the event (see figure 11-14).
3. At the annual recreation department barbecue, the Game Organizing Committee divided VMC's 60 departments into 24 teams, which selected their name, captain, and motto.
4. The games began.

Figure 11-14. Rules of the Game

The Games
A Program Designed to Promote Service Excellence
and to Recognize and Reward
the Outstanding Performance and Contribution of the
Employees at Santa Clara Valley Medical Center

"The most important thing in the Olympic Games is not to win but to take part, just as the most important thing in life is not the triumph but the struggle. The essential thing is not to have conquered but to have fought well." (Olympic Creed)

Playing the Games

1. Who, When, and Where
   A. The games begin at 12:01 A.M. on August 1, 1989, and end at 12:01 A.M. on January 31, 1990.
   B. The venues for the games will be VMC, SYC, CHABOYA EYC, and the institutions.
   C. Participation is voluntary for all YMC employees, physicians, and volunteers.
   D. Scores will be posted in the cafeteria biweekly.
2. Getting Started
   A. All teams must select a name, colors, mascot. Cheerleaders or mottos are optional.
   B. All teams must select a captain. Cocaptains are optional.
   C. It is suggested that routine method(s) of communication between captains, cocaptains, and their teams be set up.
3. Events
   A. The "Most Valuable Player" program.
      1. Employees observed demonstrating the House Rules are eligible to become an MVP at VMC.
      2. The observing individual must complete an MVP coupon and forward it to the Games Headquarters.
      3. If players are on the same team, one (1) point will be earned by the receiver. If players are on different teams, both observer and receiver will receive one (1) point.
      4. Upon receipt of the coupon, the Games Headquarters will notify the acknowledged employee.
      5. All employees who are recognized will be eligible for periodic drawings for prizes.
   B. Player of the Week
      1. Each week one player will be selected by the committee for his or her outstanding service excellence.
      2. The selection will be made by the Games Committee and will be determined from the MVP coupons submitted.
      3. The player of the week will earn two (2) points for his or her team.
   C. Innovative idea program
      1. Teams may earn additional points for initiating a new process or procedure for making their department or work between departments more user-friendly.
      2. The selection will be made by the Games Committee and will be determined from the MVP coupons submitted.
      3. Innovative ideas will earn between one (1) and ten (10) points as determined by the Games Committee.
   D. Fan Letters: Any team member or department receiving a complimentary letter from a patient or family of a patient will receive five (5) points for the team.
   E. Additional events will be added throughout the games.
   F. The Rules
      1. All rules of the games will be interpreted by the Games Committee with final determination by the Commissioner.
      2. All appeals and questions are to be forwarded by team captains to the Games Headquarters (Ext. 6176).

Created by Alliant Health System in Louisville, Kentucky, the "All-Star Quality Rally" is based on an idea developed at Milliken and Company. Alliant's rally recognizes large numbers of employees during a quarterly daylong event featuring team activity and presentations, as well as fun and food. Individuals are nominated to be "Quality All-Stars," who are then recognized at the rally with accolades and credit toward Alliant Quality memorabilia. According to Mary Newby of Alliant Health System, this rally successfully integrated recognition of teams and individuals for contributions to Alliant's quality philosophy, while also providing team building, games, and spirited celebration.

Following are some additional ideas for recognition activities:

- *Spotlight the exemplary people:* Give exceptional employees a chance to speak at orientation sessions on what excellent service means to them. Appoint them to high-visibility spokesperson positions, such as master of ceremonies at events, TV appearances on behalf of your organization, press interviews, or tour guides. During new employee orientation and service refresher programs, invite outstanding employees to present key service components.
- *Reward service innovations:* Offer rewards for service improvements that increase your customers' positive experiences in your organization. For example, try a "User-Friendly Contest":
  - Discuss with department heads the importance of service excellence and positive customer relations as an objective of every department in the organization.
  - Write articles for the employee newsletter about user-friendly behaviors and systems and ways departments and people can think and act in a more user-friendly manner.
  - After the groundwork has been laid, promote a contest that rewards departments or units that initiate the best user-friendly improvements. Such improvements should enable that department or unit to better serve its internal or external customers.
  - Include in your publications and on bulletin boards pictures of the winning group and articles highlighting the people and their achievement. Add to this a gift for the group; for example, a microwave oven, new lounge chairs, a luncheon, $300 to spend as they wish.

☐ Final Suggestions

Even though recognition strategies have great potential, they need to be carefully designed to fit your unique requirements. Keep these points in mind:

- *Not every reward and recognition program should come from the management:* Grassroots programs are most powerful.
- *Neither you nor your management team can second-guess employees on which rewards they find meaningful:* Ask them.
- *The more involved, the more invested, the more effective:* Plan your reward strategy in advance and solicit reactions from key people before implementing it. Reevaluate your mix of strategies periodically, for the same tactics will not be valued forever.
- *Trial and error and close monitoring of the results are indispensable:* When you try something new, watch carefully to see if it generates better performance.
- *Avoid offending people by rewarding one group more noticeably than another:* In addition to physicians and employees, make sure that others who serve customers (directly and indirectly) are eligible. Include all shifts.
- *Rewarding global performance at the expense of specific service behavior is to be avoided:* Use your reward strategies to reinforce service excellence and to educate or remind your work force about what it entails. Celebrate often.

- *The consequence should be equal to the behavior:* Don't cheat by offering too little or too much. Go beyond Employee of the Year programs as the only formal recognition strategy, because it celebrates too few people and is highly competitive. And unhealthy competition can jeopardize a recognition strategy.
- *Executives set the pace for saying thanks:* Insist on managers and supervisors expressing appreciation every day instead of relying solely on in-house programs.
- *Cooperative teamwork is more important to service excellence than individual stardom:* Because service delivery systems are complex and rely on the group effort, err on the side of team rewards.

The reward and recognition possibilities reviewed here are only a sampling of available systems. The key is to mix your methods, attach rewards to specific feats of service excellence, and celebrate more intensely and more visibly the desirable behavior among your caregivers. Finally, check out your methods periodically to make sure employees' real responses to these incentives match your good intentions.

References

1. Lawler, E. III. Merit pay: fact or fiction. *Management Review* 70(4):50–53, Apr. 1981.

2. Lee, C. Using customers' ratings to reward employees. *Training* 26(5):40–46, May 1989.

3. Cox, H. *Feast of Fools.* New York City: Harper and Row, 1972, p. 43.

Chapter 12

Employee Involvement and Empowerment

If employees are demoralized or impeded in their efforts to perform effectively, they are hardly able, or likely, to show enthusiasm for satisfying customer needs. To sustain (and retain) a satisfied and productive employee, your workplace must foster a nourishing, safe, and comfortable environment. You need to empower employees with the tools, autonomy, and latitude needed to make key service improvements that are in the best interests of your organization and its customers.

Before reading further, take the self-test in figure 12-1. A high number of "true" answers indicates that your organization has satisfied, involved employees. It also means that your management demonstrates its belief in teamwork and values each individual's

Figure 12-1. Self-Test

Employee Involvement and Improvement. *Circle the appropriate answer. The more "true" answers, the better. "False" answers indicate areas that need improvement.*

1. Our work atmosphere is comfortable for employees and conducive to their job effectiveness.	True	False
2. Our administrative team realizes that employees who are involved and empowered have a greater stake in the organization and greater loyalty.	True	False
3. Managers here take active steps to remove obstacles that prevent employees from doing a good job.	True	False
4. Employees participate in planning for changes that will affect them.	True	False
5. Employees here have clear opportunities to become involved in making improvements.	True	False
6. Our administration periodically updates employees on the organization's goals and plans.	True	False
7. Employees feel that management cares about what they think.	True	False
8. Employees have the tools they need to serve their customers without ongoing frustration.	True	False
9. Employees here have the latitude to make decisions without undue interference by red tape, bureaucracy, or highly controlling supervisors.	True	False
Total:	___	___

---

ideas and ability to contribute. A low number of "true" answers signals cause for concern, because disengaged employees make customers unhappy, thus jeopardizing the organization's best interests.

☐ Involvement versus Empowerment

Often, *involvement* and *empowerment* are used as buzzwords without thought to their precise definitions. Here we use the term *involvement* to connote employee participation. To become involved, employees must have *opportunities* to participate—not only in performing their own work, but in influencing policies, events, and behavior that relate to, and extend beyond, their work. Participation opportunities might relate to how work processes are designed and improved, how customers are served, the quality of work life, strategies for organizational improvement, and so forth.

Involvement and participation can be significant or they can be a sham. They are significant only when leaders *act* on employee input and suggestions; they are a sham when they do not. Many organizations commit to a participative management philosophy and create extensive networks of improvement teams and employee advisory groups. Once teams produce recommendations or proposals, leaders either ignore them, reject them consistently, or permit the bureaucracy to swallow them whole, never to be heard of again. Later, they wonder why employees are disheartened by these participative mechanisms with only lackluster efforts to comply with them.

Ed Lawler explains that participative processes are key to empowerment, because they move four resources—knowledge, information, power, and rewards—downward throughout the organization. According to Lawler, employee involvement in processes differs to the extent that these four characteristics are deployed.[1]

Involvement is important, but it is not enough to support continuous service improvement, even when administrators do follow through on employee input. It is not enough because leaders retain responsibility for organizational improvement and remain the only decision makers. The result is that employees fail to develop their own judgment capabilities and their own potential to be creative and resourceful in the face of customer needs.

Ultimately, empowerment is key to continuous service improvement. Empowerment grants autonomy that is directed to serving customers, the freedom to act responsibly. Empowerment does not promote anarchy or unlimited license; nor does it promote "doing whatever it takes to make the customer happy," because that can be financially disastrous for the organization. Empowerment takes place when the employee's (or team's) level of authority matches the employee's (or team's) level of responsibility. When used as a verb—*to empower*—the term sometimes is taken to mean giving your power to someone else. We prefer this definition: to provide the direction, latitude, and support employees need in order to evolve from followers into leaders. The manager's role, then, is to unleash the employee's personal power and remove the barriers to it.

In *Managing Knock Your Socks Off Service* authors Chip Bell and Ron Zemke define empowerment succinctly: "Empowerment is the self-generated exercising of professional judgment and discretion on the customer's behalf. It is doing what needs to be done rather than simply doing what one has been told routinely to do. From the manager's perspective, empowerment is a key element in the process of releasing the expression of personal power at the front lines. It is the opposite of enslavement."[2]

The authors explain empowerment by showing what it is compared to what it is not. They cite these features of empowerment:[3]

- Something you encourage, *not* something you give
- Congruence, *not* compliance
- Consistency, *not* conformance
- Accepted, *not* assigned

- Partnership, *not* parenting
- Values oriented, *not* rules oriented
- Right things, *not* easy things
- Appropriate, *not* correct

□ Why Empowerment?

Empowerment is emerging in industries all around us. According to Block: "There is a quiet revolution taking place in many organizations. The source of the revolution is the growing realization that tighter controls, greater pressure, more clearly defined jobs, and tighter supervision have, in the last 50 years, run their course. . . . Attention is shifting to the need for employees to take responsibility for the success of our businesses, if we hope to survive and prosper."[4]

Empowerment is particularly pivotal in service-oriented organizations. This is true for these additional reasons:

- Too often employees are prevented from following their instincts to do what it takes to satisfy their customers. This occurs when they are bound by restrictive policies and procedures that might have originated to protect the organization, without the customers' needs in mind.
- In today's atmosphere of resource constraints, lean staffing, and shrinking middle management ranks, every employee, regardless of his or her level, needs to share the responsibility for satisfying customers quickly and resourcefully in firsthand interactions. Since hospitals can't afford more people, they need the people they do have to take on more responsibility. Empowerment and responsibility are related; that is, more empowerment requires more responsibility.
- Customers are impressed when employees have the power to satisfy their needs without having to check with supervisors and policy manuals. They think more of the employee and they think better of the organization.

□ Increasing Empowerment Using the Six-Factor Formula

To move managers and staff toward higher levels of empowerment, it helps to break down the phenomenon of empowerment into its component parts. To do this, we use the empowerment formula shown in figure 12-2. You can then identify methods for strengthening weak components, resulting in a positive effect on the product. The formula is based on multiplication, not addition, of these factors because without any one of the six, the product is zero. All six factors are a prerequisite to empowerment. Factors of the empowerment formula are defined below:

- *Autonomy:* Latitude to act without permission. Employees need some latitude to act in the best interests of their customers. Hidden resources are disclosed when an individual is free to assume responsibility instead of being restricted by strict and confining instructions and policies. Imagine that your organization has no

Figure 12-2. Empowerment Formula

Empowerment = Autonomy × Direction × Opportunity × Proficiency × Support × Personal Responsibility policies that restrain staff; then start from scratch and ask, "What do we *really* need?"

- *Direction:* Goals, vision, and purpose. These lead to commitment. People are empowered when they know how their work contributes to a higher purpose and share a vision of what it means to achieve that higher purpose. Consider the age-old tale of three stonemasons. When asked, "What are you doing?" the first said, "I'm laying bricks." The second said, "I'm making a wall." The third said, "I'm building a cathedral." Who do you think felt best about his work? In an atmosphere where empowerment is valued, your best protection against anarchy is shared vision.
- *Opportunity:* To act empowered, staff need occasions for interacting with customers, access to resources so they have options in these interactions, and, in some cases, structured situations that help them increase their level of responsibility (such as improvement teams and task force service).
- *Proficiency:* To become effective in their actions and to build supervisors' trust in their judgment, staff need proficiency in creative problem solving. They also need to be capable of making decisions that balance the interests of the customer with those of the organization. Skills are key, and in many cases empowerment skills need to be developed because the employee's previous experience has not cultivated them.
- *Support:* Supervisors need to validate staff. They need to give them attention and care, know what they're doing, and let them know that their efforts are important to the organization.
- *Personal responsibility:* This factor entails esteem for one's own contribution and impact and a realization that "nothing happens unless I make it happen." Employees who take personal responsibility are also prepared to take the consequences for their decisions without unduly blaming other people or circumstances where things don't work as expected. Personal responsibility exercised in the name of excellent service has as its prerequisite shared information. Without information one cannot take responsibility; with it, one cannot avoid taking responsibility. The challenge is to create an environment that cultivates responsibility. A bureaucratic work environment interferes with this goal, robbing the individual of direct and immediate impact on customers and quality.

☐ Strategies for Increasing Employee Involvement and Empowerment

Other chapters have already identified strategies for building empowerment. For example, chapter 7 ("Problem Solving and Process Improvement") described various approaches (such as suggestion programs, improvement teams, a service assistance line) that provide opportunities for employees to act with a sense of personal power. This chapter focuses on the following selected strategies, which relate directly to empowerment in improving service:

- Demonstrate administrative behavior that encourages empowerment
- Consider employees as partners and take steps to acknowledge and respect their needs
- Help managers and supervisors exercise less control over employees
- Help department managers engage staff in a transition to greater empowerment
- Equip all employees to engage in effective service recovery
- Help staff develop a strong sense of personal responsibility
- Remove barriers to empowerment

Demonstrate Administrative Behavior That Encourages Empowerment

Administrative behavior is mirrored at every level. If administrators support and empower their people, then others will follow their lead. To prove this statement is more than rhetoric, let's look a little more deeply at the way administrators use their *power*.

The traditional organizational structure of most health care facilities is like the pyramid shown in figure 12-3. Trustees are at the top; administrators report to them; and middle managers report to administrators. The key to success for administrators is in satisfying the expectations of trustees; for middle managers, the key to success is satisfying the needs of administrators; and so on down the line. Customers and their needs are at the bottom.

In a service-oriented organization, this pyramid needs to be inverted, as shown in figure 12-4, with customers and their needs at the top, serving as the facility's driving force. The measure of success for frontline employees becomes their effectiveness in satisfying customer needs. The measure of success for middle managers becomes their effectiveness in supporting and enabling their staff to satisfy customer needs. And the measure of success for administrators is their effectiveness in supporting and guiding middle managers in their efforts to help frontline staff meet customer needs.

This inverted pyramid has dramatic implications for the administrator's role: Instead of excelling at directing, controlling, and monitoring, the empowering administrator establishes a sense of direction, communicates key information, delegates clearly and effectively, removes barriers that impede staff ability to serve customers, and coaches staff to exercise increasing autonomy and make effective judgments in fulfilling their expanded roles. Figure 12-5 lists 14 essentials that middle managers say they need from their bosses in order to embrace their leadership role and act as empowering managers.

Administrators need to take a hard look at what they can do to enable their employees to better serve their customers. For department heads to be responsive and helpful to their employees, administration needs to be responsive and helpful to department heads. Administrators can and should involve middle managers in developing concrete action

Figure 12-3. Traditional Organizational Structure

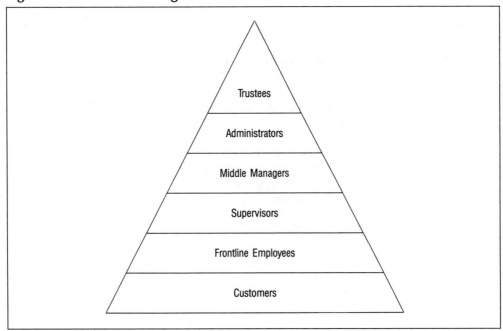

Trustees

Administrators

Middle Managers

Supervisors

Frontline Employees

Customers

plans for improving service. This effort includes goal setting with individuals, skill-building plans, periodic campaigns, and special events.

Employees also need to know that administrators are doing what they can to identify and solve problems that interfere with great service delivery. Such problems include poor signage, a scarcity of wheelchairs in key areas, poor scheduling systems that produce long waits for patients, broken phones, and much more.

To succeed with service excellence in the long run, management must establish support systems that give employees the power to serve the customer. Developing support systems for gathering input, solving problems, and keeping lines of communication open are the job of top managers. Only they have the clout to create such systems and to make them work to everyone's benefit.

Figure 12-4. Organizational Structure That Empowers Employees to Satisfy Customers

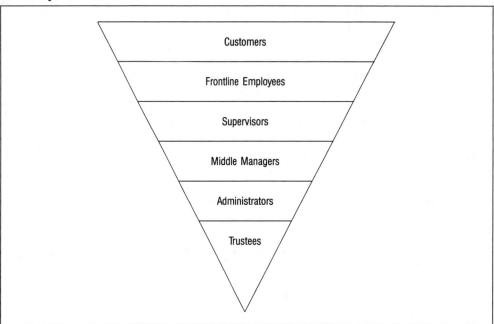

Figure 12-5. What Do Managers Need from Their Bosses?

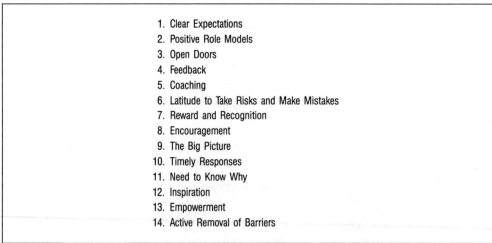

1. Clear Expectations
2. Positive Role Models
3. Open Doors
4. Feedback
5. Coaching
6. Latitude to Take Risks and Make Mistakes
7. Reward and Recognition
8. Encouragement
9. The Big Picture
10. Timely Responses
11. Need to Know Why
12. Inspiration
13. Empowerment
14. Active Removal of Barriers

Reprinted, with permission, from The Einstein Consulting Group, Philadelphia, Pennsylvania, 1990.

Administrators also need to keep employees and physicians informed if they expect their commitment, dedication, and salesmindedness. Truth telling about the organization's goals, challenges, strengths, and weaknesses fosters individual respect and builds people's identity with the organization. Administrators must be honest and forthright with them and avoid the temptation to shelter or exaggerate. Otherwise, employees and physicians resist taking personal responsibility to satisfy customers for the sake of the organization.

Consider Employees as Partners and Take Steps to Acknowledge and Respect Their Needs

Investment, commitment, partnership—these words have little meaning to employees unless the organization communicates appreciation for staff as key contributors to customer satisfaction. Employees with customer satisfaction skills won't necessarily use those skills unless they understand what the words imply. Employees need to be *willing*, not just *able*, to satisfy customers, and this willingness emerges when they feel respected and connected to the organization's mission. The employee's job needs to satisfy his or her needs while also satisfying those of the organization. That's why, as noted earlier, the premier strategy to advance employee empowerment and involvement entails treating employees like valued partners, whose needs deserve attention and consideration. This derives from the management philosophy "Employees are your first customers. If you treat employees well, then they care about the customers and organization enough to act in an empowered way."

Instead of making assumptions about what employees need and want, management should employ the traditional tools of market research and segmentation to find out from the employees themselves what they value and how they perceive key workplace dimensions (work atmosphere, working conditions, policies and procedures, mission, quality of supervision, compensation and benefits, job definition, for example). Regular survey techniques, personal interviews, questionnaires, focus groups, or rap sessions can yield useful learning about employee perceptions of these dimensions. In many large corporations— for example Lockheed, General Electric, Minnesota Power and Light, Kaiser Aluminum, and GEICO to name a few—executive managers sit down with small groups of employees and do what is called *deep sensing*, that is, they simply solicit employee concerns and address them.

A more analytical explanation about what employees need and want is to be found in Abraham Maslow's classic *hierarchy of needs* as discussed in *Motivation and Personality*.[5] Maslow claimed that basic needs for survival (food and shelter) need to be largely satisfied before a person's needs are activated at the next level. (No wonder, then, about the fuss during the night shift when no food is available or when only fattening foods are available for dieters.)

Then comes the need for safety and security. Traditionally, health care workers chose their profession because of its inherent stability and its focus on the giving of comfort. Now, suddenly, with changing reimbursement practices, marketplace whirlwinds, mergers and acquisitions, and hospital closings, caregivers have become tense and insecure in this uncertain atmosphere. On another level, safety and security needs also emerge for the employee who walks from the car to the hospital (and vice versa), down empty hallways, and to and from public transportation.

The next level of needs has to do with belonging and group identification—or social needs. Witness the growing malaise of the middle manager or overworked nurse who is increasingly isolated from peers.

The next level of needs involves status or ego. This level includes the need for appreciation, respect, and esteem in the eyes of others. The cry for the simple pat on the back, for recognition of individual accomplishments in a sea of people, and the preoccupation with promotions to "get what I deserve" all reflect these needs.

The final level of need, self-actualization, emerges when the other needs are largely satisfied. The needs at this level include the quest for job enrichment, opportunity, growth and education, creativity, the thrill of risk and innovation, employee participation in solving the stickiest organizational problems, and the chance to take on challenges.

All of these needs are present in varying degrees at different times with different employees. If your organization lacks a variety of ways to fulfill these needs, you cannot expect employees to act empowered or take advantage of opportunities for involvement, even if you think they have the latitude and opportunities to do so. By creating a high quality of work life tailored to respect employees as key contributors, you can spark in your staff the stamina, dedication, commitment, and emotional generosity you want them to extend to your department's external customers. Promoting employee empowerment through enhanced quality of work life and a sense of partnership is explored in the next two subsections.

Improving the Quality of Work Life

Quality of work life involves many factors, including work satisfaction, clear expectations, a positive relationship with the boss, opportunities to get ahead, feedback on job performance, adequate pay and benefits, and comfortable and safe working conditions. Departments and other work groups need to devote attention to making continuous improvements in the quality of work life for employees to feel that their satisfaction is important to you. Too many organizations focus their employee satisfaction tactics on the organization as a whole, which inevitably leads to "big brother" or "gimme" approaches that have employees pressing for more money and benefits and the organization struggling to provide them globally. Ironically, employee satisfaction is much more related to factors closer to the employee's needs, factors the employee can share responsibility for improving.

At the department or work-group level, employees need to be involved in creating the quality of work life they want. This starts with identifying their satisfaction criteria and periodically monitoring satisfaction levels according to those criteria, then feeding back the results to managers and staff who engage in improvement efforts. To improve quality of work life across the hospital, consider this approach.

1. Form a volunteer committee of employees from different departments to serve for a period of 6–9 months to identify quality-of-work-life issues. These ombudspeople use as their primary source the issues information generated by quarterly employee surveys. The committee facilitator should be someone who can remain objective and impartial and can grasp clinical and nonclinical issues.
2. Have the committee separate issues into meaningful categories (for example, those dealing with amenities/benefits, supervision/management, policies/procedures, bonding/celebrations, systems/space, and job expectations).
3. Have them prioritize the issues within each category to identify solvable problems.
4. Ask them to make recommendations to administration or refer problems to other more appropriate teams.

Treating Employees as Partners

Numerous methods exist for satisfying employee needs and showing that your institution thinks of them as valued partners. Here are just a few:

- *Employee relations committee:* If you don't already have one, form an employee relations committee composed of a core group of interested employee advocates who can identify employee needs and develop approaches to meeting them. This group continuously takes the pulse of employees at large and feeds relevant information to the larger committee for review and action. Employee relations committees tend to reveal sagging morale in a specific department, systemwide frustrations, gaps in service to employees, and the like. In some organizations, they have pressed for a new look at benefits, formation of employee assistance programs, development of annual events, and so forth.

- *A service excellence subcommittee called the Fun Committee:* Some hospitals include as part of their service strategies a subcommittee devoted to building employee spirit and well-being and organizing morale-boosting events—contests, for example. The idea is to address needs creatively so that employees feel better about work, are more energetic in serving customers, and are more at peace with themselves and their coworkers. Sometimes the Fun Committee defines its task as developing team-building experiences that develop an organizationwide sense of family.

- *"We care about you" gestures:* Does your management take the time to recognize promotions, send plants to hospitalized employees and their families, give birthday cards or a small birthday gift to employees, offer free ice cream sundaes after a hectic week, honor retirees, conduct exit interviews, hold welcome receptions for new people, honor security guards with a Security Day, recognize volunteers during National Volunteer Week, and so forth? In all these little ways managers say "We care about our employees here. You are our partners in fulfilling our important mission. We do not see you as replaceable or dispensable. We do not take your commitment or contribution lightly."

- *Participation opportunities:* Does your organization have vehicles for involving employees in problem identification, problem solving, and decision making? Whether you have process improvement teams, task forces, ad hoc problem-solving groups, work teams, or whatever, these participation opportunities cater to an employee's need for a sense of belonging.

- *Specific employee services:* When your facility plans to construct a new building, is an employee lounge or fitness area or a comfortable snack bar an automatic consideration? When you promote free health screenings to your patient community, do you take special steps to do the same for your employees? Do you make provisions for night shift personnel to be escorted to their cars? Do you offer an employee assistance program (for example, stop-smoking programs or weight loss clinics), aerobics instruction, or on-site college courses for the convenience, health, and well-being of your employees even if these programs do not generate additional revenue?

- *Programs on caring for the caregiver or energy renewal:* Today's health care environment breeds employee insecurity, and the pressure to be productive and adaptive to dramatic change can weigh heavily on them. Do you devote resources to programs that help your employees maintain their emotional balance in such a climate? Stress management, anxiety clinics, support groups, and employee renewal programs all reflect concern for the employee's well-being in the hyperstressful health care environment.

Treating employees as valued partners and customers is still hard for many managers to swallow. After all, they reason, aren't employees being paid to do a job? The fact is, a paycheck is not enough these days, and the concept of employee as partner refers simply to a workplace variation of the Golden Rule: Do unto your employees as you want your employees to do unto all your customers. The result of following this rule is high-quality service and self-respecting, productive employee-partners who demonstrate energy and empowerment in the service of your organization.

Help Managers and Supervisors Reduce Control over Staff

The need for employee involvement in service improvement is escalating, along with the need to empower employees to take independent action to satisfy their customers.

Without employee involvement, few problems reach adequate solution because few people work on problem solving. The unfortunate outcome is missed opportunities and waste.

If employee involvement and empowerment are so important, why do managers resist them? If you ask them, they offer compelling responses:

- "They threaten my authority."
- "My subordinates might outshine me."
- "My subordinates might see that they don't need me."
- "I might be left out of important decisions."
- "It bothers my ego."
- "I've never done things that way, and you can't teach an old dog new tricks."
- "Decisions take longer when you involve employees."
- "These employees aren't smart enough to make good decisions—and they're irresponsible."
- "I just don't see what's in it for me."

From years of experience and learning from role models, many managers and supervisors share a common belief. That is, "If staff have more power, then I have less." Consequently, they resist initiatives designed to involve and empower staff.

Figure 12-6 shows the inverse relationship between management control and empowerment. When managers retain all control and authority, there is no employee empowerment. As managers relax their authority and control, employee empowerment increases. Committing to employee involvement and empowerment requires a shift in the manager's mind-set from authoritarianism to leadership, to giving employees the tools and information they need and the leeway to adapt and innovate as needed. Strict supervision doesn't work in a customer-focused organization where flexibility and responsibility are the keys to customer satisfaction.

Power is not a fixed and finite property that cannot be shared. Managers need to recognize that power is increased all around when sharing it produces positive results. By relaxing their control over employees, managers and supervisors:

- Free staff and themselves to accomplish more. Employees become less dependent and act without the need to "check in" for approval at every step.
- Enable staff to become innovative. Even though they may fail in some of their efforts, the benefits of experimentation and innovation are invaluable.
- Encourage employees to support one another instead of leaning on the supervisor for support. This leads to better enhanced teamwork.
- Strengthen staff commitment to their jobs, because they develop a strong personal stake in their work.

Consider instituting management development and support systems that help managers and supervisors adjust their mind-set so that they embrace involvement and empowerment as powerful, positive routes to achieving service excellence. After defining the management mind-set prerequisite to empowering staff, managers may need help dealing with fear of losing control. Two strategies help in this area: defining boundaries for staff and building trust in employees' independent judgment by coaching them on decision making.

Defining Boundaries for Staff

Empowerment leads to anarchy only if no boundaries have been clarified and no limits set, a kind of negative and counterproductive empowerment. Productive empowerment sets parameters for action that are as broad as possible, defining the latitude employees have to take initiative and risks. This is another way of saying that productive empowerment establishes rules for making decisions.

Managers and staff can work cooperatively to clarify employees' latitude for taking action. One process might be the following:

1. Have staff fill out a "responsibility map" (see figure 12-7). Taking into account a department or work group's current way of operating and key responsibilities, identify the specific responsibilities that fall into each quadrant.
2. Ask which tasks could (and should) be shifted:
   - From the boss to individuals (for example, scheduling)
   - From the system to the boss or to individuals (for example, department orientation, interviewing job applicants)
   - From the boss or individuals to the system (certain paperwork that should be automated)
   - From employees to no one (an obsolete or outdated process, policy, or responsibility)
3. Consider the actions needed to shift responsibilities as indicated above.
   - Brainstorm potential roadblocks (for example, training needs, scheduling issues)
   - Assess interest/skill levels of participants by asking them to fill out a readiness chart (see figure 12-8)

Figure 12-6. The Control–Empowerment Relationship

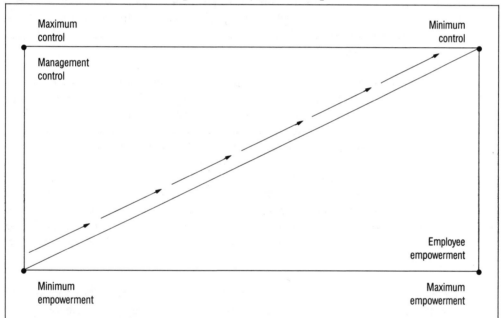

Figure 12-7. Responsibility Map

Things the boss is responsible for	Things employees are responsible for
Things someone else is responsible for	Things no one is responsible for

Figure 12-8. Readiness Chart

Tasks	Readiness 1 2 3 4	Interest 1 2 3 4

1 = High interest/readiness . . . 4 = Low interest/readiness

4. For responsibilities targeted for shifting to employees, work with staff to clarify the boundaries (or latitude) employees will have regarding their new responsibilities. One way to accomplish this is to make three lists: "Not OK to Do," "OK to Do," and "Gray Area."

  • Identify with staff what is *not* permissible (policies and practices that they are not to violate under any circumstance), what is clearly permissible (alternatives clearly available to them if they judge the alternative appropriate in a specific situation), and the situations that fall into the "gray area" (actions an employee is not sure he or she is allowed to take without permission). For additional clarity, the manager needs to list the "not permissibles," the "clearly permissibles," and gray-area actions.

  • Then the manager, perhaps with staff input, decides whether each of the actions in the gray area is or is not permissible. The gray area list should be cut down as much as possible, because that's where problems occur. To reduce the gray area, manager and staff discuss the specific situations and clarify the conditions or boundaries within which it is OK to engage in an action.

If managers and staff work through this kind of process together, all end up feeling clearer about what constitutes permissible action. This kind of discussion needs to take place frequently because, as managers come to trust staff judgment over time, they will voluntarily loosen the boundaries on permissible staff action.

Coaching Employees on Decision Making
Managers should adopt a coaching style that promotes employees' self-management, individual responsibility, and sound judgment in situations that involve choices. Supervisors who don't trust employee judgment will not expand the latitude employees have to show initiative and act independently. To build this prerequisite trust, supervisors must shift their style from control to coaching so that over time they build trust in employees' judgment and can "let go." Employees should ask themselves these questions:

  • Is my preferred action in the best interest of my customer?
  • Is my preferred action in alignment with our organization's values?

- If my preferred action satisfies a customer but interferes with a policy, is the explanation for that policy compelling? (If not, do what I think is right and I probably will be right.)

Figure 12-9 shows a model for a supervisor–staff coaching process that supports employee empowerment. With this approach, supervisors keep the responsibility for decision making in the hands of staff while fostering independent thinking and resourceful problem solving.

In addition to using this model to coach employees in the real situations they face, managers and trainers can accelerate the development of good judgment through group

Figure 12-9. Model for Coaching That Fosters Empowerment

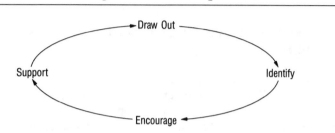

Draw Out: Assist the employee to see and describe the situation/problem.

- What's the difficulty causing dissatisfaction?
- What do you think is contributing to this problem?
- How do you know that there is a problem?
- What about this situation is causing you concern?
- What are you, personally, contributing to the situation?

Listen, Listen, Listen

Identify: Guide the employee to see possibilities and an ideal future state.

- What will happen if the difficulty doesn't change?
- What would you like to see different?
- How would you know if the problem or difficulty were resolved?
- What has to change in order for you to see improvement?
- What do you have to do differently?
- What do you have to stop doing?

Listen, Listen, Listen

Encourage: Support the employee to have confidence in him- or herself and his or her ability to achieve a solution.

- What about this situation feels like a personal risk to you?
- Is it truly a risk?
- What qualities do you personally possess to deal with the situation?
- Is there anyone else whose support you need?
- What do you need from them?

Listen, Listen, Listen

Support Action: Focus the employee on taking action.

- What are some actions you need to take to resolve this situation?
- What else?
- What actions will you ask of others?
- By when do you want this situation to improve?
- What's the first action step you need to take?
- When are you going to take it?

Listen, Listen, Listen

practice. The hypothetical situations in figure 12-10, for example, can be used in training sessions or staff meetings to develop the thinking and decision-making skills that allow staff to become more resourceful and act appropriately in situations where choice is involved, and that engender more trust from their supervisors. As each situation is explored, it is important to examine in detail the degree to which the employees can bend rules, bypass red tape, and take special initiatives to satisfy their customers. Many employees have great ideas about how to handle situations, but they feel constrained by rules, regulations, policies, procedures, approval processes, and the confines of their job descriptions to act.

After examining these situations, ask employees to recall real situations that they found difficult to handle. Discuss alternative solutions, clarifying boundaries on the employee's latitude to act in the situation and the elements that constitute good judgment.

Help Department Managers Engage Staff in a Transition to Greater Empowerment

To further empowerment through partnership with employees, managers can identify empowerment as an explicit objective that they work toward with staff. Figure 12-11 shows a 14-step strategy, developed by The Einstein Consulting Group, to increase empowerment and involvement. Because this strategy is extensive and time-consuming, it is most appropriate if the department manager identifies employee involvement and empowerment as a breakthrough objective for advancing service quality.

Figure 12-10. Hypothetical "Sticky" Situations That Develop Staff Decision-Making Skills

Instructions: Divide the group into pairs or trios. Give each group a sticky situation and ask them to generate appropriate ways to respond. The small groups then share their approaches with the large group and get feedback, reactions, and additional ideas. The supervisor or trainer then offers additional guidelines and suggestions.

Practice Situations

1. Ninety-year-old Helen Johnson has serious heart trouble and has been admitted to the hospital several times in the past year. Her daughter signed a Do-Not-Resuscitate form each time and you are aware that both the patient and daughter have asked the physicians involved not to use extreme measures if Mrs. Johnson experiences heart failure. Mrs. Johnson has been admitted today and you notice that the DNR form has not been signed.
2. Your superior asks you to evaluate two vendors' services and to recommend the better vendor. After investigating both, you really don't like the services of either one.
3. You need an O-ring for an elderly patient. You called the storeroom and found out that they are on order. You called other floors to see if they had one and found that none was available. Your patient really needs this.
4. Mr. Harris's daughter is upset with you because her father's personal belongings have disappeared. Mr. Harris isn't your patient and his nurse is on vacation.
5. You are a supervisor in Environmental Services. One day, because of absenteeism, you find that you don't have enough staff to set up rooms for all three special functions scheduled that day.
6. You work in Maintenance. You stopped into a room to fix a window latch and the patient asks you for a stronger light bulb for a lamp. Policy dictates that you need a work ticket to change a light bulb.
7. You are a radiologic technician. Suddenly your equipment breaks down. There are many patients waiting. You can't find a supervisor.
8. Bob Smith has been admitted through the ER. His clothes were ripped and covered with blood when he arrived in the ambulance. They've been thrown out.
9. Jim Rush has been at his father's bedside since he was brought into the hospital. Every time you suggest that Jim take a break to get some food or coffee, he refuses. You know he hasn't eaten in at least 6 hours.
10. A patient has traveled a long distance for a test. Unfortunately, according to the department's schedule, this patient is not scheduled until the next day.

Figure 12-11. Departmental Strategy to Encourage Employee Involvement and Empowerment

Actions/Results	How/Method	When	Results
1. Assess personal readiness for and vision of empowerment. • Where am I with employee involvement/empowerment? • What will this take from me? • What do I need to learn?			
2. Assess departmental readiness. • Where are we now as a department? • Are the employees "on board" with our business/service mission?			
3. Communicate to staff commitment to building an empowered and aligned work force.			
4. Reconfirm departmental service mission. • Who are our customers? • What service do they expect?			
5. Build a shared vision of how you want to work together to actualize your service mission.			
6. Develop a supportive work environment by creating and instituting coworker norms.			
7. Take stock of current reality re: responsibility map.			
8. Identify key areas to transfer accountability.			
9. Implement delegation plan for each area.			
10. Develop skills in self-management. • Monitoring devices • Feedback skills • Coaching support			
11. Design and implement problem solving and support structures. • Support groups • "Sticky situation meetings" • "Fix, bury, cheer" • Appreciation devices			
12. Track and monitor performance outcomes. • For individuals • For the department			
13. Celebrate achievements. • For individuals • For the department			
14. Do it all again. • Set the stage. • Assess current reality. • Create a vision of the future. • Develop a plan for continued involvement and empowerment.			

The tactics described in this strategy all involve department managers engaging in conscious and deliberate steps to foster employee empowerment. To overcome managers' psychological resistance to letting go of some control over employee actions, the transition to empowerment must be handled carefully, and managers and supervisors must be provided with the tools and training necessary to replace their old controlling methods with methods that allow for and foster an empowered work force.

Equip All Employees to Engage in Effective Service Recovery

Although most hospitals hire dedicated staff such as patient representatives to handle complaints, these people aren't the *only* ones who need to develop and demonstrate expertise in service recovery. Every supervisory and nonsupervisory employee needs to accept his or her role as problem solver for customers and learn to fulfill this role effectively and willingly. If managers always intervene in an employee–customer conflict, both employee and customer are kept at arm's length, which prevents employees from developing the skills they need to handle tough issues. As a result, they feel less committed, less proud of their own abilities, and less invested in the outcomes of their actions. Anyway, managers can't always be around to put out fires. Their time is better spent planning improvements that prevent future fires.

Complaint management is difficult and takes substantial skill building. As a result, many hospitals with service excellence strategies use professional trainers to teach complaint resolution skills. However, you can train your own people to develop complaint management skills, which they can then pass on to their staff.

Melrose–Wakefield Hospital in Massachusetts, St. Luke's Hospital in Racine, Wisconsin, and Duke University Hospital in Chapel Hill, North Carolina, have trained every employee in their organization to cope effectively with complaints. Their reasoning was that they never know when, where, or to whom complaints will be voiced. In all three hospitals, managers and supervisors not only become involved firsthand in complaint management, they also train their staff to handle complaints effectively and to see complaint management as a critical and positive element of their jobs. To equip their people to handle complaints effectively, managers and supervisors watch out for the "it's-easier-to-do-it-myself" pattern that works against allowing their employees to recognize problems and take the initiative to solve them.

Your organization can make every staff member a member of your service recovery team by taking these steps:

- Develop organizationwide policies and procedures that make explicit the primacy of customer satisfaction; the need for every staff member to engage in service recovery; the limits you want staff to go to in order to achieve it; and the record-keeping system you want to track problems, complaints, and their resolution.
- Select one model for effective complaint handling and make it the focus of training in service recovery. Helpful resource material can be found in the booklet *Complaint Handling in Health Care*.[6]
- Train all managers in service recovery, complementing classroom training with a system of peer problem solving and troubleshooting that helps managers across functional lines to learn together about available resources and creative solutions.
- Train a small team of the most skilled managers to become service recovery trainers who train the rest of the organization.
- Equip all managers and supervisors with staff meeting and individual coaching formats that help them help staff become increasingly effective in service recovery in a nonthreatening learning environment. For instance:
  - Develop a repertoire of typical complaints heard by their department, use these case studies to teach new employees about complaint management, and review skill refinements with veteran employees.

- Do role plays until people are comfortable handling complaints in a welcoming, nondefensive manner.
- Let employees see their managers solving sticky customer service issues. Then review the steps and discuss the techniques used.
- Define boundaries for decision making using the approach detailed above.
- After incidents in which a customer problem was not resolved effectively, go back over the steps and ask open-ended questions to look at better alternatives.
- Create a rotating "supervisor on call" so that staff, not necessarily supervisors, practice helping one another resolve complaints and problems.
- Institute methods of recognizing and rewarding employee efforts and reducing fear of reprisals.

As managers work through this learning process with their employees, they need to believe that there's more than one right answer. People learn from their mistakes, and what may appear to be a heavy investment in training now pays off later.

Help Staff Develop a Strong Sense of Personal Responsibility

Managers and supervisors can create the conditions that foster staff empowerment, but the *feeling* of empowerment comes from within. Staff need to embrace the power available to them, viewing themselves as leaders, decision makers, and problem solvers, not followers who wait for instruction to act.

Often managers are the root cause of employee passivity and reticence because of tight controls on employee autonomy. But many employees frustrate managers who expect and want them to act more autonomously and decisively; these employees do not see themselves as the source of decisions and actions. Instead, they see themselves as "good soldiers" who do as they're told or—even worse—as oppressed victims of circumstances beyond their control.

To an extent, this worldview on the part of some employees (and managers) flies in the face of empowerment and involvement. Even if they're provided with opportunities to act empowered and become involved, and if they have a manager who coaches and supports instead of directing and controlling, some employees still resist the responsibility that comes with autonomy. If this pattern is rampant in your organization, your service strategy needs to include personal skills tactics for helping employees alter their mind-set of powerlessness. The Harmony program, developed by the Nursing Services Department of the Albert Einstein Medical Center and The Einstein Consulting Group, is an example of a growing number of programs available to help employees examine their own inclination to take or avoid personal responsibility for the way they do their job, the way they interact with others, and the results they get with customers and coworkers.

The Inner Action Model in figure 12-12 drives the personal skills employees learn in the Harmony program. Employees examine their own inner cycle of thoughts, feelings,

Figure 12-12. Inner Action Model

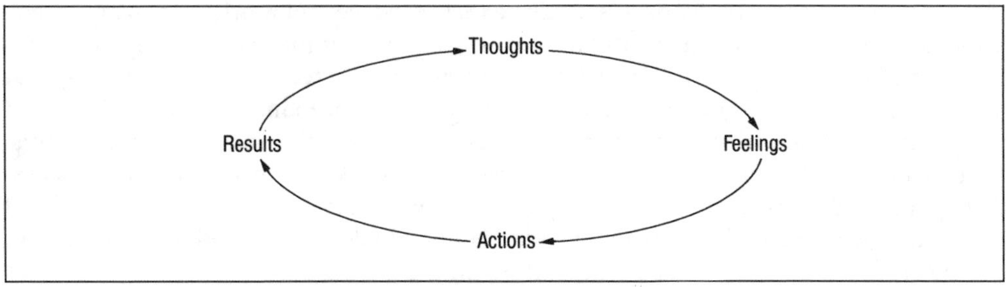

Reprinted, with permission, from Albert Einstein Healthcare Foundation, Philadelphia, Pennsylvania.

actions, and results and practice changes they can make in any part of this cycle that will have positive ripple effects for other parts of the cycle. For example, a nurse who sees a difficult doctor approaching and thinks, "Dr. X is going to make my day miserable, as usual" generates with this thought feelings of resentment and fatigue. These feelings translate into avoidance behavior or veiled hostility (actions). It's not surprising, then, that the physician is short-tempered with the nurse and fulfills the nurse's expectation (results).

In this example, the nurse could use personal skills to reverse the cycle. For example, upon seeing the doctor, the nurse could think, "Dr. X is here to see how the patient is doing; maybe I can help." The feelings are experienced as "interest" and "challenge" rather than resentment or veiled hostility. As a result, the nurse behaves differently, greeting the physician warmly and asking, "Is there any way I can help you this morning?" Because of this behavior, the nurse will likely get a different reaction from the physician.

Employees need help recognizing the power they have to affect results by controlling and *choosing* their thoughts, feelings, or actions. An employee can become more effective by experimenting with personal changes at any point in this cycle. This kind of experimentation helps employees recognize and use the power they have as doers, not victims or passive observers. Taking personal responsibility for results is a key ingredient for empowerment. Your organization might need to formalize an approach that helps staff recognize and accept personal responsibility for their effectiveness and their effect on customers and coworkers. Such an approach would help staff learn valuable skills such as positive self-talk, reframing, and personal stress reduction.

Remove Barriers to Empowerment

We've already discussed how unclear boundaries and management resistance to loosening control impede empowerment. In addition, if the following four barriers sabotage empowerment, intervention may be needed:

1. Managers who feel disempowered exemplify powerlessness to their staff.
2. The organizational culture may breed fear of failure or reprisal.
3. Red tape and layers of permission policy restrict action.
4. Constraints on communication across levels and department lines prevent employees from using resources needed to solve a customer problem.

Alleviating Manager Powerlessness
Powerlessness felt by managers is contagious among staff who witness it and conclude that the organization simply does not permit initiative and risk taking. Like their manager, they become reactive or passive, resorting to memos, asking permission, and other tactics intended to shield them from responsibility for anything that goes wrong. Top executives need to address rampant lack of initiative among managers and rethink their expectations of and reactions to managers who take initiative.

Overcoming Fear of Failure
Related to manager powerlessness is a culture that breeds fear of reprisal. In many organizations, only lip service is paid to *empowerment* because employees fear repercussions if they make a "wrong" decision, even if they've never tested it. Sometimes they fear repercussion because they've seen it happen. All layers of management need to audit their behavior when managers make decisions or take initiative that top executives disagree with *after the fact.* Executives and administrators need to relabel failures as learning opportunities: Instead of reprimanding people whose decisions or initiatives did not work out, they need to thank them for caring enough to take action and then coach them so they learn from the results of their efforts and can make more effective judgments in the future.

At Lexington Medical Center in Columbia, South Carolina, CEO Ken Shoal distributed "Get Out of Jail Free" cards to entice managers to take risks without fear of reprisal. He promised that if they acted without permission and their action later was deemed inappropriate, they could turn in their card and be absolutely protected against repercussions. This clever gimmick brought fear of reprisal into the open while at the same time allowing the administration to communicate clearly that it preferred risk taking with occasional undesired outcome over no risk taking. Shoal asserted that the total absence of risk taking and initiative constituted high-risk management behavior.

Cutting through Red Tape

The third barrier to empowerment, bureaucratic red tape, poses a distinct hazard. Process improvement is one way to test the boundaries and see whether convoluted organizational practices that impede customer satisfaction are really necessary. Through individual and team process improvement efforts, people identify "clogs" in their systems that restrict employee action or slow down response time. They then redesign these processes to eliminate the blocks.

Employees faced with having to plod through layers of permission and tedious paperwork to fulfill a customer need are discouraged from action. Furthermore, they are encouraged to pass the buck. Managers need to ask employees: "What gets in the way of acting to satisfy your customers? What policies and procedures slow down your ability to respond effectively? Specifically, what do I do that gets in the way of your being more productive?"

Communicating across Departments and Levels

Much has been said in other chapters about the need to cut across turf lines to fulfill the service mandate and need only be briefly revisited here. For staff to be resourceful in solving problems, they need to know who can do what within the organization, and they need to have ready access to these resources. To accomplish this, managers need to expose staff to broader spheres of influence (take them to meetings, introduce them to people, put their names on their work, for example). Doing so helps them form strategic networking relationships and connects them with important sources of information.

☐ Final Suggestions

Three spheres of influence foster empowerment: the individual, the individual's manager or supervisor, and the organization. Figure 12-13, from the booklet "Basics of Employee

Figure 12-13. Questions for Gauging Your Organization's Level of Empowerment

---

The empowered individual:

- Does the individual seek and accept responsibility?
- Does he or she take risks?
- Does he or she "own" his or her work?

The empowered supervisor:

- Does he or she gather and share information?
- Does he or she recognize the expertise of subordinates?
- Does the supervisor train, facilitate, and coach subordinates?

The empowered organization:

- Do procedures recognize and reward risk taking and ownership?
- Does it support facilitation and coaching?
- Has it established boundaries within which supervisors and employees operate?
- Does it foster climate-changing activities by altering administrative processes?

Empowerment," is a checklist summary of forces that need to be in place for your organization to rate high on the empowerment scale.[7]

Management folklore has a saying: "The good manager has sense enough to pick good people to do what needs doing, and self-restraint enough to keep from meddling while they do it." Many managers breed dependence by looking over employees' shoulders and giving unsolicited advice, even in situations where the employee could have managed the situation responsibly and felt gratified because of it.

There is a lengthy continuum of empowerment, ranging from broadened individual responsibility, to process improvement teams, to self-directed work teams. Over the next years, health care workers will be experimenting energetically to move practices up the continuum of empowerment. After all, provision of excellent service requires mobilization of all of the organization's dwindling resources. By confining individuals to tight circles of specialization, a deathblow is wielded to individual initiative and problem solving. This creates a self-fulfilling prophecy of health care burnout. We see employees playing narrow roles and therefore don't trust them to handle wider responsibilities and help the organization meet its broader challenges. It's time to think of employees as "hired heads," not "hired hands," to expand their latitude to act, and to provide them with the opportunity to demonstrate their potential toward the end of satisfying customers.

References

1. Lawler, E. *High Involvement Management*. San Francisco: Jossey-Bass, 1986.

2. Bell, C., and Zemke, R. *Managing Knock Your Socks Off Service*. New York City: AMACOM, 1992, p. 157.

3. Bell and Zemke, p. 157.

4. Block, P. *The Empowered Manager*. San Francisco: Jossey-Bass, 1987, p. xiii.

5. Maslow, A. H. *Motivation and Personality*. New York City: Harper and Row, 1970, pp. 1–48.

6. Leebov, W. *Complaint Handling in Health Care*. Chicago: American Hospital Publishing, 1990.

7. American Society for Training and Development. Basics of employee empowerment. *Info-Line* (booklet) 105:12, May 1991.

Chapter 13

Reminders and Refreshers

I f you've developed a service mission, set service standards, provided training and development opportunities, and installed ongoing monitoring and feedback mechanisms, it is likely that employee awareness of your service priority is ingrained in daily operations. If you do not remind people, however, of the priority you place on service quality improvement and keep them reminded with updated goals, new approaches, and employee success stories, the progress made toward a service quality improvement and customer awareness will fade.

Before reading further, take the self-test in figure 13-1 to determine how high-visibility your service quality mission is. Many "true" answers means that your organization keeps

Figure 13-1. Self-Test

Reminders and Refreshers. *Circle the appropriate answer. The more "true" answers, the better. "False" answers indicate areas that need improvement.*

1. In our organization, the importance of a service consciousness and customer orientation is understood by most employees. — True False

2. At least annually, programs are offered to all employees to revive their energy and commitment to service quality improvement. — True False

3. We sponsor contests or events focusing on service themes to keep people energized. — True False

4. In staff meetings, managers often focus staff attention on service issues. — True False

5. Our employees recognize that our service quality improvement must be ongoing, not a flash in the pan. — True False

6. Whether an employee has been with us for 20 years or one year, he or she well aware of our commitment to improve service. — True False

7. There's visual evidence of our service commitment in this organization (signs, posters, complaint boxes). — True False

8. Managers talk to employees about service and customer satisfaction in their everyday interactions. — True False

9. Managers regularly share and discuss customer feedback with staff about their department's service performance. — True False

Total: ____ ____

---

its service quality mission at the forefront. If your score resulted in more "false" answers, consider implementing visual reminders, energizers, and refresher programs to rejuvenate employee awareness and involvement in continuous service improvement.

Regular reminders and refreshers are essential because so many other priorities compete with attention to service issues and behaviors. To revive enthusiasm, it also helps to capitalize on the powers of novelty and repetition to keep employees mindful of the service mandate. Memory triggers and skill enhancers sharpen this awareness day after day, month after month, and year after year.

Employees tend to be highly creative and enthusiastic when called on to participate in developing "excellence reminders and refreshers" for your organization. To get them started, this chapter describes five strategies used successfully by organizations to keep service excellence high on the list of hospitalwide priorities:

1. House Rule of the Month campaigns
2. Posters, paycheck stuffers, pins, and other visual reminders
3. Events and celebrations
4. Staff meetings to improve service
5. Service lending library

□ House Rule of the Month Campaigns

A large part of your service excellence strategy involves installing and maintaining clear service expectations for all employees. Your managers will be involved in incorporating service dimensions into job descriptions and making these requirements an important aspect of an employee's performance review. Consider using as the foundation for reminder campaigns your Service Excellence House Rules, that is, your explicit set of behavioral expectations related to service. Because the House Rules are a lot to absorb, it helps to break them down and, over time, go into each one in greater depth.

Several hospitals have accomplished this by highlighting one house rule each month. Figure 13-2 shows an example of a memo Rutland Regional Medical Center in Vermont

Figure 13-2. House Rule of the Month Memo

Please Post!

To: Senior Managers, Medical Staff, and Administration
From: Laurie Loveland
Subject: House Rule of the Month: #14 **Keep It Quiet**

We know that noise annoys, but there are some interesting facts about how noise affects us:

Patients:
- Increases their perception of pain
- Interferes with their sleep
- Leads to irritability and anxiety
- Triggers high blood pressure, a major cause of strokes and heart attacks
- Is interpreted as an insult

Coworkers:
- Creates stress, a major cause of illness
- Makes people irritable and argumentative
- Makes people lose patience
- Reduces concentration and problem-solving ability
- Makes people less sociable and more aggressive
- Promotes accidents and mistakes

As you can see, our efforts to reduce noise levels can, and will, have a positive effect on all of us and our patients.

---

used to kick off its House Rule of the Month campaign. Other organizations highlighted particularly troublesome service issues, using a media mix of posters, lapel pins, tent cards in the cafeteria, newsletter articles, and contests. For example, Roanoke Memorial Hospitals in Roanoke, Virginia, developed several awareness campaigns including one on confidentiality. To heighten sensitivity to the need for confidentiality and privacy, RMH used paycheck stuffers, posters, a videotape, and ear signals. The video reviewed hospital policies and portrayed confidentiality as the important professional ethics issue that it is. The silent tugging of the earlobe was set forth as a socially acceptable way that every employee and physician could use to signal others they perceived to be threatening confidentiality. Also employees were invited to sign the Confidentiality Commitment statement in figure 13-3.

The University of Virginia Medical Center in Charlottesville, Virginia, also developed the T-CAT campaign (figure 13-4) built around their mascot T-CAT (Talk with Tact, Care And Thoughtfulness), which included these components:

- T-CAT buttons and explanatory letters were sent to 500 randomly selected employees.
- Employees were asked to wear T-CAT buttons without explaining their meaning. Fliers posted around the Medical Center said "T-CAT is coming."
- Letters were sent to managers explaining the campaign.
- T-CAT posters were delivered to departments.
- *Draw Sheet* (employee newsletter) and other house publications included new pieces on confidentiality.
- New ideas began "raining cats and dogs" in staff discussions of how to improve confidentiality.

Lake Hospital System in Painesville, Ohio, sought to raise employee awareness by presenting a Service Excellence Fashion Show. Organized by the Client Satisfaction Standards Subcommittee of the hospital's service excellence effort, the fashion show launched a set of guidelines for professional dress. Three stores provided business attire for men and women that reflected varied styles and prices. Lake Hospital team members volunteered to serve as models. To enliven the show and raise awareness of the standards even further, volunteers modeled inappropriate clothing as well as appropriate clothing. More than 250 employees attended.

Figure 13-3. Confidentiality Commitment Statement

CONFIDENTIALITY COMMITMENT

I have read the following information on Confidentiality:
Confidential File: For Your Ears Only
Paycheck Stuffers:
    Confidentiality: Why Is It So Important?
    Confidentiality: How Can It Be Broken In Hospitals?
        Parts I and II
    Confidentiality: How Can It Be Improved?
I have viewed the videotape "Confidentiality: How Do You Plead?"

I understand the importance of Confidentiality in the healthcare setting and will practice it.

_____
signature

_____
department

Figure 13-4. Talk with T-CAT

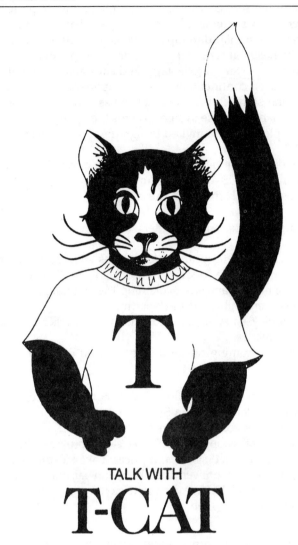

T-CAT is here! T-CAT is here! T-CAT?

He's a new cat on the scene with a serious mission. This feline is here to remind us in a catchy way about an important patient right.

T-CAT brings new life (nine actually) to Hospital Policy 0021. This policy on patient confidentiality states "information regarding the patient's admission, diagnosis and treatment, as well as personal and financial affairs, is confidential and must be rigidly respected."

T-CAT's message is simple: when discussing patients, talk with Tact, Care And Thoughtfulness (T-CAT).

Since his arrival, T-CAT has **CAT**-scanned the medical center to assess how we are doing with this responsibility.

In the cafeteria last week, he couldn't help but overhear two health care workers who were talking loudly about the catatonic Mrs. Tabby in room 212. Later, a conversation in the lobby about Mr. Tom's catheter awoke T-CAT from a catnap. Laugh if you will at T-CAT's "findings," but these incidents aren't too far from reality.

That's why the patient relations committee created T-CAT. He serves as a mascot to spearhead the new confidentiality awareness campaign. It's a light way to make a serious point.

Signs of T-CAT's presence abound: buttons, paw prints and posters. These reminders serve the **purr**pose of keeping his message alive.

So be the cat's meow, help to **cat**apult this campaign to success by remembering to "Talk with T-CAT!"

Reprinted, with permission, from "Draw Sheet," University of Virginia Medical Center, 1988.

To reinforce their house rule "Pick it up, toss it out," Roanoke Memorial Hospitals developed the "Clean Team" program to encourage staff to strive more actively to make every work area and public area clean and neat. Grounded in the philosophy that housekeeping is everyone's job, the Clean Team concept was supported by constructive competition, Clean Team Awards, paycheck stuffers, and miniature standup photos of employees picking up trash. Every department received standup photo cutouts for display in their department. Three paycheck stuffers, distributed every two weeks for six weeks, communicated the concept of the Clean Team to employees. Each area of the hospital was eligible to be recognized as an official "Clean Team" (see figure 13-5). Selected "inspectors" randomly walked through assigned areas and recommended that the area receive a Clean Team Award if it fulfilled these criteria:

- Projects an image pleasing to the public.
- Hallways and other public areas are free of clutter and litter.
- Bulletin boards are neat and orderly.
- General housekeeping is maintained.
- Dishes, trays, and other items are returned to their proper locations.

With the inspiration of Peg Schorle and her Noise Campaign Committee, Riverview Medical Center in Red Bank, New Jersey, developed a campaign around noise reduction (see figures 13-6 and 13-7).

Awareness campaigns like these offer opportunities to explore service issues and behaviors in greater depth and with large numbers of people all paying attention to one focal issue at a time. They can also be very powerful in boosting morale.

☐ Posters, Paycheck Stuffers, Pins, and Other Visual Reminders

Consider posting visual reminders on walls, doors, or bulletin boards. Posters, cartoons, slogans of the week, and the like all remind staff of the importance of service and communicate visibly to your customers that your organization makes service a priority. Also, posters aren't too expensive and they dress up the environment while communicating your service excellence message. Adorn key areas in your facility with eye-catching posters about customer relations, generic posters about the human ingredient, posters highlighting specific behaviors, and those showing your staff relating to people. Work with your public relations department to create your own posters. Hold an employee poster contest with prizes. If you lack the in-house resources to produce your own posters, then buy them.

Change posters periodically so that employees don't get so used to them that they fade into the woodwork. Some hospitals create novelty by having a *poster of the month*, which they rotate to 30 different locations where permanent frames are installed. Some hospitals also create a stunning *gallery* of posters to adorn an entire wall in a lobby, cafeteria, or waiting area. Also, you can have a poster lending library, making posters available to departments and individuals upon request. Here are other suggestions:

- *Wall murals:* Once you have identified a set of service expectations for employees, focus on one each month. Create a changing wall mural with the expectation written at the top and a blank space below for write-in comments, examples, and appreciation statements.
- *Calendars:* Greater Southeast Healthcare System in Washington, D.C., created a wonderful calendar (see figure 13-8). Opposite each month are two photographs illustrating a negative and a positive example of a House Rule in action and featuring employees.

Figure 13-5. Clean Team Paycheck Stuffer

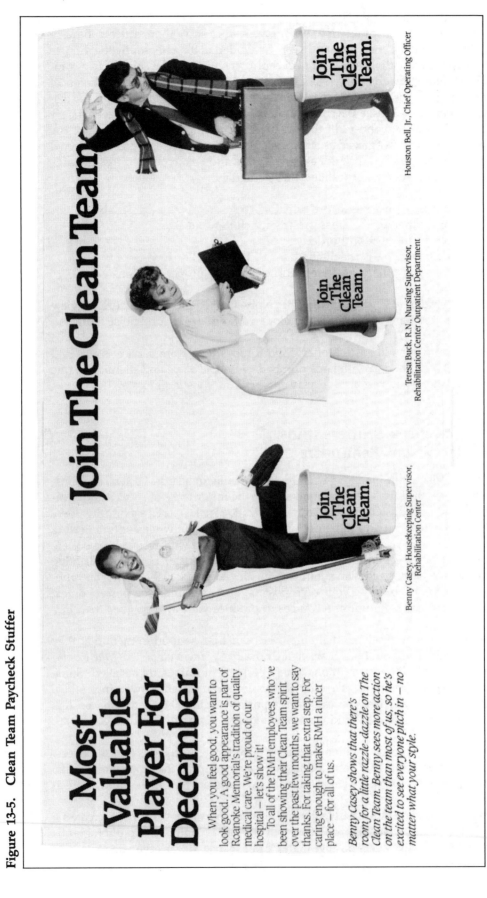

Reprinted, with permission, from The Packett Group for Memorial Hospital, Roanoke, Virginia, 1987.

Figure 13-6. Noise Reduction Campaign

Goals

- Improve patient satisfaction levels by offering a quieter and more restful environment.
- Improve productivity and increase concentration levels by providing a calmer and less chaotic atmosphere for staff to work.

Two Specific Objectives (identified by root cause analysis)

- To improve awareness of conversational noise
- To fix equipment

Promotion

- Kickoff of campaign to be done at the yearly Managers' Retreat
- Fliers and buttons to be handed out by Department Manager to all employees, along with goals and objectives of campaign
- Posters, buttons, articles distributed throughout RMC
- Present in graphical form the scores from the Press, Ganey report
- Blinkie messages each week include statement on noise
- Balloons distributed to all areas
- Mobile Symbol hung throughout the medical center
- Articles in Newsletter (Update) periodically on how we are doing
- Recognize the areas that show improvement

Measurement Tools

- Patient satisfaction survey with results posted on bulletin boards
- Observation checklist by visiting staff (They will post report cards and ideas for improvement in these areas.)

Recognition

- Department/Unit that achieves desired satisfaction level and implements improvement ideas receives special recognition on bulletin board, Blinkie, and bouquet for display
- Individuals who give a workable suggestion receive two tickets to cinema

Results

- Out of 15 Patient Care Units, 7 Units surpassed the target score
- All increased their scores
- Overall hospital noise rating went up two points

Reprinted, with permission, from Riverview Medical Center, Red Bank, New Jersey, 1990.

Figure 13-7. Antinoise Poster

Shhhhhh!

Quiet Heals

Service Excellence

at Riverview

Medical Center

continues . . .

Reprinted, with permission, from Riverview Medical Center, Red Bank, New Jersey, 1990.

Figure 13-8. Calendar Illustration Showing Negative and Positive Examples of One House Rule

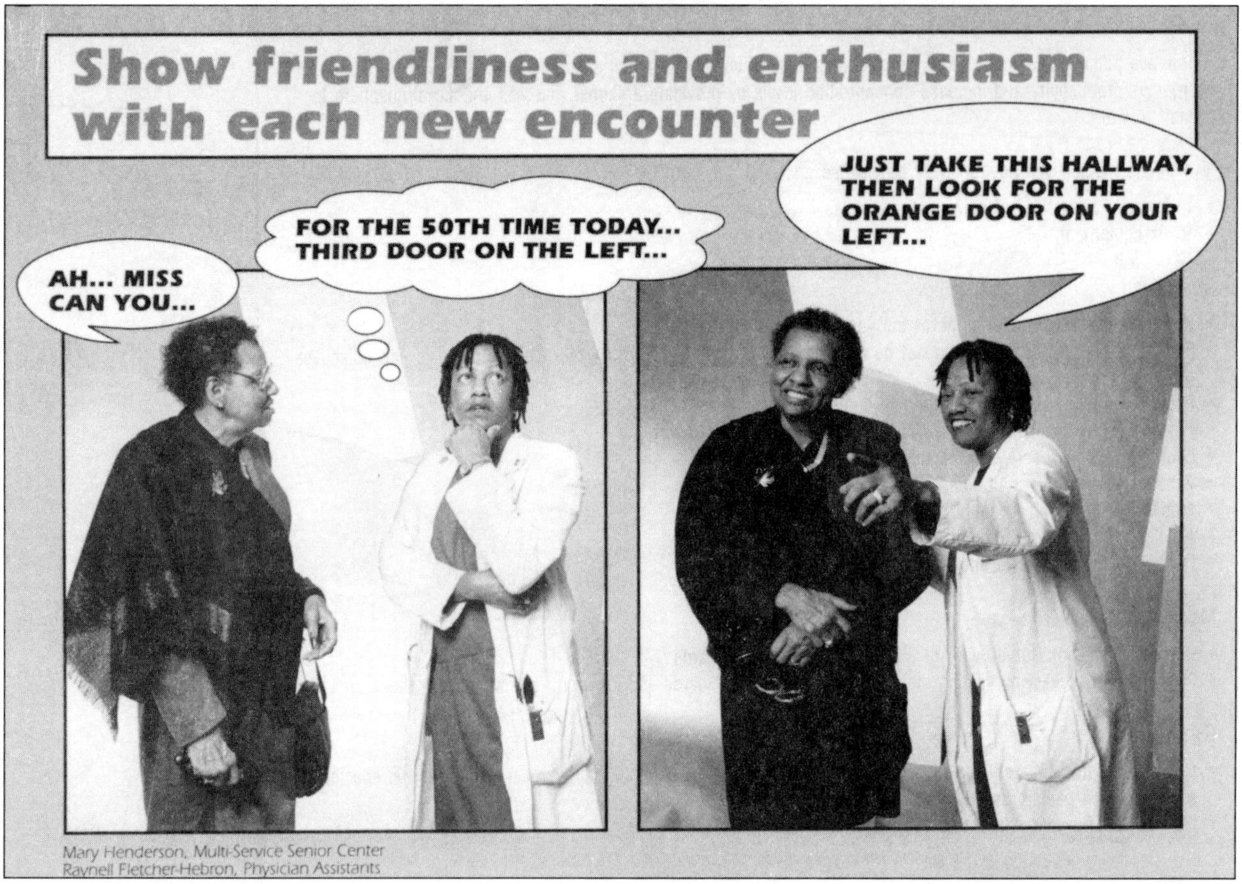

Reprinted, with permission, from Greater Southeast Healthcare System, Washington, DC.

- *Poster-a-month:* Each month locate a poster that focuses on a service-related theme or message (see figure 13-9).

Also consider displaying clippings from your employee newsletter or other in-house communication vehicles. Hang articles, slogans, and skill-building material for all to see. A helpful resource for such items is *Clip 'N Copy: 101 Camera-Ready Items to Communicate Your Service Message* (published by The Einstein Consulting Group).

Finally, a paycheck stuffer can be distributed each month with employee paychecks. Figures 13-10 (p. 252) and 13-11 (p. 253) show examples of the text of two such stuffers used as reminders of specific house rules.

□ Events and Celebrations

Another reminder and refresher tactic is use of special events and celebrations. For example, you may have an annual "Patient First Day" or a special speaker at a luncheon for middle managers. Following are descriptions of a few possibilities:

- *Be it resolved:* Baptist Medical Center in Oklahoma City held a ceremony to renew employee commitment to the center's ongoing TLC Plus effort.
  - A written statement, called "Commitment to Caring," was developed on the hospital's purpose.

Figure 13-9. Poster Used as a Reminder of Service Priority

You are this medical center

You are what people see when they arrive here.

Yours are the eyes they look into when they're frightened and lonely.

Yours are the voices people hear when they ride the elevators and when they try to sleep and when they try to forget their problems. You are what they hear on their way to appointments that could affect their destinies. And what they hear after they leave those appointments.

Yours are the comments people hear when you think they can't.

Yours is the intelligence and caring that people hope they'll find here. If you're noisy, so is the medical center. If you're rude, so is the medical center. And if you're wonderful, so is the medical center.

No visitors, no patients can ever know the *real* you, the you that *you* know is there—unless you let them see it. All they can know is what they see and hear and experience.

And so we have a stake in your attitude and in the collective attitudes of everyone who works at the Albert Einstein Medical Center. We are judged by your performance. We are the care *you* give, the attention *you* pay, the courtesies *you* extend.

Thank you for all you're doing.

Reprinted, with permission, from Albert Einstein Healthcare Foundation, Philadelphia, Pennsylvania.

- —A press conference was arranged to cover the signing of the commitment by the hospital's president and board.
- —At the ceremony, the signatures were affixed to a parchment scroll with the "Commitment to Caring" statement on top.
- —Afterward, at a reception, the employees signed the scroll and received a copy of the commitment and a special mug with a similar slogan.
- —The scroll was placed in a specially designed display case to be installed in the hospital lobby. Copies were framed for hanging in every department and unit in the hospital.
- —The "Commitment to Caring" statement was reproduced as a full-page ad for the local newspaper.
- *Entertainment through employee theater:* Several hospitals are rejuvenating service awareness through original theater events developed by an employee theater troupe. At Einstein Medical Center, two theater extravaganzas boosted morale like nothing else Einstein ever tried.

Figure 13-10. House Rules Paycheck Stuffer

Flap 1: As health care professionals, we have a special responsibility . . .

Flap 2: To help our customers feel respected, appreciated, confident, and secure—in our competent and caring hands.

Flap 3: Even if our patients and their families are not consciously aware of what constitutes high-quality service, they know when they get it, and they certainly know when they don't.

Facts:
- When patients are dissatisfied with service, they tell 20 relatives and friends.
- When they're satisfied, they tell only 5.

That means we have to satisfy *four times* as many people as we disappoint, just to stay even in our reputation. Said another way:
- It takes $10,000 to get a customer.
- It takes 10 seconds to lose one.
- It takes 10 years for the problem to go away. The fact is, our behavior toward our patients is the most powerful marketing strategy we will ever have.

Flaps 4 and 5: What do patients and coworkers want? (Insert your House Rules here)

Flap 6: Back

Consumers base their health care choices on service criteria. After all, that's what they know best. Do your part in making our service a symbol of hospitality and source of pride for all of us. Help our patients feel at home when they wish they were.

In the original musical "Not Just Another Day," written by Gail Scott of The Einstein Consulting Group, hospital employees acted out three versions of one patient's hospital visit: the horrible experience, the ideal experience, and the achievable realistic experience given the stresses on staff. Another musical, "What's Good about Now," tells the story of a disillusioned hospital employee who seeks employment in a baby food company and, in the process, rediscovers what it was that first attracted her to health care. She returns to her job with a new mind-set and renewed vigor.

- *Walk a day in my shoes:* Interdepartmental visitation programs or role-swapping programs can become annual rituals to refresh people's service priority.

☐ Staff Meetings to Improve Service

At department head meetings, equip managers with several formats for conducting staff meetings to refresh and advance service quality. Staff meetings provide a natural forum for refreshing the service mind-set. You already have people together, and it's good management to infuse staff meetings with work on key departmental priorities. Following are examples of two such formats that can be used repeatedly and with effective results:

Meeting Format 1: "From Good to Great"

Spend 20 minutes per month on "from good to great" exercises in order to accomplish the following:

- Help your staff recognize the difference between "good" and "great" service behavior.
- Inspire staff toward "greatness" by helping them to identify and seize previously missed opportunities to satisfy customers.

- Provide much-needed practice in achieving excellence in everyday service interactions.

Here's how it works:

- Explain the purpose of moving from "good" to "great" (heightened customer satisfaction, a positive grapevine about service quality, staff pride).
- Divide staff into small groups of three or four.
- Give each group a card that describes briefly an everyday situation that arises between people in your department and a customer. You can progress from simple to complex exchanges, starting with exchanges like "greeting a patient warmly" to more complex situations like "entering an AIDS patient's room to find the mother of the sleeping patient sitting there crying." Brainstorm situations in advance with staff—one list will last for months!
  Examples:
  −Changing a light bulb in a patient's room
  −Helping a lost person find his or her way
  −Explaining a long wait to a radiology inpatient
  −Delivering a food tray to a patient with arthritic hands
  −Greeting a physician at the front desk
  −Responding to an angry physician
  −Receiving a phone call that was meant for another department
  −Saying no to a patient request that's beyond your ability to fulfill
  −Handling a complaint about your department's biggest systems problem
- *The task:* Each group is to plan two, one-minute skits. The first should show their situation performed very poorly. The second should show their situation performed

Figure 13-11.   Telephone Skills Paycheck Stuffer

Flap 1: When you're on the phone . . .

Flap 2: Our reputation is on the line.

Flaps 3 and 4:

Be a Telephone Pro

1. *Answer quickly:* When people are waiting, every moment is forever.
2. *Greet warmly:* Take a breath and smile before you pick up. Introduce the organization or department and yourself. Sound welcoming. ("Nursing, Pat Harris, may I help you?")
3. *Call the caller by name:* Ms. or Mr. until the caller suggests a preference. Make the caller feel important and respected.
4. *Listen and show understanding:* Allow callers to have their complete say. Tune in and shut out distractions. Repeat back what you heard and communicate empathy. It reassures and calms the caller.
5. *Do all you can to help:* Follow through and keep your promises.
6. *Reveal your plans and actions:* Tell the caller exactly what you intend to do and when he or she can expect a response and a result.
7. *Take careful messages:* Help your coworker by writing down the caller's name, number, purpose, and level of urgency.
8. *Transfer calls skillfully:* If callers haven't reached the right party, tell them who they've reached and help them get where they're going. ("This is Radiology, not Obstetrics. Let me transfer you to Obstetrics, but in case you get disconnected or hear a busy signal, the number is 555-7777.")
9. *Apologize and act:* When you hear a problem or complaint, be our goodwill ambassador. Do all you can to make things right and apologize on our behalf.
10. *Close warmly:* At the end of a call, say something that leaves a cordial last—and lasting—impression, like "thank you for calling." And let the caller hang up first.

Flap 5: Be a ringer! Earn the merit award for outstanding phoning. Your customers and coworkers will appreciate you for it. And you'll earn their goodwill on our behalf.

with "greatness." The idea is to define the two extremes on the behavior continuum for that situation.

- After the five-minute planning period, have the groups perform their skits for one another. Post on the wall the two questions people should consider after seeing the two skits related to each situation.
  - What behaviors were great?
  - What *other* behaviors might have made the employee's performance even better?
- Reconvene the groups and ask: "How easy (or hard) was it to be really great?" Comment that it's not hard to be good—and most people are. But, being *great* involves consciously working to identify missed opportunities, figuring out the behavior that will seize these opportunities, and then integrating that behavior into your everyday behavior.

Meeting Format 2: "Taking Stock of Service Quality"

At least once a month, devote a portion of a staff meeting to discussion of how staff think your department is doing with regard to service to key customers.

Here's how it works:

- List your key customers.
- Divide people into pairs. Ask them to discuss with their partners the two important service strengths they observed during the past month in relation to each customer group, as well as two service problems that bothered them. Encourage them to consider individual interactions they witnessed, patterns of complaints, or the like. Create an "anything goes" atmosphere.
- After pairs have talked for a few minutes, reconvene the group and ask people to share their results. As they do, write down on a flipchart key words for each customer group.
- After all have shared, invite people to draw conclusions by asking:
  - "What should we feel great about regarding our service?"
  - "What do we need to pay special attention to this month in order to improve our service?"
  - "What one problem do you wish we could tackle once and for all?"

☐ Service Lending Library

Skill building is an important component of any service excellence strategy. Since managers and employees simply cannot get away from their jobs for extensive training, one solution is to create a lending library stocked with support material to reinforce service skills and awareness. Following are some examples:

- Books and articles on service management (see bibliography at end of book)
- Films and tapes on service-related topics, such as dealing with difficult people, communications skills, phone techniques, and service recovery
- Training videos. Some hospitals have created simple in-house "trigger" films, using their staff development departments. These films can address such skills as nondefensive listening, counseling, giving direct feedback, frontline skills for employees, and so forth. They could be as basic as a role play, showing a good way and a bad way to handle a tough situation with a customer.

Create a system that enables managers and supervisors to sign out these resources, show/use them at staff meetings or with employees, and take them home to play on their own VCRs.

☐ Final Suggestions

In your efforts to maintain, refresh, and advance awareness and skills related to service excellence, take the following precautions:

- *Don't fail the taste test:* Make sure that any visual items you develop are appropriate to a health care environment. In their eagerness to develop eye-catching, attention-getting visuals and events, some hospitals forget to examine their materials and ideas from the customer's point of view. For example, one hospital kicked off a program with a big reception for all employees in the hospital's front lobby and hired a person in a gorilla suit to entertain. When distraught family members walked through on their way to visit their dying mother, naturally they were horrified by the carnival environment.
- *Don't fail the credibility test:* Some posters may look convincing to the public, but employees will see through them and feel disgusted with the people who created and approved them. They blame the new "PR mentality" and concern for "image" at any cost and call attention to what they perceive as hypocrisy on the part of the administration. Make sure the messages in your awareness campaigns and events are credible.
- *Avoid the machine-gun approach:* In their enthusiasm to produce refresher programs and visual campaigns, service strategists and committees may develop an ambitious, many-faceted campaign and institute it too hastily only to run out of creative steam. Space out your strategies so that they have impact over the long term. A gradual, step-by-step, patient approach makes the flavor last.
- *Don't delegate to the artists:* If your organization has a public relations department, a designer or creative liaison for your house publications and publicity campaigns, be careful not to delegate customer relations campaigns to them without substantial involvement of the "nonartists" in your facility. Not only are ownership and investment shared, your strategy is less likely to be accused of being merely a cosmetic approach to service improvement. If you don't have a solid strategic function in place, don't do awareness campaigns and media events.

So many organizational priorities and everyday job demands compete for attention. To sustain a focus on service excellence so that a customer-oriented mind-set guides employee behavior, stubbornly resist letting your quality improvement priority grow stale. An ongoing, varied, thoughtful agenda of reminders, refreshers, and attention grabbers keeps awareness high and deepens sensitivity to the breadth and depth of customer-oriented health care delivery.

Part Three

Operational Strategies

Chapter 14

Planning for Service Excellence

"Young man, you certainly have a great gift. No matter what they say about you, you have developed a unique skill. Tell me," she said, "how did you get to be such a champion shooter?"

The boy answered, "There's nothing to it. First you shoot, and then you draw the target."

This quotation describes the shortcomings apparent in many organizations' service improvement strategies. To advance service quality purposefully and efficiently, you need a carefully wrought plan with an infrastructure and allocation of resources to support it. You need to decide where you're going and map out how you intend to get there.

There are four keys to effective planning. These are clear goals and direction, long-term thinking, early identification of progress indicators, and involvement of key players in the planning process.

It bears repeating—you can't develop a plan unless you know where you're going. Therefore, you must *establish clear goals and direction*. Many organizations launch strategies that mimic those of the hospital down the street or follow the generic advice heard by the chief executive officer at a recent conference—without asking these important questions:

- Is this what we want to commit to?
- Is this where we want to go?
- Is this really right for our organization?

Without clarity on goals that are unique to your organization, you're drafting a plan in a vacuum and will pay the price later when you find it necessary to backpedal in order to achieve the clear direction you failed to establish at the outset.

Service strategies must be ongoing efforts, so you need to *think long term*. Begin by imagining a three- to five-year effort and plan in detail for at least the first two years. Thinking this way will give you focus, direction, and a concrete understanding of the extent and nature of the effort necessary to advance your service vision. It will also help you maintain momentum, schedule activities in advance so you involve key players, and help staff embrace the seriousness of your commitment. Strategies that consist of activity after activity without a careful, preconceived sequence experience inordinate amounts of downtime (as people stop after each step to plan their next step from scratch) and are not viewed as serious strategic priorities.

To be clear about what key results you want and to decide how you will measure and monitor them along the way, you must *identify progress indicators early.* Many organizations launch service strategies without putting progress indicators in place, only later to try—unsuccessfully—to substantiate what they perceived to be positive outcomes. Common global indicators include patient, physician, and employee satisfaction surveys; employee retention figures; and physician utilization rates. More direct indicators include improved performance on specific service factors of importance to customers, such as "timeliness of service" (in areas like admissions, outpatient services, appointment scheduling, emergency services, radiology, discharge). You need to determine these indicators in advance so that (1) your strategy is "Ready, aim, fire," not "Ready, fire, aim," and (2) you can track results using data to guide and drive continuous improvement in your strategy.

Apart from the obvious point that you want and need good ideas and don't want to cut off any supply of energy and enthusiasm, failure to *involve key players in the planning process* can wreak political havoc on your strategy. In some organizations, hostility and sabotage resulted because the "right" people and departments were left out. Better to have considerable input and planning design sessions that yield multiple perspectives than to suffer the fallout from excluding key players whose participation, after all, may translate into commitment. Structure participation so that it is perceived as being worth the time and truly informs your planning decisions. Senior management, informal and formal medical staff leaders, trustees, department directors, and frontline staff all have a meaningful role in the planning process.

☐ Overview of a Comprehensive Planning Process

A comprehensive planning process includes the following components: groundwork with leadership, development of a vision with clear goals and objectives to guide your strategy, an organizational service and culture assessment, and feedback of results to key players and strategy planning.

Groundwork with Leadership

You can't plan for *it* without understanding *it.* Senior management and physician leaders must understand without a doubt what service excellence and continuous service improvement are *before* they begin the envisioning and goal-setting aspects of the planning process. There are many ways to build the common language and common conceptual framework that are prerequisite to an efficient planning process in which people understand each other. Some are summarized below:

- *Books and articles:* Virtually thousands of books and articles have been written about service improvement in (and beyond) health care. The bibliography at the end of this book includes many helpful resources you can use to stimulate discussion and help your top team adopt a common language. Some organizations start journal clubs (read-and-discuss groups) six months before they begin their formal planning process to build people's knowledge base.
- *Service-related conferences and workshops:* The Einstein Consulting Group hosts a Service Quality Conference every year, as do many other health care organizations and associations. These conferences provide invaluable opportunities to learn specific skills related to service improvement as well as hear best practices from

others who are several steps ahead in their service improvement efforts. This way, people hear from peers in other institutions what worked and what did not work.
- *Site visits and benchmarking:* Another powerful way to build a knowledge base about service improvement tactics is to examine, through site visits and other forms of information sharing, organizations known to have effective service strategies. To prepare for site visits:
  - Identify organizations with effective service improvement strategies; ideally these are organizations similar to your own in key attributes and objectives.
  - Determine data collection methods (for example, visits, reading of articles, sharing of plans).
  - Gather data on the benchmark organizations.
  - Compare practices and performance levels.
  - Determine superior practices and communicate about these as you develop your plans.

  Figure 14-1 lists some useful questions to help visitors focus on their purpose in exploring how others accomplish service improvement. Have several people from your organization visit sites as a group, so that during the visit you can hold structured discussions with the CEO, key physicians, middle managers, the steering committee, and selected employees. Suburban Hospital in Bethesda, Maryland, made three site visits and sent several people from their steering committee to each site. They met beforehand to identify what to look for and questions to ask and met afterward to share their findings. They learned a great deal from organizations who were open about their experience—about what to do and what not to do.
- *Consultant visits:* A more costly but helpful method is to have service consultants present educational overviews to your group. Specialist consultants can customize their presentations to your specific needs and help later to guide your planning process. By bringing in outside experts, you enable your team to learn together, achieving a common base of understanding within the context of your organization's issues and needs.

Development of a Vision with Clear Goals and Objectives

Once your key players share a common understanding of what constitutes service excellence and what it takes strategically to achieve continuous service improvement, you're ready to identify your service vision and your goals and tactics for approaching that vision.

Most organizations arrange a retreat environment in which they convene senior management, representatives of medical staff leadership, and key operational managers to develop this vision and tactics. Beforehand, each individual is asked to engage in some "prework"—to think through his or her feelings, reservations, and hopes about service excellence. Figure 14-2 shows a set of questions that can be used in this prework.

At the start of your planning sessions, you might pool results face-to-face or have someone compile results for distribution to and review by your planning team. This ensures that every individual has considered service excellence from several important angles.

Figure 14-1. Previsit Questions for Benchmarking Service Strategies

- What are your specific objectives—over what time period?
- Are you willing to share your plan with us? What are the main components of your plan?
- From your perspective, what's working and what isn't? What would you do differently? What have been your accomplishments?
- Describe the roles of senior management, medical leadership, middle managers, and frontline people.

Figure 14-2. State-of-the-Organization (Prework) Questionnaire

To help your team build a strong vision for your service strategy, please answer these questions.

1. What does service excellence mean to you?
2. What are all the reasons you feel it's important to launch a service improvement strategy at this time?
3. Think of the 3 to 5 outcomes you want to see as a result of this effort.
4. What in your organization will support this strategy? (For example, What are you doing right? What driving forces are in place to help?)
5. What are some of the roadblocks and obstacles you see ahead?

To characterize your people and your culture, please answer these questions:

1. Which employee behaviors do you want to change or strengthen? What do employees do that you wish they didn't do? What do they do that you wish they would do more often, more consistently, or better?
2. Which skills and abilities need strengthening among your executive team, managers, and supervisors in order for them to champion, lead, and support your strategy?
3. What words would you use to describe your corporate culture?
4. About employee perceptions:
   • How do employees feel about working for your organization?
   • What do employees like about your organization?
   • What are your employees' biggest complaints?
5. About physician perceptions:
   • How do physicians feel about their association with your organization?
   • What do they like and dislike about your organization?
   • What are their biggest complaints?
6. About public image:
   • Who do you see as your customers?
   • How do your customers perceive your organization?
   • Which three words describe your public image (excellent, good, cloudy, mixed, poor)?
   • Which aspects of your reputation would you like to change or improve?

The first step is to create your service vision. In a nutshell, this means imagining your organization as you want it to be. For example:

- How you want patients to be treated as customers
- How you want physicians to be treated as customers
- How you want employees to be treated as customers
- How you want the physical environment to be
- The emotional climate you want
- How you want decisions to be made and who should make them

When you meet to articulate your vision, allow participants an opportunity to think through their vision, share it with others, collect common themes and ideas, discuss areas of disagreement, and reach consensus on the key elements of the service vision to drive your service strategy. The goal is to synthesize all of this information into one clear vision statement that describes the ideal customer-focused organization you want to create. Specific design suggestions for clarifying your team's service vision are contained in chapter 4.

Organizational Assessment

The next step in planning is to do a thorough assessment of your organization to identify strengths and weaknesses related to your vision. The objective of this step is to glean a rich variety of information about your organization to help you:

- Identify the factors already in place that reflect excellent service and drive service quality improvement—from the perspectives of staff and customers

- Identify service weaknesses and barriers to service quality and continuous improvement—from the perspectives of staff and customers
- Establish priorities for improvement so that you can tailor strategy components to address these priorities

A variety of tools can help you assess your organization's service strengths and weaknesses. These include customer satisfaction survey analysis; systems assessment; complaint analysis; and qualitative methods such as focus groups, think tanks, and interviews. An organizational culture assessment is made using survey devices and qualitative methods such as focus groups and interviews. Other assessment tools are discussed in the following subsections.

Service Audits

Service audits examine service delivery as it happens and customer reactions to it. Audits are performed by a variety of measures, some of which are:

- *Customer surveys:* Listen to the voice of the customer to guide your setting of priorities. Analyze your existing customer satisfaction surveys, including organization-wide surveys of patients, physicians, visitors, employee surveys, and community image studies, as well as any department-specific surveys that are designed to solicit feedback about service quality in particular programs or departments. Examine these data to identify trends and problems that reveal service improvement priorities.
- *Systems/process assessment:* Systems and process problems make it difficult for qualified staff to extend service quality to patients, physicians, and to one another. Also, they take up time, cost money, and frustrate patients, physicians, and staff. An audit of key service systems (for example, patient scheduling, transportation, telecommunications, admissions, discharge planning, and care planning) identifies prime targets for service improvement and cost reduction.

  Bring in systems experts to examine your key service systems and identify those that, if improved significantly, would create breakthroughs in service quality. Operational Management Systems (Blue Bell, Pennsylvania) is one such company that can perform a wall-to-wall systems audit and identify not just problematic systems (because you already know which ones they are), but also root causes and the scope, time, and resources needed to yield breakthroughs in service quality if identified as focal points for improvement in your planning process.
- *Complaint analysis:* Ideally your organization tracks complaints and can provide complaint data, including dialogue with patients, to help you set priorities in your planning process. Patient representatives should be tracking these dialogues. It is helpful to understand what customers are saying about your services right now before shaping your improvement strategy.
- *Focus groups, think tanks, and interviews:* These techniques help you to obtain new, rich qualitative information about service quality from key stakeholders. If you choose to collect this kind of information using in-house people, see chapter 6 for descriptions of how these methods work. Many organizations use facilitators or interviewers skilled in these techniques to ensure that the information gained is useful and reliable.

Culture Assessment

You are already familiar with the 10 pillars of continuous improvement (introduced in chapter 3) and the variety of ways you can align your cultural practices with continuous service improvement. To identify priorities with regard to a change in culture, determine the extent to which your everyday practices are already perceived to support service excellence and continuous service improvement and then determine which ones are already being changed by individuals and task forces. A culture audit helps you to accomplish this task.

Most organizations find that many practices are already in the midst of change, although many people are unaware of it. Your planning team might identify committees that overlap with other committees, projects that are being addressed ineffectually by several groups because they have not received support as an organizational priority. You might find out that some changes that are well under way are already aligned with the direction your organization needs to move in. Learn about your existing efforts and programs before you launch new initiatives to improve practices that support service improvement. The audit shown in figure 14-3 can help.

Key Jobs Analysis

Another important component of your assessment involves examining how key service jobs/functions are being performed to identify strengths, weaknesses, and missed opportunities. One way to obtain this information by job shadowing. For example, have managers shadow a transporter and identify the behavioral and systems strengths and roadblocks along the service pathway they follow as they do their job. You can also use the "mystery" caller approach (described earlier in the book). Have committee members target a call at random times to high-volume service departments and complete a checklist that describes how the calls were handled (for example: How many rings? Did employee identify self? Did employee know answer to question?). Both approaches help in setting your goals, and they also help later in the process of customizing training to the on-the-job dynamics and skills that need strengthening among employees.

Feedback and Strategy Planning

After assessing your organization's current service performance in relationship to your service goals and vision, use this information to establish and refine your goals and objectives and develop a long-range plan for your service strategy. Your key people need to review the assessment results, define and rank your priorities, and develop your road map—complete with the sequence of events, responsible parties, needed resources, and time lines.

Key questions are: "What do we need to do to bridge the gap between where we are now and where we want to be (our vision)?" "What must we do to achieve our service improvement goals?" More specific questions follow:

- Which customer groups do we want to focus on? How do we want to attend to particular customer groups?
- Do we need to build a customer orientation among staff? Among whom? How?
- What do we want to accomplish with executives? How?
- How do we want to affect managers?
- How do we want to affect supervisors?
- What do we want to accomplish with frontline staff? How?
- What do we want to accomplish with physicians? How?
- Which services processes are top priority for improvement? How will we organize our approach to accommodate them?

Some organizations use tools of quality improvement to facilitate a group generation of elements in the plan. For example:

- Brainstorm what needs to be done to bridge the gap between today's reality and your service vision.
- Use affinity charting to cluster the activities into related items or affinity groups.
- Look at the groupings and identify which ones drive which other ones, so that you achieve a sense of sequence. Consider using Post-it™ notes so you can arrange

Figure 14-3. Culture Audit

Pillar	Methods	Results	Notes
1. Management vision and commitment • Talk vision and commitment • Role modeling	• Planning retreats • Executive development	• Managers clear on vision, direction, and commitment • Managers able to articulate these • A common language	
2. Accountability for service Quality and continuous improvement Clarify expectations: • Management expectations • Service standards and protocols • Job-specific employee expectations Build expectations into: • Hospital policy • Job descriptions • New employee orientation • Performance appraisal • Hiring practices	Work sessions with human resource specialists, committee to: • Examine current policies/ practices • Make changes as needed • Focus group with managers to debug proposed changes	• Policy that addresses service quality and continuous improvement • Behavioral expectations • Specific screening device for hiring • New employee orientation module • Revamped performance appraisal	
3. Measurement and feedback Customer feedback • quantitative • qualitative • Service standards versus actual performance	• Service report card system • Focus groups, employee meetings, interviews • User groups with internal customers • Complaint system • Process controls • Service audit • Trend charts	• Ability to track satisfaction levels • Knowledge of service strengths and weaknesses from customer/ employee perspectives • Trend charts that show expectations versus actual at a glance	
4. Problem solving and process improvement	Improvement teams: • Liaison teams • Cross-functional teams • Natural teams • Teams per customer group Interdepartmental service contracts Strategy to support experimentation	• Short list of high-impact problems to tackle at their root • Ongoing vehicle for process improvement • Experiments, solutions/answers	
5. Communication • Inform • Empower • Invest	• Trend charts • Newsletter • Bulletin boards • Administrative updates • Team building	Employees: • Less resistance to change • More invested • Better able to take organizational perspective Smoother teamwork perceived by customers	
6. Staff Development and Training • For managers • For employees	• Service management mind-set • Customer-driven management • Accountability • Employee involvement and empowerment • Process improvement basics • Complaint management • How to strengthen internal customer relationships • Awareness raising • Customer contact • Handling complaints • Coworker relationships • Dealing with difficult customers • Problem-solving tools • Telephone skills • Professional renewal	• Management focus on service quality and customers • Installed system of customer-driven management • More effectiveemployees • More efficient and cost-effective service to customers • More effective employees • More satisfied customers	

(Continued on next page)

Figure 14-3. (Continued)

Pillar	Methods	Results	Notes
7. Physician involvement	• Briefings • Improvement teams • Bridge building • User-friendly initiatives • Practice enhancement	• Greater physician cooperation and satisfaction • More patients	

8. Reward and recognition
  • Individual
 	
  • Team/group
	• Incentive pay
	• Catcher program
	• Commendations
	• Telegrams
	
	• Manager of the quarter
	• Newsletter recognition
	• Recognition events
	• Innovation/experimentation awards
		• Higher frequency desired pay
		• Increased commitment
		• More satisfied employees	

9. Employee involvement and empowerment	• Improvement teams • "Latitude" expansion • Renewal • Rap sessions/hearings • Spirit-boosting events • Service assistance line	• Organizational improvements by tapping employee talent • More satisfied employees • Improved retention	
10. Reminders and refreshers	• Feedback on service performance • Resource center • Reminder campaigns • Refresher programs	• Rejuvenated people • Enduring focus on service quality and continuous improvement	

Reprinted, with permission, from Albert Einstein Healthcare Foundation, Philadelphia, Pennsylvania.

and rearrange strategy components until you think you have the right components and the optimal sequential relationship between them.
• Use a tree diagram to fill out the key actions needed to implement each strategy component.

Figure 14-4 shows one approach to mapping strategy components.

Organizations tend to fall into four traps during this planning phase: (1) they overlook key players; (2) they plan to do too much too soon; (3) they view their service strategy in isolation, apart from their overall strategy plan and business priorities; and (4) they adopt a plan that worked in another organization instead of tailoring a plan to their own needs.

As discussed earlier, all managers need to be involved in the planning process, or they resist the plans they're expected to carry out. *Overlooking key players* also applies to medical staff leadership. People who generate the plan have no "buy-in" problem later, because you don't have to sell them the plan.

Many organizations develop a plan that calls for too much to happen early on. *Doing too much too soon* causes organizational overload because it requires too much time and resources, given everything else the organization is doing (such as instituting a new information system or opening a new ambulatory center). It helps to post a huge calendar and place all known activities on it before you schedule your strategy components.

Your service strategy can't be considered a program, but a strategic priority. You need to help employees understand how your strategy fits into your organization's big picture and how it relates and supports other initiatives. *Viewing your service strategy in isolation* is inadvisable.

Figure 14-4. Example of Mapping Strategy Components

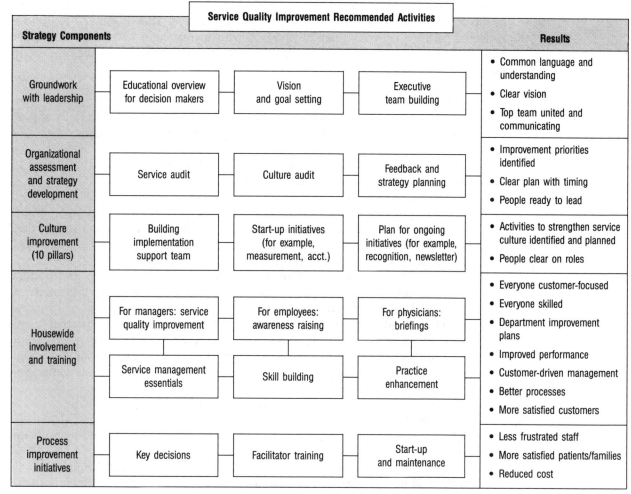

Service Quality Improvement Recommended Activities			
Strategy Components			**Results**
Groundwork with leadership	Educational overview for decision makers — Vision and goal setting — Executive team building		• Common language and understanding • Clear vision • Top team united and communicating
Organizational assessment and strategy development	Service audit — Culture audit — Feedback and strategy planning		• Improvement priorities identified • Clear plan with timing • People ready to lead
Culture improvement (10 pillars)	Building implementation support team — Start-up initiatives (for example, measurement, acct.) — Plan for ongoing initiatives (for example, recognition, newsletter)		• Activities to strengthen service culture identified and planned • People clear on roles
Housewide involvement and training	For managers: service quality improvement — For employees: awareness raising — For physicians: briefings Service management essentials — Skill building — Practice enhancement		• Everyone customer-focused • Everyone skilled • Department improvement plans • Improved performance • Customer-driven management • Better processes • More satisfied customers
Process improvement initiatives	Key decisions — Facilitator training — Start-up and maintenance		• Less frustrated staff • More satisfied patients/families • Reduced cost

Reprinted, with permission, from the Albert Einstein Healthcare Foundation, Philadelphia, Pennsylvania.

Some organizations adopt a plan that worked for another organization or a comprehensive plan more extensive than this organization needs or can handle. It is important to tailor any plan that you adopt to fit your particular organization's needs. *Using a canned approach* is not recommended.

☐ Examples of Plans Tailored to Particular Organizational Needs

Following are examples of eight hospital plans that vary to match the unique circumstances, needs, and goals of their institutions. Use these examples to generate your own strategy.

Hospital A

Hospital A is a mid-sized community hospital that had no previous service or guest relations strategy. This hospital has traditional, conservative management, with a hierarchical, bureaucratic structure that makes for slow decision making and we–they turf lines. Over the past several years, the administration has provided no skill development for staff or managers.

Hospital A must now redesign its service processes, which are cumbersome and cause long delays. They need to help staff feel connected to the hospital and cognizant of the organization's challenges and strategies for success. They also need to build a sense of partnership with their physicians, who increasingly have been admitting patients to other hospitals. Despite this fact, patient satisfaction levels have been fairly good.

The leaders don't see the need for a change in culture. Top management needs substantial education, especially on how to achieve service and quality improvement. They need to become more visible and assertive as role models of teamwork and unity of purpose. Hospital A's plan for improvement encompasses the following approaches:

- One-day team building with executives to outline their vision and goals and to assess, clarify, and agree on their leadership role.
- Two-day team-building retreat for top and middle management. On the first day, they identified new norms for management focusing on customer orientation, teamwork, empowerment, continuous improvement, and so forth. On the second day, they provided an overview of what it takes to achieve service quality improvement and build a common language and framework for change.
- Managers then developed a steering committee consisting of top and middle managers and physician leaders. The initial focus was to examine improvement of internal communication.
- They then conducted hospitalwide workshops designed to build a customer orientation and to focus everyone on the challenge of service excellence and continuous improvement. All employees and physicians were exposed to the following:
  - An overview of the organization's challenges and how service quality improvement would be a key success strategy
  - Discussion of why service excellence is important
  - Specific service skills
- All managers attended "Service Management Essentials," a skill-building program for managers, executives, and supervisors.
- High-visibility frontline staff attended a training program on customer relations skills, and their supervisors worked together on how to follow up with support through coaching, job-specific expectations, and recognition.
- Physicians attended a briefing on the organization's strategy and were invited to help identify processes that needed improvement because of their impact on the user-friendliness of the hospital and patient satisfaction.

Hospital B

Hospital B has experienced dramatic management turnover and with it a change in management philosophy. Employees and physicians don't know whom to trust; people feel abused by what they perceive as precipitous layoffs; medical staff are angry. Patients perceive employees as inhospitable and they notice ill will and a lack of teamwork among staff. Under previous management, this organization had pursued several organizational change programs, but staff claimed they all failed. Their plan was as follows:

- Senior managers held a retreat devoted to team building. They recognized the need to unite behind a common mission and set of objectives and to build communications to lead the organizational change initiative.
- Senior managers then held a trust-building retreat with middle managers, acknowledging the problems that had existed and inviting communication about them in a way that showed people the possibility of change.
- Hospital B's executives then held round-the-clock updates for all employees to share their mission and goals and to reveal plans for how they wanted everyone to help

achieve them. This session shared the organization's big picture, thus encouraging people to contribute.

- Starting with managers, then supervisors, then frontline staff, workshops addressed *internal* customer relationships. The premise: If people in the organization didn't take care of each other and work cooperatively across functional lines, they couldn't possibly serve their external customers well.
- They then formed a steering committee that focused on longer-term strategies for improving internal customer relationships. This committee identified several "experiments" that departments could join in to improve their relationships with other departments. Some chose development of service contracts; others chose formation of liaison teams; and others developed survey feedback devices so they could tackle problems important to their internal customers.
- A team-building committee was also formed to identify strategies to further enhance trust and communication throughout the organization. The committee redesigned management meetings; identified responsive complaint systems; and developed communication forums between executives, physicians, and various levels of staff.
- A physician relations task force formed to consult physicians, identify their key expectations, and target a small number of improvements that would contribute greatly to meeting their key expectations.

Hospital C

Hospital C has a rush of new programs in place, which lead people to think a great deal is happening at once. Change is epitomized by a massive building campaign that signifies active growth. Some employees and physicians are excited by it; others are distrustful and fearful. Still, people perceive the future as exciting. Senior management is cohesive and has been working hard on teamship so as to provide unified, strong leadership for the organization. Their plan is as follows:

- Senior management provided an update on all the strategies in place and how they fit together into the organization's grand plan. They communicated pride, optimism, and excitement about the future.
- Because there are already many task forces and teams working on specific projects, hospital C decided to focus its energies on training all managers to institute customer-driven management and work with staff to develop excellence protocols for interactions with customers. Their reasoning was that under a customer-oriented management, people in all corners of the organization would make continuous service improvement without complicated strategies or executive oversight.

Hospital D

Hospital D has watched other hospitals engage in organizational change strategies for years, not quite knowing what they wanted to do or how they wanted to do it. They finally decided to institute an ambitious wall-to-wall approach to service improvement. Their plan is as follows:

- Hospital D started with building management commitment and selecting a philosophical framework and common language to drive their strategy.
- Teams of managers were sent to visit other hospitals that had similar approaches.
- The hospital set up and provided training for a steering committee that mapped out major components of their approach.
- They began with wall-to-wall awareness raising about customer orientation and the power of service quality and followed employee sessions with briefings for physicians.

- The hospital took the time to provide substantial management development for department directors and supervisors on "Service Management Essentials."
- Administrators clarified expectations for managers and supervisors regarding service management in their own departments and work teams.
- Three areas that needed strengthening—employee accountability, satisfaction measurement systems, and start-up of improvement teams chartered by the steering committee—were targeted.
- After plan implementation, the organization set up a certificate program in customer relations skills for frontline staff.

Hospital E

Hospital E had a previous customer relations strategy that received mixed reviews. It was too successful to throw out and start over, but not good enough to make the lasting changes that the management still sought. Their plan:

- Senior management retreated together to identify their disappointments and missed opportunities with their previous strategy. They also crystallized their strengths and decided how to talk about these in ways that credited people who had helped to achieve them. They then solidified their unfulfilled hopes in the form of new expectations for middle managers.
- With newly clarified management expectations, they held a retreat with middle managers, explored these expectations, and identified support systems that would help managers fulfill these new expectations.
- One support system was a management development system that addressed accountability skills, the service quality improvement process, how to facilitate effective process improvement teams, and how to strengthen internal customer relationships. Managers also developed peer teams that coached each other through the changes needed to get customer-driven management up and running.
- More sophisticated customer feedback systems were installed so that progress could be monitored and improvement opportunities identified department by department.

Hospital F

Hospital F had a reputation for comprehensive service strategies. Outsiders looking at its ambitious schedule of activities were impressed with all the hospital had done, but they saw no results. Furthermore, middle managers seemed to be bad-mouthing the quality of the effort. Top management perceived that middle managers had never fully embraced the need to change their ways, so that the many activities the organization had launched had no long-term effects. The hospital decided to develop a management revitalization strategy. Their plan:

- The senior management conducted focus groups on the middle management role and identified role shifts that managers needed to make to achieve continuous service improvement.
- The organization presented the expectations to managers and then provided a tailored training program that developed management skills for each of the key role shifts expected of them. Classroom training was enhanced by extensive "applications" homework between sessions and by follow-up meetings with senior management to provide coaching and ensure implementation.
- Managers also formed peer support groups that helped them through the change process.
- Management meetings were designed to focus on presentations by individual managers and teams who would describe their improvement initiatives, learning, and progress—with substantial acknowledgment from the audience.

- A team of middle managers developed a system for recognizing and providing incentives for service improvement initiatives and experimentation, so that people would be encouraged to "get off the dime."
- Every meeting between a manager and his or her supervisor began with "What have you changed lately?" and "What are you working on improving?"

Hospital G

Hospital G's previous service strategy had achieved visible improvements in patient and physician satisfaction as a result of improved behavior on the part of employees in their interactions with customers. However, relationships among staff were perceived to be weak. Some also believed that staff members were taking out their stress on each other. Their plan:

- They focused on internal customer relationships.
- They installed an internal customer satisfaction survey and provided quarterly feedback to every department about the quality of its services to its internal customers.
- Each department had to target three other departments with whom they established service contracts.
- They also started an interdepartmental visitation program, so that staff could see how their counterparts in other departments spent their time and understood their challenges, routines, and frustrations.
- After training process improvement team facilitators, they started a number of crossfunctional improvement teams focused on improving processes that cut across department lines.
- Frontline staff attended workshops on "coworker relationships" and in their work teams held at least one meeting a month focused on taking stock of coworker relationship quality and making necessary agreements for improvement.

Hospital H

An ongoing customer relations strategy was considered very successful at Hospital H, but employees and physicians remained frustrated by disabling systems. These injuries were epitomized by long waits for admission, test results, procedures, payments, and so forth. Their plan:

- Hospital H held a workshop for managers that expanded the definition of service quality to include not only service *behavior* but also efficient, timely, and streamlined service *processes*.
- Three key processes were targeted: ancillary scheduling, patient care planning, and patient transportation. A consulting firm called Operational Management Systems was brought in to help them redesign these systems using design teams consisting of managers in the departments involved in each process. They focused on these systems intensively until the redesigned systems were up and running and working well—which took six months given the intensive attention devoted to them.
- They then trained facilitators of design teams and created a system for chartering improvement teams to tackle processes needing continuous evolutionary—not revolutionary—improvement.

After identifying the components of your plan, it's helpful to integrate them and show this integration visually. For example, visuals from various hospitals often serve as road maps and checklists connecting each point along the way with the next one and charting the organization's progress. Figure 14-5 shows a Gantt chart that a large metropolitan teaching

Figure 14-5. Gantt Chart of Hospital Plan

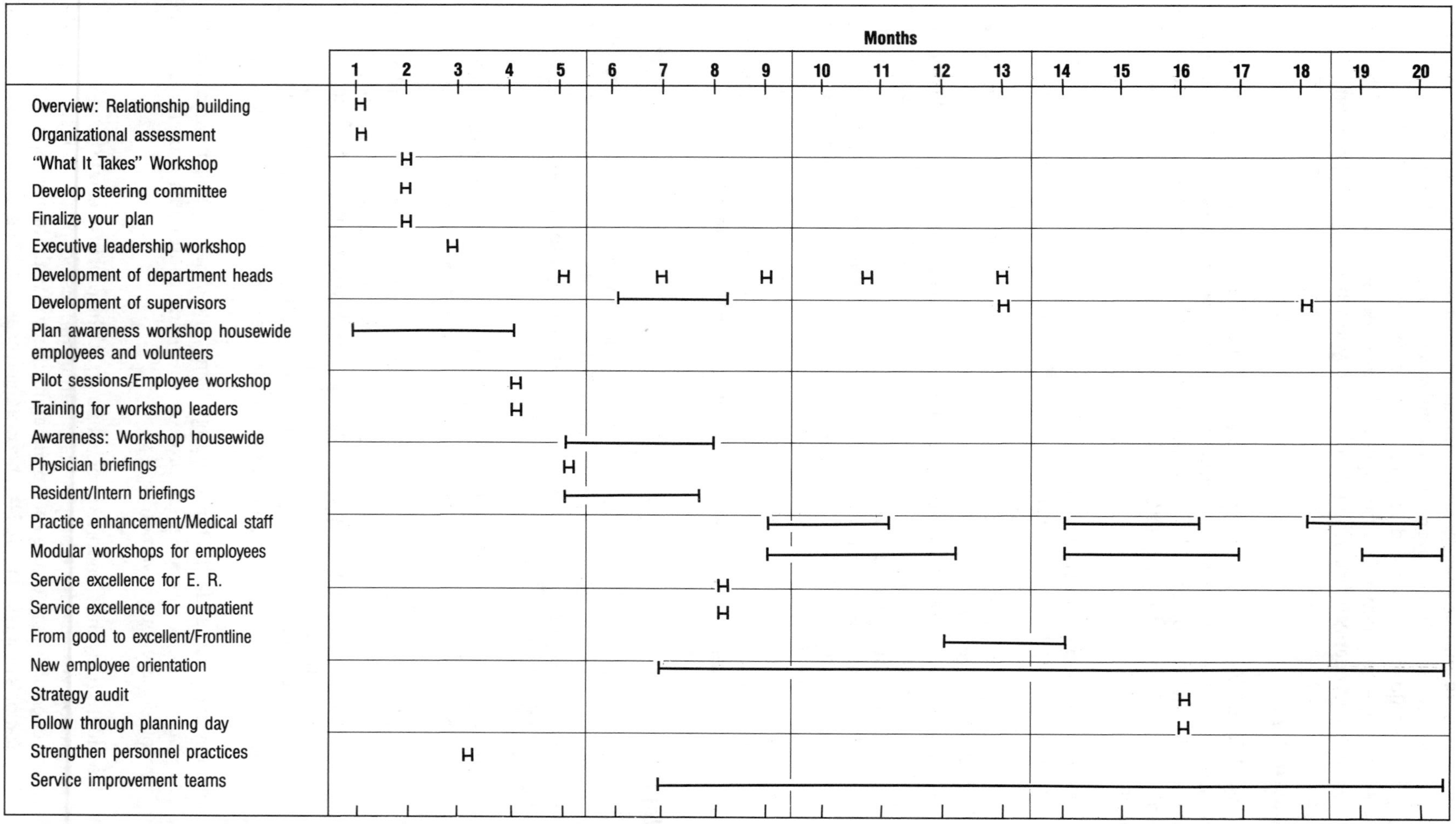

Reprinted, with permission, from The Einstein Consulting Group, Philadelphia, Pennsylvania.

hospital used early on to chart its course. The chart shows (left-hand column) the key components in the service improvement strategy and the time line for each across a 20-month period. Figure 14-6 shows a storyboard used by another hospital to show the flow of events and their interconnections in the service of their vision. Figure 14-7 shows graphically the plan from Oconomowoc Memorial Hospital in Oconomowoc, Wisconsin.

□ Why Plans Fall Apart

Once you've drafted your plan, test it to ensure that you've avoided the following eight common pitfalls:

1. *No shared vision:* The plan is either not fully developed or not communicated. This is clearly a problem because "If you can't see where you're going, how will you know when you get there?" *What to do:*
   • Consider an executive "vision" retreat that starts at the top.
   • Develop a new organizational mission statement for service quality improvement and roll it out at a department head meeting in discussion groups.
   • Reintroduce the terms *service excellence* and *continuous improvement* and talk about what these mean.
   • Reintroduce mission and goal statements from service quality improvement programs and annual reports.
2. *Turfism at the top:* Some planning teams have political infighting or undertones that result in a plan that is built on personal agendas and control needs. This results in uneven *commitment* from executive team members and therefore uneven support for implementation.
   What to do:
   • Hold an off-site executive retreat to develop your team, group support, acceptance, and team commitment.
   • Focus on middle management development and squeeze the top and middle layers together.
   • Make "operations" responsible for your strategy and clarify each VP's support role.
3. *Something the top tells the middle to do for the bottom:* Some plans provide massive work for everyone in the organization *but* the executives. It's as if the executives are saying, "You/they need this," not "We are all in this together." Continuous improvement must become everyone's course, and building a culture of continuous improvement begins with each individual and each team, including the executives and the executive team.
   What to do:
   • Stress the inverted triangle model. Have the CEO get feedback from his or her VP "customers." Have the VPs get feedback from their department head customers and have department heads solicit feedback from their supervisors.
   • Hold an executive/management retreat to explore this team's own team process improvement.
   • Conduct a skills and needs assessment for all managers.
4. *Fragmented activities:* Many organizations' plans include activity after activity but lack the glue that a strong service mission, vision, and progress indicators provide. "The more activities, the better" is an approach that leads to organizational overload and eventual skepticism about the payoffs of their strategy. During the planning phase, it's helpful to ask continually, "How can we simplify this?"
   What to do:
   • Build an integration/steering committee.
   • Create a czar to oversee all program components.
   • Hold a one-day unification and reenergizing program to integrate the pieces.

Figure 14-6. Storyboard Used to Show Flow of Events

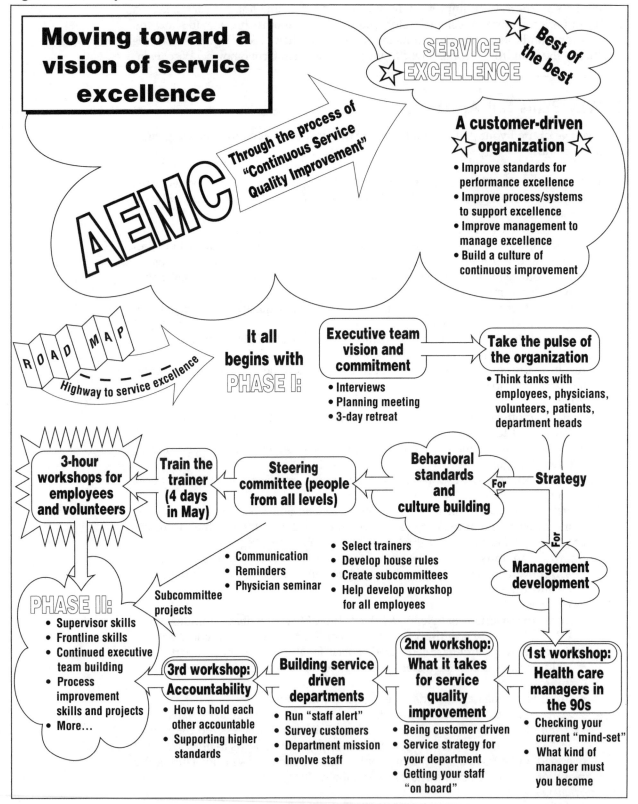

Figure 14-7. Chart Showing Plans of Memorial Hospital at Oconomowoc

Activity	Responsibility	F	M	A	M	J	J	A	S	O	N	D	J	F	M	A
Steering committee meetings for trainer selection and 10 pillars		x	x	x	x	x	x	x	x	x	x	x	x	x	x	x
Planning consultant support for steering committee			x													
Planning next steps for physicians and management development			x													
Management development "What it takes for CQI"			x		x			x					x			
Trainer selection for wall-to-wall vision workshops						x										
Vision slide show and workshop design							x									
Train the trainer (4 days)							x									
Facilitator and team training for process improvement																x
Accountability system implementation and workshop design									x							
Accountability workshops for managers and supervisors										x						
Executive team building retreat						?										
Practice enhancement workshop for physicians and staff											?					

x indicates one day that month

? estimated time

Reprinted, with permission, from Memorial Hospital at Oconomowoc, Oconomowoc, Wisconsin.

5. *A "fix-it" versus "learning" orientation:* Some plans are fix-it plans that focus on glaring problems. The hidden assumption is, "If we could only fix these, we'd be much better off." The people involved with these glaring problems are on the hot seat and feel blamed. This contrasts with a "learning" orientation that focuses not on what's broken but on how we can do important things better and better and how can we learn from our experience at every step. Continuous improvement involves learning and must be never-ending, not one-shot.
   What to do:
   • Form ongoing learning support groups for managers.
   • Engage in an appreciative process to build on "what's right" and how we can continue to build on what we do well.
   • Celebrate learning as part of the mission statement.
6. *One right way paralysis:* Some planning teams are paralyzed because they can't agree on "the right plan" or "the perfect plan." The fact is that after making your best guess at a plan, you need to adopt an experimental attitude regarding the plan itself. Start it, monitor how you're doing, and redesign your plan as you go along. But start somewhere and learn along the way. There is, after all, no one right way. Some strategies have worked from the top down; some have started from the middle; and some have started at the grassroots. All approaches can fail or work depending on whether you make course corrections along the way.

What to do:
- Hold a workshop on experimentation and risk taking.
- Sponsor a "just do it" and "learn" campaign.
- Set up small experiments.

7. *Empowerment before alignment:* Some teams get excited about their many plans and start moving ahead before they have adopted a common direction and sequence. The result is many canoes paddling in different directions.
   What to do:
   - Go back to building a shared vision.
   - Write out the overall mission for your change strategy and tighten the infrastructure for all subgroups by creating specific purpose statements for each group.

8. Consultant-driven plans: Some organizations adopt plans but don't build the infrastructure they need to implement these plans with their own energy. Instead they delegate ownership and responsibility too extensively to external consultants, one internal change agent, or one project leader. The result is that the leadership doesn't own the process. It is an add-on activity, not driven by operations.
   What to do:
   - Work on your own or with a different planning consultant to help you plan your next steps and how you'll determine what training or consulting you'll need to support *your* strategy.
   - Fire your consultant and use different groups.
   - Make all management accountable for specific action steps.

☐ Final Suggestions

As you plan your service strategy, keep the following in mind:

- Avoid a flash in the pan. You need to develop a long-range plan for service excellence that reassures your employees that the emphasis on service excellence is not a short-lived enthusiasm. This reassurance is especially important if your organization has a history of starting programs with a bang and then letting them fizzle. Show people a staged, carefully sequenced strategy that goes on year after year.
- Start by clarifying your vision. Remember this from *Alice in Wonderland*: " 'Cheshire Puss,' she [Alice] began, 'Would you please tell me which way I ought to go from here?' 'That depends on where you want to get to,' said the cat." Be sure you know exactly where you want to go.
- Involve a wide array of key people from the start. Dwight Eisenhower said that plans are nothing, but planning is everything. Eisenhower knew what he was talking about when he emphasized the power that the planning process has in building commitment and in ensuring clarity of purpose and a shared sense of direction among people whose cooperation is key to making things happen.

The planning process is tedious and complex but also necessary. A good planning process is necessary if you want to minimize resistance and maximize results. As usual, prevention is easier than the cure and less costly. Consider the tedious, complex planning job as an investment that reduces false starts, dead ends, and risks and increases the chance that your vision will become reality.

Chapter 15

Building the Infrastructure for a Service Improvement Strategy

Although service improvement is everybody's job, there must be in place an infrastructure of people who guide the strategy and take overall responsibility for its ongoing assessment, planning, and the initiation of course corrections. The appropriate mix of people to be responsible for the activities, processes, and decisions for the strategy and to meet the demands of the strategy as it evolves must be identified. No service strategy can thrive unless it has at least four support features: (1) executives at the helm who assert their leadership continually (not just at the outset); (2) at least one person respected in the organization who coordinates the strategy; (3) human (that is, people) resources available to that person; and (4) an active steering committee, task force, and subcommittee structure tailored to the particular components of the strategy. The functions of each component are described in the following section.

☐ Typical Functions of Infrastructure Personnel

Regardless of what form your infrastructure eventually takes, the following entities and their respective functions are a given:

- *Executives at the helm:* Many strategies fall apart because organization leaders (CEOs) launch the strategy with lots of hoopla—vociferous commitment, strong leadership, and aggressive attention—but then moved on to other priorities. Service excellence doesn't happen unless leaders revamp their everyday functions to include "walking the talk," facilitating process improvement efforts, reviewing customer and employee feedback, and using it to identify improvement priorities. Leadership of a service excellence strategy cannot be fully delegated, even to the most gifted internal consultant, organizational change expert, or coach.
- *Coordinators (directors, facilitators, or coaches):* These persons are the "process owners" of your service strategy and must report to a respected administrator with clout (preferably the CEO). They certainly need secretarial support (at least) because, in reality, most cannot serve this function *on top of* their full-time responsibilities unless their priorities are radically shifted or support staff is added to help. In some

situations, a dynamic team devoted part-time to the effort can manage a comprehensive strategy. Many organizations, however, deploy an entire existing department to manage the service strategy, focusing the lion's share of their time and energy on it. In other words, instead of adding the service strategy to other functions, coordination of the strategy becomes their job, reflecting the organization's shift in priorities to service improvement as "the right thing" to spend time on.

- *Human resources (administrators, managers, supervisors, all other employees):* All employees must understand that service is still *everyone's* responsibility, despite the fact that certain people have been given overt responsibilities for coordinating service improvement activities.
- *Active steering committee, council, or task force:* This group should be comprised of people from many different functional areas throughout the organization and should represent opinion leaders who can, by the intensity of their involvement, spur others to become involved proactively.

Flexibility is needed to deploy people to participate in process improvement teams, task forces, and subcommittees that have the built-in ability to *terminate at will*—that is, with shelf lives that suit their mandates.

☐ The Consultant Relationship

Outside consultants can be helpful, but organizational change must come from within. Consultants can guide you through or facilitate the process of mission clarification, team alignment with the mission, and strategy planning. They can also provide state-of-the-art expertise in training, measurement, and other specialties key to strategy installation, process design, and continuous improvement. But when they leave, your employees must be fully equipped to carry on, building on the practices initiated by the consultant. Long-term reliance on consultants for such activities as measurement, feedback, and training indicates hesitation to truly change your everyday practices and processes to support service improvement.

☐ An Internal Shadow Organization

In his excellent book *Busting Bureaucracy,* Kenneth Johnston of Kaset International describes the need for a "shadow organization."[1] A shadow organization is a second, informal organizational structure, superimposed on your existing structure, that can introduce changes that cut across stable functional lines. Shadow organizations are more flexible, elastic, and adaptable than the organization's basic structure. They can adjust with the need, creating new entities and dissolving those no longer needed. A basic structure for a shadow organization (shown in figure 15-1) includes a senior management team, a steering committee, several task forces, and any number of action teams. Johnston emphasizes the need to tailor your shadow organization to suit the strategy, goals, plans, politics, and culture unique to your facility.

As emphasized in chapter 14, it makes no sense to set up your shadow organization—your strategy's infrastructure (lines of reporting, span of authority, number of staff needed, and the like) before you have a set of goals and a plan. After assessing service strengths and weaknesses; diagnosing what change in the culture is needed; and setting goals, objectives, tactics, and desired time line, you can make rational decisions about what infrastructure to install. Remember, form follows function. Two forms, or models, are discussed next.

Figure 15-1. Structure of a Shadow Organization

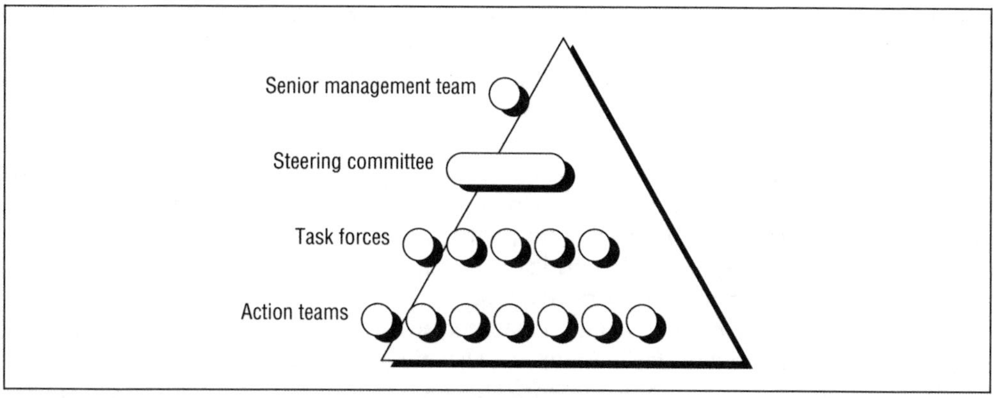

Reprinted, with permission, from Kaset International, Tampa, Florida.

☐ Two Common Models

The following two models, or approaches, have been used by various organizations to implement the functions described earlier:

- *The coordinator approach:* In this model, the organization creates a "coordinator" (sometimes called "director," "facilitator," or "coach") position that reports to a key administrator.
- *The departmental approach:* The organization establishes a department (or redefines the function of an existing department) to manage the service strategy. The department usually consists of two or three professionals and support staff dedicated to service strategy implementation.

Both models have advantages and disadvantages. In the *coordinator model,* the coordinator is usually perceived as a political appointment in a very key position—the right arm of the administrative champion of the service strategy. This perception often helps the coordinator get the cooperation needed to orchestrate the strategy. On the other hand, the components of a comprehensive service strategy often exceed the capability of one individual. This is especially true if the coordinator has other functions in the organization as well. Also, if the coordinator is not the right person for the job, the strategy suffers because he or she does not have complementary coworkers who share responsibility for the strategy oversight.

In the *departmental model,* the department typically includes a director (with the title director, vice-president, associate vice-president, or assistant vice-president); training and organization development professionals; and secretarial/support staff. On the positive side, allocation of several people to orchestrate the service strategy sends a powerful message about the extent of leadership commitment to the strategy. Employees and physicians perceive the strategy as a serious, long-term effort because a functional group has been created with the sole purpose of making sure the process unfolds according to plan. Also, an extended department will have the resources to serve as internal consultants to managers and physicians who can help with a variety of service-related projects, such as team building or service protocol development with staff groups.

On the downside, the department model runs the risk of undermining investment in the service strategy by people in other departments who might think, "The service strategy is that new department's job, not mine." Furthermore, creating a new department risks generating turf problems with other departments, especially those that initially vied for a visible leadership role in the service strategy. Whole departments tend to be especially vulnerable when financial strains produce pressures to make budget cuts. The key to success with a department model is to ensure that the department uses its energies to involve people beyond its own members.

Is one model better than the other? It depends on how ambitious your goals and plan are. The approach that works extremely well in our own large urban medical center is the departmental approach, in which members of our Department of Organization and Staff Development serve as coaches, facilitators, and internal consultants to executives and all line managers in their quest to improve service. Our department personnel neither drive the strategy nor police other people's actions in relation to it. Instead, their role is to serve other departments and leaders in their pursuit of service improvement.

Ideally, your department of service/quality improvement will be staffed by people experienced in organizational change, customer advocacy, project management, training, process improvement facilitation, constructive feedback and negotiation, and troubleshooting for service improvement. The staff should also include people skilled in physician relations and support staff who do the administrative work.

Recognizing how people with unique skills in group facilitation, culture change, and organization development can contribute to their particular strategies for change, hospitals are increasingly developing departments like this to facilitate their quality improvement strategies. These new departments are the wave of the future because expertise in organizational development and organizational change can help health care facilities make the ongoing changes needed to respond to the ever more complex internal and external health care environment.

☐ The Coordinator/Director/Coach

Regardless of which model you choose, you will need a credible strategy coordinator, director, or coach who should report to an effective administrator with clout, an administrator who can make things happen for the sake of advancing service improvement. Unfortunately, in some hospitals an ineffective administrator oversees the service strategy because service is seen as a "soft" area of health care delivery. This kind of "oversight" can indeed prove to compromise your strategy. All too soon, the service strategy becomes just another weak program with a short life. Other administrators, and many employees, label the strategy a failure and disband it because, they conclude, "you can't make headway with service." However, what really happened was that the strategy never had a chance because the organization failed to put the necessary vision, push, and clout behind it.

The coordinator/director/coach mobilizes the various players to install and continuously improve your service strategy. Continuing with the pillar metaphor presented earlier in the book, the coordinator/director/coach is your contractor who coordinates people, committees, and subcommittees to ensure that together they build strong pillars to support service excellence and continuous improvement.

Figure 15-2 lists elements of a sample job description for a strategy coordinator. Some of these elements may already be part of existing positions. Although few individuals could adequately fulfill all of these job responsibilities by themselves, all the functions listed have to be served in some way, either by internal or external human resources.

Instead of creating a new position and posting or searching for the right person in the usual fashion, Georgetown University Hospital in Washington, D.C., tried an innovative approach to filling the job. Believing that a respected and senior employee would be best received as the director, the administration advertised a one-year sabbatical. The "winner" would take a leave from his or her current position to serve as service strategy director. The following criteria were used in selecting the director:

- The candidate should be able to articulate his or her understanding of the service program, its importance, and his or her plans for implementing it throughout the hospital.

Figure 15-2. Job Description for Service Strategy Coordinator (Director or Coach)

Major Job Responsibilities

1. Works with the organization's leaders to develop, coordinate, and evaluate the implementation of a long-range plan for improving patient, visitor, employee, and physician service, including complex scheduling, writing correspondence and reports, recruiting of employees to act as workshop leaders, and related duties.
2. Supports the leadership council or steering committee and several subcommittees to develop, implement, monitor, troubleshoot, and make continuous improvements in the service strategy.
3. Develops and implements methods for monitoring staff concerns, obtaining staff input on problems, and feeding back responses and actions taken.
4. Develops and implements or works with others to implement methods of:
   - Monitoring patient, visitor, and physician satisfaction with various hospital practices and services
   - Serving as a catalyst in follow-up
   - Communicating results to appropriate parties
   - Forming teams that improve key service processes that result in heightened customer and staff satisfaction
5. Intervenes and serves as group facilitator to engage administrators and other key individuals and departments to solve problems that interfere with customer satisfaction.
6. Develops strategies that build employee morale and commitment to service excellence.
7. Conducts meetings and provides training and group facilitation services for teams, physician and employee groups, Council planning activities, and more.
8. Manages the time line for the service strategy, by coordinating the work of various people and departments, including human resources, patient/customer relations, physician relations, marketing, training and organizational development, nursing, and others.
9. Ensures feedback and communication about strategy components, their outcomes and problems, providing this information to the various people and groups with responsibility for making course corrections.
10. Ensures celebration of milestones in service improvement.
11. Handles an array of other duties as required.

- The candidate must receive the endorsement of his or her supervisor, who must indicate how the candidate's present responsibilities would be handled if he or she were selected.
- The candidate must be able to demonstrate a proven ability in verbal and written communication skills.
- The candidate must be able to demonstrate good judgment, maturity, and an understanding of the hospital's operating systems.
- The successful candidate must have significant managerial responsibility including, but not limited to, that of a department head.

As it turned out, after a successful year on the job, the person stayed on as the service strategy director. Luther Hospital in Eau Claire, Wisconsin, developed the job description for Director of Customer Relations shown in figure 15-3.

The service strategy coordinator (or director or coach) must be a booster and flak catcher. In a hospital setting, there are always some people who resist organizational change; some cooperative people who fail to keep their promise; some who are enthusiastic and want more to do; and some who see your director as a Pollyanna, complaint department, cynic's respite, and lightning rod for every spark that flies between people. So, in addition to the characteristics of an effective director described so far, your coordinator also needs to have these attributes: concrete, finely tuned communication and facilitation skills; guts; thick skin; aplomb; acceptance; assertiveness; *more guts*; flexibility; self-confidence; and dogged, unflinching persistence.

If you have a strategy in place, someone in your organization already has faced this reality firsthand. If not, here's a smattering of the details that most coordinators have to handle early in their tenure—for example, when they set up training sessions on service management or process improvement. This example focuses *only* on *one* of many components in their overall work: preparation for the training of workshop facilitators. To prepare to train workshop leaders, the coordinator has to:

- Identify, probably with the help of a subcommittee, the training approach that best suits the organization—drawing on external and/or internal sources
- Organize and implement the process for selecting workshop leaders
- Communicate the results of the leader-selection process to those chosen as well as those not chosen, and to the rest of the staff
- Schedule the training for your workshop leaders and notify them and their supervisors of the time involved
- Reserve adequate, consistent, reliable, conducive space
- Order lunch and morning and afternoon refreshments
- Arrange for audiovisual equipment; make sure it works and is there on time
- Prepare and duplicate materials
- Develop a list of workshop leaders' names, departments, and telephone numbers
- Ensure administrative involvement

Figure 15-3. Job Description for Director of Customer Relations

Main functions: Develop, coordinate, and evaluate a long-range plan for improving patient, visitor, employee, and physician customer relations. Identify areas of concern and communicate interdepartmentally to improve service quality.

Responsibilities:

1. Monitor customer perceptions and expectations of quality service and communicate the results to appropriate staff.
2. Develop strategies that build employee morale and commitment to service excellence.
3. Identify obstacles that interfere with customer satisfaction and act as catalyst to initiate problem solving and follow-through to improve service quality.
4. Coordinate education programs to increase awareness and build commitment and personal responsibility for excellent service among staff and volunteers.
5. Develop a mechanism to document and follow through on customer complaints.
6. Develop a process that encourages employees to identify and participate in solving problems that interfere with the delivery of excellent service.
7. Coordinate appreciation programs that identify and recognize employees and volunteers who provide excellent service.
8. Promote communication and cooperation with physicians to improve service quality for patients and physicians.
9. Measure and document customer satisfaction as an indirect measure of quality service.
10. Advise the vice-president of marketing concerning customer perceptions and expectations that affect customer satisfaction, retention of talented staff, and financial viability.
11. Participate in planning and presentation of Hospital orientation to communicate service behavior expectations to new employees and volunteers.
12. Act as an enthusiastic, positive role model for all staff and volunteers to demonstrate the Luther Touch and the established service excellence behaviors of Luther Hospital.

Qualifications

A. Professional
   1. Bachelor's degree in health care or human resource emphasis
   2. Membership in ASDVS, NSPRCA, and other related professional organizations
   3. Supports the mission and philosophies of Luther Hospital
B. Personal
   1. Possesses excellent communication and problem-solving skills
   2. Able to establish and maintain good interpersonal relationships
   3. Possesses excellent organizational and project management skills
   4. Demonstrates self-motivation for professional and personal growth
   5. Demonstrates maturity, tact, judgment, and sensitivity to people
C. Experience
   1. Five years in a health care setting with good knowledge of health care delivery systems
   2. Experience in management and supervision
   3. Experience in adult education involving training and motivating adults

Reprinted, with permission, from Luther Hospital, Eau Claire, Wisconsin, 1991.

- Ease prospective leaders' concerns, fears, and last-minute cold feet
- Participate in the training sessions, working to develop a supportive relationship with the workshop leaders
- Arrange just-in-time training for workshop leaders who must learn to use the audio-visual equipment or group facilitation tools; create time, place, and structure for supervised practice
- Become expert in the tools and equipment to be used, in order to troubleshoot when needed
- Monitor or create a system for monitoring the training sessions to ensure consistent quality and maintain an evaluation and redesign process whereby these sessions can be improved continuously
- Plan for the recognition of workshop leaders
- Plan and help implement communication opportunities designed to communicate improvement stories, strategy progress, and feedback that can drive improvement
- Develop frequent, nurturing support systems for facilitators/trainers

These are just a few of the details or subtasks associated with only one small facet of the coordinator's role, that of preparing workshop leaders for team meetings or training workshops. The list of details and subtasks associated with every other element of a service strategy tends to be just as long. That's why the strategy coordinator has to be a special, committed, multitalented person or team of people. You need to do all you can to make sure people appreciate the complexity of the role and the extreme dedication, stamina, and skill that the person (or persons) who fills that job must have.

Your organization's leadership must make sure that they are steering the strategy. They must then carefully select the internal coordinator, who should be a systems thinker, an effective project manager, a role model of excellent service behavior, and a person trusted, respected, and able to communicate with the diversity of constituents key to your strategy's success.

☐ The Steering Committee or Service Quality Council

A service quality council or high-level steering committee is essential, because people from every aspect of organizational life must drive the strategy to make personal investment and energetic implementation contagious. Such a committee is the central vehicle for ensuring widespread, substantive involvement of people who represent and have the potential to communicate with the entire organization.

You may already have such a service advisory committee, steering committee, or council. If so, make sure you have the right people on it. If you have no such body, consider developing one. Without such a leadership team, your coordinator will feel isolated, swamped, and probably bereft of appropriate leadership support. The council or steering committee should do the following:

- Clarify your service vision and mission.
- Assess your service strengths and weaknesses and set goals and objectives for your strategy.
- Design the long-term plan for your strategy, complete with strategy components, goals, criteria for effectiveness, methods of monitoring, and responsibility charting.
- Communicate your service mission.
- Review feedback about your progress and about specific strategy components and revise your strategy continuously to ensure ongoing course corrections.
- Ensure ongoing communication about activities, responsibilities, successes, and problems—keeping communication lines open, well oiled, and well used.
- In short, keep your strategy on course.

283

The question of who should be on this steering committee is controversial. In our experience, the best councils/committees are heavily weighted with administrators and augmented with other senior managers who have critical components of the service strategy in their areas of expertise and responsibility (for example, a training specialist who can help with training programs and a human resources expert who can help improve accountability devices). This group should also include the *lunatic fringe*—the visionaries and mavericks at all levels of the organization who are willing to stick their necks out to achieve service excellence.

In short, enthusiasts must be mixed with people who have the authority to make things happen, in case these categories are nonoverlapping. If you don't have power in the group, the enthusiasts fast become frustrated cynics.

☐ Subcommittees and Functional Teams

The service quality council oversees the strategy and keeps it on course. Beyond this group, you might also consider subcommittees, "think tanks," or "planning and implementation teams" that focus on particular functions that need to be served to make your strategy successful. Many hospitals develop 10 subcommittees, task forces, or "pillar teams" that closely parallel the 10 pillars of continuous improvement described in earlier chapters. Each team is chaired by a member of your steering committee/council and consists of people with knowledge, experience, and credibility related to that team's charge.

These teams develop blueprints for aligning organizational practices with their service mission. Their intense work is typically short term (four to six months) and their members are a diverse group of executives and managers. The job of each team is to determine what the organization needs to do to bring practices related to their assigned pillar into alignment with the organization's service mission. Several teams are briefly profiled in the following:

- The *management vision and commitment team* identifies the particular management expectations and actions needed in order to champion, model, and advance the organization's service mission and strategy.
- The *accountability think tank* determines what needs to happen to your performance appraisal system, job descriptions, and personnel policies to support alignment with your service mission and foster continuous service improvement by individuals.
- The *measurement and feedback team* determines how to measure how you're doing on service dimensions, so you can celebrate accomplishments and identify service improvement opportunities, and figures out how to feed back the results so that data drive improvement.
- The *problem-solving and process improvement team* identifies structures and methods needed to respond effectively to customer problems and complaints, to use multiple data sources to identify service problems and snags, and to make process improvements that affect customer satisfaction.
- The *communication team* examines your mix of methods of written and face-to-face communication and figures out how to augment them or to alter their content to better support service excellence and continuous improvement. This team also identifies bridges and other teams that need to be built among people within your organization in order to "sing one tune" about service.
- The *staff development and training team* outlines the content and approach to training that will help executives, managers, supervisors, frontline staff, and physicians develop the competence and confidence to live your service commitment.
- The *physician involvement team* figures out how to draw the multiple layers of physicians to your service improvement strategy.

- The *reward and recognition team* identifies ways to strengthen your reward and recognition practices to align with and advance service excellence by individuals and teams.
- The *employee involvement and empowerment team* identifies strategies for harnessing employee talent, energy, and ingenuity in making service improvements and in intervening directly with customers to meet their needs.
- The *reminders and refreshers team* identifies methods for keeping service issues at the forefront of people's awareness, so that your service strategy doesn't fade because people stop paying attention to it.

If you plan to form teams to do your organization's thinking and planning related to bolstering these pillars, use the questions in figure 15-4 as a guide. Throughout the process ask, "Which other pillar teams do we need to consult with because of potential overlap between our plans and their plans? (For example, the training team might want to consult and work with the recognition team for some kind of recognition to be attached to the completion of a training program.)

After these teams develop the blueprints for changing your organization's cultural practices to support and advance service quality, the steering committee or council integrates these specific plans into the ground plan for your strategy and determines who in the organization is best equipped to implement them. Often organizations develop implementation teams that work together to complete particular projects. For example, an accountability team might outline the particular practices an organization needs to enhance or change in order to make those practices advance service quality (such as an accountability policy, job descriptions revised to include service expectations, and a revised performance appraisal process that heightens the attention to service performance). Several implementation teams might then be formed—one on job descriptions, one on

Figure 15-4. Questions to Guide Pillar Planning Teams

---

1. What in the organization's current practices relates to this team's focus (pillar)—both formal and informal practices?
   - *Use brainstorming:* The technique of "brainstorming" involves getting people to generate as many of their thoughts as possible aloud without stopping to criticize or compliment along the way. By encouraging rapid flow of thoughts without discussion, people are encouraged to speak up and think quickly.
   - *Use interviews or focus groups:* Consult employees/physicians to determine the practices they perceive.
2. Related to our team's focus, to what extent do our current practices align with and advance our service mission and continuous service improvement?
   - What *are* our current practices?
   - How aligned is each with our service mission?
   - Which need to be strengthened? Maintained as is? Eliminated?

   Conduct interviews or focus groups with staff to find out which practices have positive vs. negative effects on service quality. There may be practices that *seem* to advance service, but don't really because they don't have the desired effect on staff.

   Do "Force Field Analysis." The logic that underlies the technique of Force Field Analysis is this: To move toward alignment, you have to challenge the status quo. You can do this in two ways. You can:
   —Strengthen the practices that are currently pushing toward excellent service and continuous service improvement (the driving forces), or
   —Weaken or eliminate the practices that are impeding excellent service and continuous service improvement (the restraining forces).
3. Related to this team's focus, if we were to start from scratch to build practices that align with and advance our service commitment, which practices would we want to institute?
4. Given everyday realities and the resources at hand in our organization, what do we propose as priorities for strengthening this pillar so that it supports continuous service improvement?
5. Related to each priority, specifically what needs to be done?
6. What human and material resources are needed to accomplish our proposed plan?
7. Propose a reasonable time line for achieving the priorities.

---

recruitment and hiring, and one on performance management and appraisal. These implementation teams would then take responsibility for making the changes and reporting progress back to the council.

□ Where Service Strategy Leadership Belongs in the Organization

There is no one place for service strategy leadership. The right place depends entirely on your organization's structure and politics. Some organizations locate the service function within an existing department. Others create a department of service quality and then decide to whom it should report.

Although some believe that service should report to the CEO or a key administrator, we've seen the service leadership function managed successfully from a surprising variety of areas, including the quality improvement area, nursing, patient relations, marketing, risk management, training, and human resources. The key is not the department name but that wherever you locate the coordination function for your service strategy must accommodate it as having primary, not secondary, importance. And, it also needs to be tied closely to a key administrator. The best "home" for the everyday management of your service strategy should be one that is:

- Clearly patient-oriented
- Able to devote resources to service without creating a conflict of interest
- Filled with people who are credible from a service point of view; for example, if the human resources department is notoriously out of touch with employee concerns, don't put the service function there. If the marketing department is known only for its ad campaigns, don't put your service function there.
- Willing to coordinate the strategy and include others in the process. Going it alone will destroy the potential of widespread employee and physician involvement and its ultimate infusion into the entire organizational culture.

The model we've described (which includes the coordination function, executive leadership, a steering council and "pillar" teams) translates into the organizational chart shown in figure 15-5 for a service strategy. The organizational structure presented in figure 15-6 shows a somewhat different structure designed by Pacific Medical Center in San

Figure 15-5. Organizational Chart

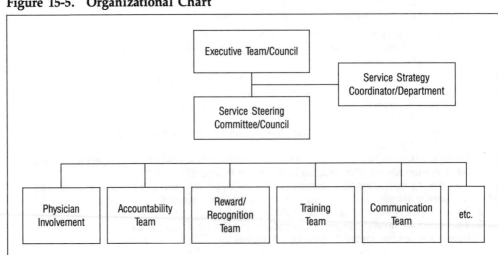

Figure 15-6.   Organizational Structure That Integrates Quality and Service

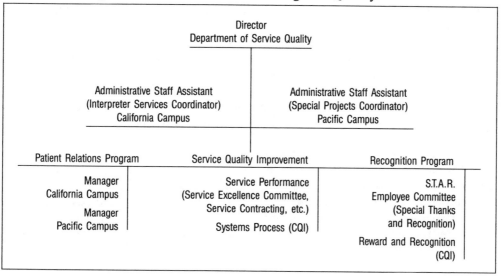

Reprinted, with permission, from California Pacific Medical Center, San Francisco, California, 1990.

Francisco that addressed their intention to integrate the new emphasis on quality improvement with their long-term and highly credible service excellence strategy. The lower middle portion of the structure shows the integration of both their service performance emphasis and their newly added systems/process emphasis.

☐ Final Suggestions

As you make (and remake) decisions about staffing your service strategy, beware of these traps:

- *"It's not my job"*: On the one hand, you need a coordinator who holds together your service strategy and nurtures the other people involved. On the other hand, once you name a person as the overseer of your strategy, others in the organization might sigh with relief that the service responsibility is now taken care of. Your organization's leaders must make it clear that service excellence is *everybody's* job and that every manager, supervisor, physician, and employee at every level is expected to make bold and continuous moves for improved service.
- *"You can handle it alone, I'm sure of it"*: So often, one person is assigned responsibility for ambitious implementation of an ongoing service strategy but is given no support staff. The service coordinator must have clerical support and a squad of collaborators.
- *"I trust you to run with it, now don't bother me with it"*: Delegation to a fault is what this sentiment reflects. Some administrators delegate service responsibility to a hyper-responsible person in the organization and hope (and expect) that the administrative team can thus avoid being bothered with it. When the coordinator approaches them for help, authority, resources, and the like, the higher-ups make the director feel inadequate to the task. Service excellence needs to be a pervasive systemwide priority. A coordinator can manage the strategy but cannot be expected to make it all happen without substantial administrative backup and leadership.
- *Short-sighted screening for the job:* Sometimes the enthusiast gets the coordinator job, but perhaps isn't the right person for it. Even an enthusiast can lack the mix of skills (leadership, energy, organizational ability, and an obsession for detail)

needed to accomplish the job efficiently and effectively. Make sure that your key people have the mix of energy, credibility, and skill needed to carry out their mandate effectively.

- *Out on a limb, alone:* The mover-and-shaker coordinator is frequently left stranded with an enormous responsibility, perhaps in a one-person department without a strong bond to a mover-and-shaker administrator who pulls strings for them. The isolation that results is intense and diminishes ability to do the job. Administration needs to position the service coordinator in a place that reflects its priority on service excellence and links the coordinator to the powers that be.

Ultimately, the infrastructure for your service strategy needs to be the same as the infrastructure for your organization. In the early years of your strategy, a shadow organization is needed to break your organization's old habits and quickly circumvent structural barriers to service improvement. But in time, as every manager and executive comes to employ customer-driven management processes as the everyday way of managing, your infrastructure for service improvement will become your organization's new infrastructure for continuous improvement.

Reference

1. Johnston, K. *Busting Bureaucracy.* Homewood, IL: Business One Irwin, 1993.

Chapter 16

Aligning Departments and Programs with Your Service Mission

The sustained success of your strategy depends on your middle managers' commitment to and skill in ensuring excellent service in their own departments and programs. If your organization equips middle managers with the processes and tools they need to accomplish this, you can help them institute a management system that ensures ongoing service improvement and holds them accountable for results.

Two frameworks or models are recommended for achieving departmental alignment: customer-driven management (see figure 2-5, p. 22) and the 10 pillars of continuous improvement described in chapter 3. Each department and program in your organization needs to ensure continuous service improvement that is customer-driven and informed by the use of sound measurement/feedback and quality planning parameters. Each department also needs a service-oriented culture with everyday practices that focus attention on customers and service quality and that provide incentives to staff to act in the customers' behalf.

Departmental alignment activities that spring from the application of these two models are two-pronged. Although ideally the two paths can be pursued simultaneously, department managers have found it easier to start up departmental alignment by working in a more linear fashion, focusing first on staff attention to service quality and continuous improvement; then on developing plans for improving the departmental culture; and finally on installing and sustaining a cyclical system of measurement, planning, and implementation that constitutes customer-driven management. Figure 16-1 outlines a model detailing the sequential steps managers can take to bring their departments' service delivery and departmental culture into alignment with the organization's service mission. Managers who followed this process have reaped the benefits of continuous, documentable service improvement in their departments and programs.

At every step of this process, employee involvement is key. As emphasized throughout this book, all staff need to know who their customers are, what their customers want, and how their everyday processes and actions are a means to fulfilling or exceeding customer expectations. They must also understand the importance of monitoring customer satisfaction and operational effectiveness and identifying and pursuing improvement opportunities continuously. By involving staff in every step of the department's service improvement process, staff become the drivers of service improvement, not the "tools of production" management uses to achieve it.

Figure 16-1. Departmental Alignment Process

1. Communicate to staff both personal and organizational commitment to service excellence and continuous improvement.
2. Identify your department's key customer groups.
3. Create with staff the department's service mission.
4. Engage staff in assessing the department's service strengths and weaknesses.
5. Establish a department steering committee for employee involvement in service quality improvement.
6. Assess the department's service culture related to the 10 Pillars of Continuous Improvement.
7. Create plans for strengthening weak pillars in the department's service culture.
8. Consult each key customer group to determine their main expectations.
9. Establish measures of customer satisfaction and service performance and collect baseline data.
10. Create departmental and job-specific performance expectations for all staff that will ensure customer satisfaction; communicate them to staff and build them into job descriptions.
11. Develop plans for improving service delivery.
12. Stick to a continuous plan-do-check-act improvement cycle.

This process requires substantial commitment and a long-term effort on the part of managers. In chapter 9 on staff development and training, three models for management development were provided to help managers start up this process and develop the habits they need to sustain an *ongoing* cycle of continuous improvement—including measurement, identification of improvement priorities, tactical planning, and implementation over the long haul.

This chapter provides guidelines and techniques for implementing each step of the departmental alignment process. Hopefully, managers will find it a helpful resource as they wend their way through the service improvement process.

☐ Communicate a Personal and Organizational Commitment to Service Excellence and Continuous Improvement

To involve staff early on, department managers need to express their own and the executive team's commitment to service excellence and the organization's service strategy and their intention to involve everyone in pursuing service improvement at the department level. Before expressing their personal commitment, managers can use the following format to think through and plan what they want to say:

- What is our service strategy about?
- What is my feeling about it (excitement? relief? enthusiasm? optimism?)?
- Why do I want it/care about it?
  - For patients?
  - For family?
  - For physicians?
  - For staff?
  - For our department?
  - For myself?
- Have I acknowledged the difficulties and barriers?
- Can I provide a statement of commitment and optimism despite these roadblocks?
- Can I, in all good conscience, request that staff seriously consider joining in on this commitment and giving service improvement their all?

If the manager is lukewarm about the service strategy and secretly satisfied with merely inoffensive or adequate service quality, there is no point whatsoever in moving forward with departmental alignment.

☐ Identify Your Department's Key Customer Groups

Department management and staff need a clear focus on customers. They need to identify and reach consensus on who their main customer groups are, both internally and externally. Key questions that help in customer identification are:

- What services or products (outputs) do we produce in this department?
- Who are our customers?
  - Who receives each of our outputs?
  - Who uses them?
  - Who pays for them?
  - Who evaluates them?
- Which external parties (for example, payers, patients, their families, referral sources) rely on our outputs, services or products?
- Which internal people or departments rely on our outputs (other departments, physicians, and so on)?

☐ Create with Staff the Department's Service Mission

With customers clearly in mind, staff and management should develop and reach consensus on the department's service mission, articulating this in words and using it as the standard against which performance is compared. This mission spells out this particular department's contribution to the organization's overall service mission. Department managers might consider using the worksheet in figure 16-2 to guide their mission-building process with staff. Following are some examples of departmental missions developed through this process:

- Unit management: "Our department's mission is to provide helpful and dependable service to all of our customers. Our employees view themselves as well-trained, reliable professionals who are pivotal in helping others deliver quality patient care in a timely, positive manner."
- Human resources department at Albert Einstein Healthcare Foundation: "Our purpose is to inform, develop, value, and support Einstein employees, managers, coworkers, and applicants. We pledge to accomplish this by creating an atmosphere of respect and advocacy in which:
  - We are knowledgeable, customer-oriented, and accessible
  - We provide timely and honest responses
  - We ensure fair treatment and confidentiality
  - We do all we can to improve employee performance, job satisfaction, and morale."

☐ Engage Staff in Assessing the Department's Service Strengths and Weaknesses

In that staff members have a history of interactions with customers and with the department's service processes, it's both respectful and enlightening to solicit their perceptions of the department's current service strengths and weaknesses in relation to each key customer group. By inviting their input on a regular basis, managers will gain top-notch information needed in service quality monitoring and improvement. Not only that, they'll be practicing participative management—a management style that is key to making your service commitment and accountability contagious among staff.

The following sections discuss three tools—service quality audit, employee brainstorming to identify problems, and scavenger hunts—that are helpful in gathering input

Figure 16-2. Mission-Building Worksheet

---

1. Define the services and products provided by your department.
   Example: Security Department
   - Primary service: to ensure a safe and secure environment for all guests and employees of the medical center.
   - Secondary services: open doors for people, provide escort services after hours, give directions and information.
2. Identify all of your key customer groups. To whom do you provide each of your services and products?
   Example: Security Department
   - External customers: patients, visitors, vendors, doctors.
   - Internal customers: all employees.
3. Identify the service features each group of customers want from your department. What are their main service requirements?
   Example: Unit Clerks
   - For Doctors:
     —Keeping all paperwork/charting user-friendly.
     —Making sure all tests are scheduled properly.
   Expectation: orderliness/timeliness
   - For Nurses:
     —Keep station well stocked with supplies.
     —Update nurses on all new orders, patient needs, physicians' needs.
     —Become the eyes and ears of the station and know at all times what needs to be done.
     —Become the "extra pair of hands" in emergencies.
   Expectation: courtesy/concern and attention
4. Identify what your department believes in. What are the values that you want to drive service delivery by your staff?
   Example: Unit Clerks
   Values: dependability and professionalism
   Unit clerks interface with a large variety of internal and external customers. They wear many hats and manage multitudes of tasks and information. Others need to know that these clerks are completely dependable, that they manage tasks with accuracy and speed and make sound judgments when they need to. They are pivotal in patient care and need to act in a professional manner at all times.
5. Identify what is unique about your department's contribution. What does your department want to be known for?
6. Formulate a service mission that says, "Here's what we do, here's why we do it; this is what we believe in and what we want to be known for."

---

from employees and engaging them in the service assessment and problem identification process. The instructions are written with the department manager in mind.

Service Quality Audit

The service quality audit is a systematic process for obtaining employee assessment of a department's strengths and weaknesses and identifying opportunities and suggestions for improvements. This operational audit looks at the entire inner workings of the department and has employees identify barriers that cause time delays, frustrations, hassles, efficiency breakdowns, and added stress for employees, patients, families, visitors, other departments, and physicians.

To conduct this audit, managers can set up an ongoing series of staff meetings. We recommend beginning with a 15-minute introduction to the service quality audit, followed by three, 1-hour meetings spread over no more than six weeks.

At the introductory meeting, the purpose of the audit is explained and worksheets are distributed and explained. Employees are told that this service assessment is the first step in an ongoing improvement process—a brick-by-brick improvement strategy in which they'll be key players. Managers let them know that the problems they identify are likely to fall into four main categories:

1. Problems that can be fixed immediately
2. Problems that are more complex and will need to be investigated further in order to understand the root causes and best course of action (These may require administrative approval if solutions involve large dollar expenditures)
3. Problems that involve one or more other departments and will require an inter-departmental problem-solving approach, which you and your group can initiate
4. Problems that may not be solvable because of factors beyond your control; for example, space or staffing constraints

After the introductory meeting, the manager posts the audit worksheets and date and time of the next meeting, which should be held about two weeks later. Figure 16-3 provides a recommended meeting process and examples of the two worksheets.

Employee Brainstorming to Identify Problems

With this technique, the manager explains to staff members, "We're going to spend 20 minutes brainstorming all the problems that interfere with our customers' satisfaction." The manager invites them to brainstorm problems—suggesting as many as they can as fast as they can, using any of the following categories as triggers:

- People problems
- Staffing problems
- Cumbersome procedures
- Policies/procedures that are difficult to enforce
- Problems caused by other departments
- Problems causing staff frustration
- Problems causing patient dissatisfaction
- Problems causing physician dissatisfaction
- Problems causing visitor dissatisfaction
- Problems that waste time
- Problems that cause other departments dissatisfaction
- Problems that cause unnecessary cost
- Problems jeopardizing quality care
- Problems that generate complaints

A healthy list is the result, along with commonalities that indicate a shared interest in several of the problems generated.

Scavenger Hunts

Two other favorite feedback methods, which we call scavenger hunts, are described below:

- The manager identifies several service issues on which feedback is required. Focusing on one issue for a week at a time, the manager develops four questions tapping customer perceptions related to that issue. Employees are then asked to pose these questions of every 10th customer on two selected days of the week. Afterward, they feed back the results to staff and discuss the implications.
- The manager generates service-related questions on which he or she wants feedback. Each staff member receives one question to ask of customers. For example, "Overall, how would you rate the quality of service provided to you by our department?" Or "What do you see as our strengths? What are we doing right?" Or "What do you see as our weaknesses? What are we doing that needs improving?" Or "What suggestions do you have to improve our department?" Each staff member

Figure 16-3. Service Quality Audit Meeting

- Introduce the meeting by explaining its purpose: "We are about to begin the Service Quality Audit, which I introduced to you recently. If you recall, the objective is to identify those problems within our department that are barriers to customer satisfaction for our patients, visitors, physicians, and for other departments, as well as barriers to our own job satisfaction and sense of accomplishment. We're going to begin working in smaller groups, filling out the Audit Worksheets that I showed you earlier."
- Divide total group into small groups of three. Counting off works best so you can ensure random mixing.
- Pass out Worksheets #1 and #2 of the Service Quality Audit to each of the small groups. Ask each group to identify one recorder. Tell recorders not to worry about spelling or sentence structure but just to jot down the basic ideas.
- Allow approximately 35 minutes for small groups to complete the Worksheets. Make yourself available to help.
- After 20 minutes, remind people to move on to Worksheet #2.
- Give a five-minute warning when time is almost up.
- After 30 minutes, ask each small group to report back to the large group on their "problems/consequences/recommendations" for Worksheets #1 and #2. Next, in round-robin fashion, hear one problem from the first group, then go to the next group and keep going around until all issues have been shared.
- Collect the worksheets from each small group and thank the group for their hard work and valuable input. Explain to participants the process for follow up.
- For future meetings, apply the Worksheets to additional customer groups.

Worksheet 1: Service Quality Audit

Service Quality Problems That Affect _____(Customer group)_____

What specific systems, procedures, or conditions seem ineffective in meeting the needs of these customers when they interact with our department? Pinpoint these, identify their consequences, and provide your recommendations or suggestions.

System/Practice/Conditions	Consequences	Recommendations
1.		
2.		
3.		

Worksheet 2: Service Quality Audit

What specific policies and procedures related to our department operations are difficult for our customers to use; i.e., hard to enforce, hard to understand, generate complaints, cause dissatisfaction? Answer this question for each of our department's key customer groups.

Policy/Procedure	Customer Group	What's the Problem?
1.		
2.		
3.		

asks the question of 20 people during a one-week period. After everyone has done their one-question interviews, a staff meeting is held in which staff report their findings and discuss ways to follow up.

☐ Service Alert: Combining the First Four Steps

To streamline the first four steps in the departmental alignment process, managers can consolidate their work with staff into one special staff meeting that we call Service Alert. The manager:

- Communicates his or her service commitment to staff
- Asks who internal and external customers are
- Asks what the department's unique service mission is
- Asks what the current service strengths and weaknesses are

Acting as meeting facilitator, the department manager can use the following staff meeting format to launch the departmental service improvement process:

1. Introduction
   - Share your commitment to service quality and continuous improvement
   - Outline what you consider to be the organization's commitment to service excellence
2. Discussion of service excellence
   - Define service excellence
   - Invite staff to share examples of what it looks like in other organizations and in your own
3. Engagement of staff in articulating the benefits of service excellence for:
   - Patients
   - The organization
   - The department
   - Physicians
   - Themselves
4. Engagement of staff in developing the department's service mission by asking:
   - Who are our internal and external customers?
   - What do they want?
   - What are our current strengths and weaknesses in providing what they want? Use the Service Quality Matrix (figure 2-3, p. 18) to invite staff to generate current service strengths and weaknesses in relation to the expectations of each department's key customer groups.
   - Where do we want to be? What is our service mission?
5. Examine the department's service culture
   - Explain the 10 pillars of continuous improvement and cite your intention to strengthen the culture to advance service
6. Explain subsequent steps in the department's development of a service strategy
   - State your intention to work with staff to launch a process of consulting customers to pinpoint their expectations and to identify and improve weak service behaviors and systems that interfere with meeting these expectations
   - State your plan to score the Culture Check and work with staff to strengthen weak pillars that interfere with continuous service improvement in the department.
7. Identify future steps:
   - Describe the idea of forming a service steering committee for the department and invite people to volunteer.
   - Describe your plans to feed back survey results, ideas, and the like to staff, so that they remain key players in driving your service improvement strategy.

The department's management team should form a service steering committee that will crystallize the department's service mission and devise the plans for all other steps in the departmental alignment process. This group will identify improvement priorities for the department and guide and coordinate improvement initiatives. Figure 16-4 provides a suggested format for this committee's first meeting that builds on the input received from the first four steps or at the "Staff Alert."

☐ Assess the Department's Service Culture Related to the 10 Pillars of Continuous Improvement

As is true in your organization's macrostrategy, culture has a powerful impact on the degree to which a department or program engages in continuous service improvement. With the help of their steering committee, department managers need to ensure that the pillars of continuous improvement are strong in their departments.

The "Service Quality Culture Check: Department Version," provided in the appendix to this chapter, is a helpful tool for collecting perceptions of the degree to which effective practices are in place in managers' departments, so they can establish priorities for strengthening their service culture. This questionnaire needs to be completed by all department managers and supervisors and by a sample (5 to 20) of frontline staff.

Figure 16-4. Departmental Service Steering Committee Meeting

1. "What's the ideal committee? What should its reputation be?" Record comments on the flip chart. Expect to hear reactions such as:
   - Everyone participates
   - People like coming to meetings
   - Meetings aren't long; time is not wasted
   - The committee is effective
   - It has the power to make change
   - People speak their minds
   - You're not penalized for what you say
   - Decisions are quickly implemented
   - There is shared leadership
   - No one dominates

2. Ask the group: "If we want to operate like the ideal, what rules or norms will help us?" Challenge people to help set norms that will make this group effective.

3. Help the group discuss possible norms for a few minutes. Challenge their sincerity. Push for consensus on a small number of group norms that people agree to adopt. Record these on a flip chart under the title "Operating Rules."

4. Mention your enthusiasm about these rules. Move on to reach an understanding of future meeting times and location.

5. Committee Meetings:
   - Discuss the frequency of meetings needed. Start with a recommendation (for example, a weekly meeting for an hour and a half or an initial three-hour meeting).
   - Lead a discussion on the best methods for communicating meeting times, results, content and decide on methods of notification, minutes, agenda setting, and so on.

6. Where do we go from here? Reaffirm your service vision of the department and why, personally, you believe this will be good for everyone, employees and customers alike. Remind everyone of the importance of their involvement in getting the strategy going. Announce next meeting date, time, and location.

7. Reflect on the meeting: Ask everyone to share one thing they appreciated about today's meeting. Everyone takes a turn in sharing a thought or a comment about the meeting. This is a positive way to close the meeting and provide a low-risk way for establishing the norm that positive comments are good and healthy for the group.

☐ Create Plans for Strengthening Weak Pillars in the Department's Service Culture

Consulting staff and the results of the departmental Service Quality Culture Check, work with your steering committee to identify top-priority pillars that need to be strengthened to support service improvement in the department. Most committees find it helpful to select one or two ambitious, long-term, culture-building objectives and two to four shorter-term ones. For example, one nursing unit developed these objectives:

- Long-term objectives:
  - (Regarding pillar 8 on reward and recognition): Institute recognition methods that ensure that every nurse and every medical secretary are recognized for their unique contributions by peers and supervisors.
  - (Regarding pillar 6 on staff development and training): Work with the training department to establish a regular schedule of training opportunities in customer service for refreshing staff skills in relation to patients, families, and physicians.
- Short-term objectives:
  - (Regarding pillar 2 on accountability): Clarify the service dimensions of every job on the unit and establish these as expectations.
  - (Regarding pillar 3 on measurement and feedback): Have every staff member on the unit rate every other staff member on service behavior. Provide this as confidential feedback to each person to help them set improvement goals as part of their personal development plans.

Many organizations create small subcommittees related to each of the top two or three weak pillars. A member of the department service steering committee chairs each subcommittee, so that the subcommittee's work stays on course and is communicated accurately back to the steering committee.

Once the steering committee selects these culture-building priorities and builds an appropriate implementation plan, it should present the plan to staff and invite feedback to ensure that these objectives are valid from the points of view of staff, who are the customers of your culture-building tactics.

☐ Consult All Key Customer Groups to Determine Their Main Expectations

Managers need to engage staff in consulting customers to determine their main expectations and to solicit their perceptions of the service quality currently provided by the department. They need to establish the criteria each customer group uses to evaluate service quality. Too often departments assume they know what customers want, or they don't think about it at all, because they've been providing service the same way for years. The result is that they tailor their services and behavior to incomplete, inaccurate, or nonexistent pictures of what customers want most.

Managers often need opportunities to learn methods they can use to identify customer expectations, including interviewing, focus groups, and survey techniques. They need to learn how to ask open-ended questions ("What do you need most from our department?"), to probe for clarity ("What do you mean by that?" or "Can you give me an example of what that might look like?"), and to help the customer move to other important issues ("Is there anything else you need from us related to technical skills, or the environment, or interpersonal behavior, or our systems?"). Finally, after the customers have discussed their expectations, the manager needs to know how to help them select their priorities, because the department will have to pinpoint and focus on the customers' most important expectations ("From all that you've discussed, what are the two or three things you want most from our department?").

Engaging staff in consultations with customers to determine their requirements reinforces a customer consciousness at the department level. The process described in figure 16-5 is one way in which small teams of staff members can accomplish this in meetings with various customer groups, particularly with internal customers. After such a meeting, staff should compare their own perceptions of customer priorities with those identified by the customer. The following questions might be helpful:

- Does our view of the customers' needs match their view of their needs?
- What did we hear that was different from what we expected?
- What were their priorities compared to what we thought they were?
- Were they more or less satisfied with our performance than we thought?
- What would they most like us to improve on?
- What would delight them?

(See *The Health Care Manager's Guide to Continuous Quality Improvement*, which provides a toolbox for identifying customer requirements using interviews, focus groups, and surveys.[1])

☐ Establish Measures of Customer Satisfaction and Service Performance and Collect Baseline Data

Once customer expectations are clear, managers need to develop measurement methods they can use regularly to let them know how well they're meeting the main expectations of each customer group and process indicators that tell them how well the department's service processes are performing. Figure 16-6 shows a satisfaction measurement device developed by an admissions department after identifying physicians' office managers as a key customer group and identifying this group's top-priority requirements as courtesy, speed, follow-through, and competence.

In setting up measurement devices, managers can benefit from help in the technical design of perception indicators, such as surveys, and direct performance measures, such as checklists, time logs, and the like. Tools to accomplish this can be found in *The Health Care Manager's Guide to Continuous Quality Improvement*.[2]

Managers may need help figuring out ways to involve employees in data collection so that they "own" the information and share a stake in the results. If they are omitted from the process, valuable time will have to be spent later convincing them to embrace

Figure 16-5. Staff Method for Identifying Customer Requirements

1. Initiate and arrange a meeting with members of one customer group.
2. Explain the purpose of the meeting.
   - To strengthen the relationship
   - To better satisfy the customer
3. Ask customers to describe their needs.
   - Listen
   - Clarify without arguing
   - Focus on understanding, not reaching agreement
   - Ask customers to prioritize, distinguishing between the "must haves" and the "nice to haves"
4. Share the team's previous understanding of this customer's needs (new things might come out here); identify areas where improvement is needed.
5. Establish next steps.
   - Thank customers for providing a better understanding
   - Establish a time to share responses and plans
6. Say thanks and reiterate the original purpose of wanting to improve the relationship and service quality extended to this customer.

Figure 16-6. Device for Measuring Satisfaction with Admissions

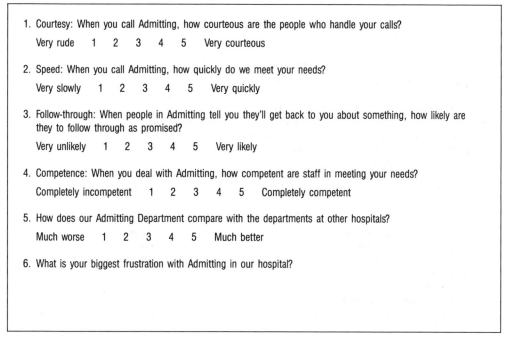

1. Courtesy: When you call Admitting, how courteous are the people who handle your calls?

   Very rude   1   2   3   4   5   Very courteous

2. Speed: When you call Admitting, how quickly do we meet your needs?

   Very slowly   1   2   3   4   5   Very quickly

3. Follow-through: When people in Admitting tell you they'll get back to you about something, how likely are they to follow through as promised?

   Very unlikely   1   2   3   4   5   Very likely

4. Competence: When you deal with Admitting, how competent are staff in meeting your needs?

   Completely incompetent   1   2   3   4   5   Completely competent

5. How does our Admitting Department compare with the departments at other hospitals?

   Much worse   1   2   3   4   5   Much better

6. What is your biggest frustration with Admitting in our hospital?

and use the results to trigger improvement. In one hospital, for example, after extensive data collection, the emergency department decided to institute a fast-track system to decrease waiting time for nonemergent customers. Having listened to customer complaints firsthand, the emergency department management team, nurses, front-desk staff, and other staff were enthusiastic about the change and worked with the hospital's marketing department to publicize the change to the community. But, unconvinced of the need to make the change because they did not hear customer needs and complaints firsthand or participate in early identification of the need to make the change, emergency department physicians did not change their ways. The physicians stuck to their old patterns of seeing patients and created havoc with the new system. Department management then had to go all out to include their physicians in listening to patients and families, designing the service, and otherwise bringing them to the point of embracing the change and cooperating with it.

This example is not unusual. Many managers shut employees and physicians out of the early process of listening to customers. Then, when they want to initiate plans to better meet customer needs, they have to "sell" the changes to staff.

To engage staff, managers need to make important data collection decisions carefully, such as which data to collect, from whom, by whom, and how often. And they need to train staff to collect valid, unbiased data. *The Health Care Manager's Guide to Continuous Quality Improvement* can be used as a toolbox in this process as it includes complete descriptions of useful customer consultation and measurement tools, provides examples, and helps managers through the planning and design process.[3]

☐ Create Departmental and Job-Specific Performance Expectations for All Staff That Will Ensure Customer Satisfaction

If your organization instituted House Rules that spelled out generic service expectations for all employees, you might need to make these more department-specific in terms of your mission. Figure 16-7 shows an example of service standards developed for a pharmacy

Figure 16-7. Quality of Service Standards Developed for a Pharmacy Department

Our department will abide by the following standards to guarantee caring and quality service is provided to our members and in-house customers.

Service standards to our members (customers):

- We will greet our members in a courteous and professional manner.
- We will listen effectively to our members' requests and promptly take the necessary actions to assist them.
- We will keep our members informed of unexpected delays in service.
- We will not engage in personal conversations while providing service to our members.
- We will call our members by name and will verify identity by means of address and/or ID card.
- We will inform our members of specific departmental procedures (e.g., refill line, last refill, mail order) to help them maximize pharmacy services.
- We will finish our encounters with our members in a courteous and professional way.
- We will respect our members' privacy and will not discuss member-related information in public.

Service standards to our in-house customers:

- We will interact with our coworkers and company staff in a courteous and professional way.
- We will not discuss staff, organizational policies, problems, or medical care in public areas.
- We will be considerate, and we will cooperate and assist coworkers, staff, and other departments to guarantee quality service.
- Telephone etiquette:
    We will answer the phone within four rings.
    We will provide our center location, our name, and our department and politely ask, "How may I help you?"
    We will listen to the caller's request and assist accordingly.
    We will direct the call to the person, department, or service needed to assist the caller.
    We will obtain the caller's permission before placing the call "on hold."
    We will end the conversation in a courteous and professional way.
    We will omit personal phone calls while on duty.

Reprinted, with permission, from Kaiser Permanente, Washington, DC.

department. Once the department's steering committee or management team has identified department service standards, management must convene staff to communicate them, explain their rationale, establish a time line for achieving them, and develop a plan for ongoing monitoring. Ultimately, managers are responsible for conformance.

Beyond these departmentwide behavioral standards, departmental alignment is also aided by developing job-specific behavior protocols. For example:

- The radiology technician helps patient after patient onto the X-ray table.
- The information desk staff greet patients and visitors day in and day out and help them find their way.
- The tray delivery worker delivers tray after tray to patient after patient.
- The billing office staff handle question after question, complaint after complaint.

Imagine employees perfecting their ways of interacting with customers in situations like these. The fact that most employees repeat some aspects of their jobs with customer after customer, day after day, presents an unbeatable opportunity to improve service quality. If employees can develop *excellent* routines for handling these repeated "moments of truth" and embrace these routines as the way the job is consistently done, they can generate powerfully positive impressions of their department and the organization with customer after customer, day in, day out.

How can managers develop job-specific expectations? Following are two processes managers and supervisors have used successfully: the staff discussion process and the service protocol design process.

Method 1. Staff Discussion Process for Developing Job-Specific Expectations

The need for job-specific service expectations must be explained: "Standards of behavior vary from position to position in this department because our customers expect different things of us depending on our particular position. Thus, in order to set standards of behavior that will move us toward service excellence, we need to first look at our different customer groups, determine what each group needs or wants from us in terms of service, and then define which behaviors can best meet our customers' needs." Then the manager leads staff through the following steps:

1. Hand out a worksheet entitled "Behaviors That Meet Customer Needs and Expectations" with the following three column headings: Key Customer Groups, Customer Needs/Expectations, and Key Behaviors.
2. Review the example page (see figure 16-8) that illustrates how such a worksheet is used. Walk employees through each column.
3. Ask your group to call out all of the specific positions in the department and list them on a flipchart.
4. Divide large group into smaller groups; one group for each job position identified.
5. Have small groups complete the three columns on the blank worksheet ("key customer groups," "customer needs/expectations," "behaviors that meet customer needs/expectations").
6. Reconvene each group and ask each to report on the behaviors they defined for their assigned position. Then invite discussion:
   • Is there anything missing that you feel needs to be added?
   • Are these behaviors realistic? Can we really do them consistently?
7. Encourage discussion; push for consensus. Be sure to get reactions from people in the specific position as to how realistic they think the expectations are.
8. Thank employees for their input, and tell them you will develop a final version of the service expectations related to their job and distribute them by a certain date.

Figure 16-8. Behaviors That Meet Customer Needs and Expectations

Key Customer Groups	Customer Needs/Expectations	Key Behaviors That Meet Customer Needs/Expectations
Patients	Prompt attention	Greet, smile, introduce, eye contact
	Reassurance	Warm words, touch
	Information	Explains delays, explain what's happening
	Easy to use systems	Explanations of procedures
		Honor appointments
		Give clear directions
Family/Friends	Questions answered	Say "I'll be happy to answer any questions"
	Distractions that ease the wait (TV, magazines)	Point out the magazines, TV, etc.
Other Departments—Especially Nursing, Transportation, Unit Management	Responsiveness	Say "How can I help you?"
	Prompt attention	Explain any delay and give accurate information on how long the request will take

Once performance expectations for each job title have been developed, the manager/supervisor needs to meet with each employee to discuss the specifics, clarify what these expectations mean for the employee, and determine what the manager can do to help move this employee from "good" to "excellent."

Method 2. Service Protocol Design Process

Managers can also work with staff to develop excellence protocols that build into every staff member's job the behaviors that will ensure customer satisfaction. The process described in figure 16-9 is a powerful way to engage staff in developing excellence protocols that become part of job descriptions, which in turn define "the way we do things around here." Many organizations have trained managers and supervisors in the use of this process, expecting them to develop and implement excellence protocols with their staff.

The film "The Other Image: Good to Excellent Radiology Service," produced by the American College of Radiology, contrasts mediocre service with excellent service in the service cycle a patient goes through in a radiology department. Use this film to demonstrate the power of service protocols to managers.[4] Managers can then document these standards and protocols as addenda to employee job descriptions and reinforce them by producing handy job aids (for example, laminated cards or posters) for appropriate employees.

☐ Develop Plans for Improving Service Delivery

Using customer expectations and your baseline data as your guide, work with your steering committee to establish improvement objectives, including objectives for staff behavior change and processes that must be refined to improve service performance.

Figure 16-9. Process for Engaging Staff in the Development of an Excellence Protocol

1. Identify a service process for which behavior of staff needs improvement and work with staff to chart the main steps in that process.
2. Engage staff in interviewing their *customers* to determine the customer's expectations of each step in the process. Focus particularly with staff on specific interactions that matter to the customer (moments of truth) and the behavior that they wish staff would extend to them in those key interactions.
3. Convene staff to develop service protocols.
   - Summarize the moments of truth that customers identified as especially important.
   - Describe the continuum of service quality from "awful" to "wonderful." Explain that the challenge is to figure out the "wonderful" approach to each key moment of truth and then to string them together into a "service protocol."
4. Divide staff into small groups. Assign each group one moment of truth.
   - Their task is to develop quickly two skits: one that shows "adequate" or "inoffensive" staff behavior in that moment of truth and another that shows "excellent" staff behavior in that moment of truth.
   - Focusing on one moment of truth at a time, the group assigned to it shows both skits and invites audience suggestions as to how to improve the "excellent" version even more, pushing people to go way beyond "inoffensive" to reflect truly "excellent" performance.
   - Someone should take notes on the behaviors that comprise the essence of the "excellent" skit.
   - Invite someone to play the patient or the customer (or invite an outsider to help you in this experiment). Line up the small groups *according to the sequence in which their moments of truth flow.* Now have the patient or the customer walk through the pathway of moments of truth that are done excellently. Afterward, find out what the patient/customer especially liked and invite their additional suggestions.
   - Draw a flowchart of the key moments of truth (steps in the process) and, within each step, note the key behaviors that reflect excellence.
5. Establish this protocol as the "way we'll do things here" from now on—so that the wonderful model is the *norm*—the expected way of serving the customer.

Managers can help structure the planning by summarizing on a worksheet (see figure 16-10) the service factors that are both important to customers and currently generate dissatisfaction. After identifying priorities, managers should work with staff to develop related implementation plans and invite staff reactions for the sake of refinement. For each objective, they need to engage in the PDCA (plan–do–check–act) cycle of process improvement reflected in the model for process improvement shown in figure 7-12 (p. 131) on problem solving and process improvement.

Managers should also be urged to involve staff in improvement initiatives. Following is an example of a straightforward meeting plan that involves staff and tends to generate service improvements. You can designate a regular time during staff meetings when you will tackle small problems or generate ideas to be considered further by ad hoc committee or ongoing teams that meet outside of the staff meeting structure. The meeting plan can be used periodically to reinforce a problem-solving mind-set, although some problems obviously require much more analysis and time.

Regular Staff Meetings Focused on Problem Solving

1. Divide your staff into groups of three.
2. Define the problem. Describe the discrepancy between actual service performance and targeted performance on an important service dimension. Communicate the consequences of this substandard performance for customer satisfaction and for departmental and organizational effectiveness.

Figure 16-10. Tool for Identifying Improvement Priorities

| Dept. Name _____ Customer Group _____ |||||
| What outputs do we provide for this customer group? (Information, services, products) |||||

| Customer needs/requirements related to these outputs? | Importance | | Satisfaction | | |
	Must have	Nice to have	High	Medium	Low

What are we now doing to meet the priority needs?

What should be our improvement priorities?

3. Define a three-part task for all trios to tackle simultaneously. Have each group select a note taker. Give people a stiff time limit (for example, 20 minutes). Alert them that after 20 minutes, you will reconvene them and ask them to share their solutions. Their three-part task is to:
    a. Brainstorm factors contributing to the problem. (It would be best to have someone in your small group list these.)
    b. Quickly brainstorm a range of possible solutions.
    c. Identify any one solution that will alleviate one aspect of the problem. (This solution doesn't have to be the grand and perfect solution, just one way to improve the situation.)
4. Draw people together after their allotted time. Invite each trio to share their solutions. Ask listeners to refrain from skeptical comments. Then, after all have *quickly* shared their solutions, go back over each solution and decide what happens next with it. Does it need to be implemented by one person or debugged by a committee? If you don't translate ideas into action plans, your staff will lose heart about devoting energy to service improvement.

If objectives target particular service processes that need improvement, consider the process improvement team approach described in chapter 7 on problem solving and process improvement. Reexamine service processes to ensure that they have the capability to consistently fulfill customer expectations. Institute improvement teams that use process analysis, flowcharting, variance control, and measurement. If objectives call for improved service partnerships with another department, consider liaison teams (described in chapter 7), or service contracting (described in chapter 17) on internal customer relationships.

☐ Stick to a Continuous Improvement Cycle

From then on, continuous service improvement is a repetitive or cyclical process that takes, above all, persistence and follow through (see chapter 7). The departmental alignment process needs to be supported by a strong service-oriented culture, consisting of recognition practices tied to service improvement initiatives and excellent service behavior, team building, and efforts to maintain and improve the quality of work life for staff. Refreshers and reminders about the importance of customers and service quality and management actions to ensure accountability are also essential.

☐ Final Comments

- The department alignment process is nothing more than quality management. It contains elements that will be redundant if department-level quality management processes are already in place. If they are not, your service strategy provides the ideal opportunity to institute quality department management as one key tactic in organizationwide service improvement.
- Most managers need a combination of training and support to move through the departmental alignment process smoothly and professionally. In chapter 9 on staff development and training, the training processes recommended for managers focus on implementing the departmental alignment process.
- Outside of a structure of accountability, some managers might find this process to be too much work. The department alignment process needs to exist within an atmosphere of organizationwide accountability. Department managers need to be *expected* to implement it, to be asked about their progress and results by their supervisors, and expected to evaluate and set development goals related to it during their performance appraisal.

References

1. Leebov, W., and Ersoz, C. J. *The Health Care Manager's Guide to Continuous Quality Improvement.* Chicago: American Hospital Publishing, 1991.

2. Leebov and Ersoz.

3. Leebov and Ersoz.

4. *The Other Image: Good to Excellent Radiology Service.* Produced by the American College of Radiology, Washington, DC, 1991.

☐ Appendix. Service Quality Culture Check: Department Version

(To be completed by all managers and supervisors in the department, as well as by 5 to 15 employees, depending on the department's size.)

Overview

Think about the climate and culture in your department. Is it supportive of great service to customers? What systems, procedures, and strategies are in place to create an environment that promotes customer-oriented actions and continuous improvements on the part of the staff?

Ten forces in your department's culture affect the degree to which your department advances customer satisfaction and continuous improvement. Called the "10 Pillars of Continuous Improvement," they are:

1. Management Vision and Commitment
2. Accountability
3. Measurement and Feedback
4. Problem Solving and Process Improvement
5. Communication
6. Staff Development and Training
7. Physician Involvement
8. Reward and Recognition
9. Employee Involvement and Empowerment
10. Reminders and Refreshers

Each of these pillars needs to strongly drive and support continuous service improvement. By strengthening weak pillars, you will have an enduring positive impact on customer satisfaction.

The department version of the Service Quality Culture Check helps you identify areas of strength and weakness that affect your department's culture. By analyzing items that reflect weakness, you know what to fix.

Instructions

1. Check "yes" or "no" in response to each question. If you have trouble deciding between these two forced choices, pick the answer that best reflects your perceptions.
2. For each pillar, count the number of "yes" responses and write this number in the column on the right.

Analyzing Results

1. Compile group results so that you can identify patterns.
2. High scores reflect strength related to that pillar. Low scores reflect weakness. To diagnose improvement needs, consider the specific items to which you responded "no" and take steps to get to "yes."

Pillar 1: Management Vision and Commitment

	Yes	No	Total # Yes
A. Managers and supervisors in this department actively seek resources needed to enhance service quality and customer satisfaction.			
B. Managers and supervisors actively advance our priority on service quality and customer satisfaction by allocating significant time to continuous improvements.			
C. Department management talks often and with feeling about service and its importance to our customers and our reputation.			
D. This department's managers and supervisors demonstrate courtesy, concern, and responsiveness in their behavior toward customers and employees—serving as positive role models.			
E. Our department managers and supervisors share a clear vision regarding service and continuous improvement.			
			1:

Pillar 2: Accountability

Yes	No	Total # Yes
		2:

A. Courteous, respectful, and compassionate behavior toward customers and coworkers is a requirement in this department, not an option.

B. Employees here have written descriptions of the service quality expectations they are supposed to meet in their particular jobs.

C. Employees here consistently receive coaching, discipline, and, when necessary, termination when they fail to meet expectations.

D. In my department, we orient new employees to our commitment to customers and the service behaviors expected of our employees.

E. People in this department know who their internal customers are and the expectations that they must meet in order to satisfy them.

Pillar 3: Measurement and Feedback

Yes	No	Total # Yes
		3:

A. Our department uses a systematic method to monitor the perceptions of our internal customers.

B. In our department, we've translated customer expectations into operational requirements that we measure.

C. Employees in our department are regularly invited to give their input in identifying service problems and generating solutions.

D. Our department has a system for "trending" or comparing our service performance from one month to another.

E. In this department, we use service performance data to identify improvement opportunities.

Pillar 4: Problem Solving and Process Improvement

Yes	No	Total # Yes
		4:

A. We have a clear, smooth-running system for handling customer complaints in our department.

B. Our department has an ongoing system for making continuous improvements in processes and systems that hamper customer satisfaction.

C. Managers and supervisors here don't hesitate to cross department lines to solve service problems.

D. Managers and supervisors in our department use effective problem-solving techniques.

E. Employees here have ample opportunities to participate in making things better.

Pillar 5: Communication

Yes	No	Total # Yes
		5:

A. Our employees are regularly informed about our department's service performance.

B. We have tools in place that help us all see at a glance how we're doing in meeting customer expectations.

C. Here, we regularly share customer feedback with our employees.

D. Managers and supervisors in our department use a variety of methods (face-to-face, written, meetings) for communicating with employees and keeping them in the know.

E. Our supervisors regularly publicize service problems, improvements, results, achievements, and experiments to employees.

Pillar 6: Staff Development and Training

	Yes	No	Total # Yes

A. Managers and supervisors in our department actively facilitate skill building with their own employees.
B. Staff here are actively encouraged to take advantage of training opportunities related to heightening service and customer satisfaction.
C. Our department has well-conceived systems for building job-specific skills that will help staff satisfy their customers.
D. Our department's new employee orientation communicates explicit expectations regarding service performance and our overriding commitment to customer satisfaction.
E. In our department, employees have the skills for making improvements.

6:

Pillar 7: Physician Involvement (if physicians interact with your department)

	Yes	No	Total # Yes

A. Physicians here are aware of our priority on excellent service to customers.
B. We ask physicians routinely how we can make our department more user-friendly for them.
C. When a physician violates our standards, that physician is confronted in a constructive way.
D. We take active steps to build cooperative relationships with physicians.
E. In our department, physicians are actively involved in generating solutions, not just identifying problems.

7:

Pillar 8: Reward and Recognition

	Yes	No	Total # Yes

A. In this department, employees who are courteous and helpful to customers are recognized for it.
B. Excellence is rewarded in our department, not just length of service.
C. Our department head and supervisors give frequent pats on the back to staff for quality service to customers.
D. Our department acknowledges, publicizes, and celebrates staff contributions to customer satisfaction and continuous improvement.
E. Experimentation and innovation are rewarded in our department.

8:

Pillar 9: Employee Involvement and Empowerment

	Yes	No	Total # Yes

A. Managers and supervisors in our department solicit and listen to employee concerns.
B. Employees participate in planning for changes that will affect them.
C. Employees have the tools they need to serve our customers without ongoing frustration.
D. Our work atmosphere is comfortable for employees.
E. Employees here have considerable latitude to take action to satisfy customers without interference by red tape, bureaucracy, or highly controlling supervisors.

9:

Pillar 10: Reminders and Refreshers

	Yes	No	Total # Yes
A. In this department, we publicize accomplishments and improvements that contribute to customer satisfaction using a variety of media.			
B. In our department, we do special things (e.g., contests and events) to keep staff energized about service and satisfying customers.			
C. When you look around our department, you can see visual reminders of the importance of service quality and customer satisfaction.			
D. In our department, staff see customer satisfaction results so they can make ongoing improvements driven by feedback.			
E. We hold staff meetings to discuss service quality and barriers to customer satisfaction.			
			10:

Personal Record and Profile of Your Score

Record your individual totals for each pillar in the space below.

Pillar	Score	Pillar Title
1	[ ]	Management Vision and Commitment
2	[ ]	Accountability
3	[ ]	Measurement and Feedback
4	[ ]	Problem Solving and Process Improvement
5	[ ]	Communication
6	[ ]	Staff Development and Training
7	[ ]	Physician Involvement
8	[ ]	Reward and Recognition
9	[ ]	Employee Involvement and Empowerment
10	[ ]	Reminders and Refreshers

On the graph below, you can plot the forces in your department's culture that advance versus those that impede service quality and continuous improvement. Using the scale on the left, fill in the space on each bar, from the bottom up, to the level corresponding to your score for that Pillar.

Department Culture Profile

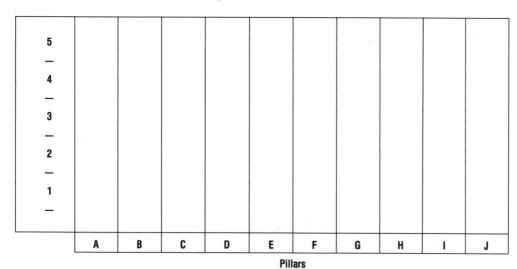

Pillars

Chapter 17

Strengthening Internal Customer Relationships

In the past decade, many hospitals have instituted service improvement strategies resulting in a heightened "customer consciousness" and improved employee behavior toward the organization's *external* customers (for example, patients, visitors, and physicians). But Hyler Bracey, president of Atlanta Consulting Group, estimates that 80 percent of all activity in a service organization involves producing outputs for *internal* customers. Says Bracey, "If this 80 percent is not high quality, how can outputs for external customers possibly be high quality?"[1]

In today's increasingly turbulent industry, where nerve-wracking competition, staffing shortages, insecurity, and rapid change are more the norm than the exception, relationships among people *within* the organization have become more strained. The result is a surge of concern about and attention to the quality of *internal* customer relationships. The underlying premise: If we take better care of each other, we'll have more to give to patients.

☐ "Partnership" Is at the Heart of the Matter

There are two traditional views of the customer-supplier partnership: the supplier (the provider) has the power and upper hand or the customer has the power and upper hand. In the first, the customer receives the service or product provided at the whim of the supplier. The customer is the victim or beneficiary, depending on the goodwill and competence of the supplier. The customer in this model lacks the power to switch to a new supplier if the current one doesn't meet expectations. The problem with this model when applied to internal customer relationships is that every internal customer is also a supplier to others (either departments or coworkers). Although it's true that the customer can rarely change suppliers (because there is only one department of each type in the organization), the result of suppliers maintaining the upper hand and not meeting customer expectations is that this customer then lacks what he or she needs to serve his or her internal customers. At worst, you have a chain of oppression in which suppliers disappoint their customers who, in the role of suppliers to other departments, disappoint them, and so on.

In the second relationship, the customer rules, defining requirements and expecting the supplier to fulfill them, usually with the threat of changing to another supplier if the current one doesn't meet expectations. This model doesn't work in internal customer relationships either. In hospitals, for example, there usually are no alternative providers available. Also, the suppliers cannot focus entirely on meeting their customers' needs because suppliers have many customers, often with competing demands.

The model for internal customer/supplier relationships needs to be that of equal partnership and interdependence. Both customer and supplier share responsibility for building the relationship and ensuring that both parties work together in an atmosphere of clear and realistic expectations, mutual trust, integrity, and accountability to each other. In such partnerships, customers need to define their needs. Suppliers need to listen. Then the two parties need to work out service agreements, monitor them regularly, and make improvements. This results in a chain of interrelating people and departments able to both serve their customers effectively and have what they need from their suppliers in order to do so.

☐ Improved Relationships by Design

Key to effective partnerships are trust, caring, and integrity—attributes that can be cultivated deliberately. Fortunately, excellent internal customer relationships don't happen by accident; they are the product of *strategy*. Two kinds of internal customer relationships deserve strategic attention: (1) interdepartmental relationships and (2) coworker relationships.

Improving Interdepartmental Relationships

Each department's mission is to transform inputs from its suppliers into outputs needed by its customers. Although only certain departments provide outputs directly to the ultimate customer (the patient), all departments provide outputs to other areas/departments. The "immediate customers" of each department, who in turn serve other customers, rely on each other to do their part to contribute to the complicated chain of activities and interactions necessary to serve patients.

Four strategies have been used successfully in health care organizations to strengthen these relationships. These are:

- Customer-driven management
- Liaison teams and cross-functional improvement teams
- Interdependent service contracting
- Interdepartmental visitation

Customer-Driven Management
To plan and install a systematic approach to satisfying the needs of other departments, department managers need first to adapt the customer-driven management process (presented in chapter 2) in developing partnerships with their primary internal customers. Specifically, each department needs to:

- Identify its internal customers and their expectations
- Translate these expectations into operational requirements, figuring out what the department needs to do internally to meet these customers' expectations reliably and consistently
- Institute regular measurements of internal customer satisfaction (for example, service report cards) and operational performance (for example, quality checkpoints)
- Use the results to drive improvement

As an example, note the following scenario: Pharmacy staff identifies nursing as one of its primary customers. Pharmacy conducts a focus group with people from nursing and identifies four primary needs nurses want pharmacy to fulfill: *timely* delivery of medications, *accuracy* in drug type and dosage, *information quality* in the face of questions, and *courtesy* in handling questions and requests. Pharmacy finds out what "timely" means to nursing and examines pharmacy's internal processes to ensure that timely delivery of medications is not only possible but a reliable output from the pharmacy's work processes.

Then, every month, pharmacy asks nurse managers to complete a simple "service report card" (see figure 17-1). Because a survey like this polls perception, not fact, pharmacy also decides to create a method for logging "fact." The department logs actual delivery times (which can be compared to expected delivery times) and the number of drug type and dosage errors (so they can track percentages and identify causes).

Pharmacy managers track the results on a trend chart so they can post them and discuss the results with staff to celebrate progress or identify problems that merit attention (see figure 17-2). Also, recognizing the value of face-to-face, qualitative feedback in maintaining a strong partnership with nursing, pharmacy employees hold what they call "user group" meetings with nurse managers at least quarterly. They ask these questions:

- How are we performing for you lately? What are we doing right? What are we doing wrong?
- You identified four major requirements you have of us. How are we doing in meeting these? Let's talk about each one.
- Where would you like to see our service or relationship with you improve? Do you have any suggestions?

In staff meetings, they review feedback from nursing monthly. Because they're committed to continuous improvement, they form a team of pharmacy staff that will investigate

Figure 17-1. Service Report Card

	Hardly Ever		Almost Always	
1. Pharmacy delivers routine orders on time	1	2	3	4
2. Drug types and dosages are correct	1	2	3	4
3. When asked questions, Pharmacy gives quality information	1	2	3	4
4. Pharmacy staff are courteous	1	2	3	4

Figure 17-2. Trend Chart to Show Nursing's Satisfaction with Pharmacy

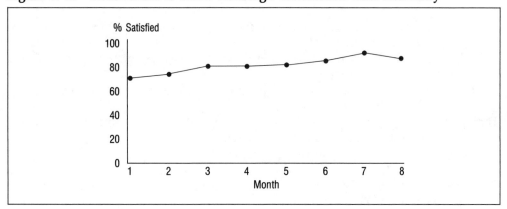

the root causes of problems and work on making process improvements to ensure improved results delivered with greater consistency and reliability over time.

Liaison Teams and Cross-Functional Improvement Teams

Liaison teams and cross-functional process improvement teams are two other vehicles for making improvements across department lines. Liaison teams are problem-solving teams consisting of representatives of only *two* departments. Cross-functional process improvement teams are multidepartmental teams consisting of people from the various departments involved in a cross-functional process.

With both types of teams, the idea is to smooth out and, if necessary, redesign the processes that cross department lines so that these processes serve internal and external customers' needs consistently and reliably. People from multiple, interrelated departments work together shoulder to shoulder to solve problems and iron out the kinks that cause breakdowns in interdepartmental processes.

For example, radiology and nursing might work together to improve their system for scheduling inpatients for radiology services. One hospital with this kind of liaison team discovered that nursing believed radiology lacked an inpatient scheduling system, causing patients to wait hours for radiology services, because nursing arranged to transport patients to radiology whenever there was a gap in the patient's schedule. In a liaison team meeting, nursing discovered that radiology was angry at nursing for not sending patients at their scheduled appointment times. It turned out that radiology created specific appointments for patients *but never notified nursing* of these times! Once the liaison team exposed the problem and cause, the team redesigned the communication loop between radiology and nursing and solved the problem—with positive results for patients and staff alike.

The potential for such teams is infinite. One hospital had as many as 18 liaison teams in action at one time—including an emergency room–admissions team, a nursing–dietary team, a radiology–nursing team, a utilization review–medical records team, a pharmacy–nursing team, and so forth.

Interdependent Service Contracting

Developed by John Rawls and Sharon Mulgrew for Kaiser Permanente Medical Centers in northern California, service contracts are a powerful tool for clarifying and strengthening service partnerships between departments.[2] Service contracts were developed as a tool for managers to reduce the "turfism" that impedes service delivery and to build service partnerships with other departments.

To produce excellent service, complex organizations like hospitals—with their highly specialized yet interconnected division of labor—need to be "seamless" in providing that service. If customer needs, complaints, paperwork, and the like fall through the cracks between departments, service suffers dramatically. For years, a number of organizations have had cracks between departments the size of elephant feet.

Service contracting is a process that helps department managers:

- Clarify their department's service mission and how it relates to the service mission of the entire organization
- Identify key relationships with other departments—their internal customers and suppliers
- Develop explicit, written service agreements between the parties involved

Through the negotiation process and the resulting agreements, the parties develop a clear system of responsibility and mutual accountability.

According to John Rawls, service contracting:[3]

- Aligns the work and performance of departments, functions, and individuals with the purpose of the organization

- Focuses managers and staff on their service mission
- Identifies and increases accountability for meeting the needs of internal customers
- Focuses managers on the most effective use of resources and processes to create and deliver the services or products to the people who depend on them
- Focuses the organization on the reality of and need for interdependence among all parts of the organization
- Builds and strengthens the infrastructure of the organization by developing "circuits and wiring" that facilitate work flow among all parts of the organization
- Makes the organization a living, viable organism rather than a mechanical structure

Interdependent service contracting works as follows:

- Before managers from the two departments meet, each manager works with his or her own staff to clarify the department's service mission and preliminary service standards that relate to the main expectations of their service partner (the other department). They also clarify the expectations they have of the other department.
- Managers from the two departments meet and share missions, service standards, and expectations of each other.
- When expectations don't match the partner department's service standards, the parties negotiate a more appropriate, more interactive level of service until expectations can be met—consistently.
- They figure out and reach consensus on how they will resolve conflicts that might arise after the contract is in effect.
- They agree on a schedule for monitoring, review, and evaluation.
- They summarize their understandings in a written "service agreement" or contract.
- In their own departments, they then improve systems, processes, and resource allocations to meet their service agreements.
- They monitor conformance in their own department and meet periodically to review progress, identify problems, work together to solve problems, and keep the communication lines open.

Generic Service Contracts

Some departments provide one type of service to multiple other departments, because it would be cumbersome and time-consuming to develop service contracts with each and every customer. For example, maintenance receives work requests from various clinical departments. Instead of developing different service contracts with each department, a generic service contract is developed to suit the primary needs of these diverse customers. In the case of maintenance, the result might be promises to internal customers about turnaround time for work requests, quality of work done (as indicated by lack of need for rework), timely explanations of delays, and clarification of a special system and criteria for rush jobs. Developing a generic contract still reaps the benefits of clarifying key internal customer expectations and communicating explicitly achievable promises about service delivery.

Specific Service Contracts

The more radical form of service contracting involves two specific departments that need a smooth, efficient, and harmonious partnership. One example at Kaiser Medical Center involved nursing and pharmacy in a service contracting process. In the course of their discussions, it surfaced that nursing wanted and expected stat medications within 30 minutes of ordering them. At first, pharmacy wouldn't agree to this because a whopping 55 percent of orders placed by nursing were labeled stat, and pharmacy couldn't possibly fill such a high volume of medication orders within 30 minutes. Furthermore, pharmacy resented the high percentage of stat orders, believing that nursing just "didn't get around to placing regular orders until the time pressure was on and then called them stat." In pharmacy's contracting meetings with nursing, people aired these perceptions and theories about cause. As a result, pharmacy agreed to the 30-minute promise if nursing would reduce the proportion of stat orders to 15 percent of total orders. Nursing agreed to keep the stat orders to less than 15 percent of total orders placed. Figure 17-3 is an example of the Nursing–Pharmacy Service Contract developed at one Kaiser Medical Center in northern California.

To make service contracting work, the following are needed:

- Clear expectations for collaborative contracting
- Continual administrative focus and reinforcement of the process, its purpose, values, and results
- Training and orientation of new managers
- Clear processes for contract renegotiation
- A redefinition of interdepartmental problems as collective issues requiring cooperative solutions
- An emphasis on negotiation of common interests versus bargaining for competing interests
- Training in negotiation skills and the contract creation process
- Employee involvement
- A mechanism for feedback after the contract takes effect to ensure compliance, refinement, and improvement

Interdepartmental Visitation

One cause of frustration in interdepartmental relationships stems from a perception that people in other departments "don't understand or appreciate what we do." How better to promote understanding and respect than to enable employees to experience, albeit for a short time, life in another department.

Waterman Health Care Systems, Inc., in Eustis, Florida, instituted Job Shadowing—a program in which approximately 40 managers and 80 frontline employees annually spend a chunk of time shadowing an employee in another department. Upon their return, they report their experience to coworkers.

At Pacific Medical Center in San Francisco, one nursing unit, under the leadership of nurse manager Greg deBourgh and charge nurse Beth Nuzzo, instituted the "5-South Ambassador Program—People Caring about People." The role of the 5-South Ambassador is to implement a planned visit and observe operations of a designated department, its workloads, problem-solving techniques, and interactions with patient care areas. An agreement is made with the designated department for its representative (ambassador) to make a reciprocal visit to 5-South. After visiting, the ambassador prepares an evaluation that describes from his or her viewpoint the issues and procedures that do and do not work well in the unit visited. After presenting the report to the unit visited, the ambassador and colleagues from the other department begin a dialogue and establish rapport that facilitates future communications and problem solving. Figure 17-4 shows the charter for this program.

Improving Coworker Relationships

Coworkers are another category of internal customers. All employees have coworkers—within and beyond their work group—as customers. They need service-oriented relationships (partnerships) with coworkers, because their relationships have a powerful effect on the quality of work life within any work group and on interactions with customers. Sometimes organizations with service strategies emphasize exclusively the need to extend courtesy, respect, and compassion to external customers, with little mention that internal customers or coworkers deserve this same quality of interaction.

Figure 17-3. Service Contract between Pharmacy and Nursing

A. Basic Contract

1. Department Name: Kaiser Foundation Health Plan Pharmacy, 901 Nevin Avenue, Richmond, California 94801

2. Manager: Franklin Choy, Chief Pharmacist

3. Administrative Designee: John Rawls, Administrator

4. Client: Chiefs of Service

5. Mission Statement: To provide comprehensive pharmaceutical service as prescribed by the medical staff and which satisfies the expectations of our patients in an efficient, cost-effective manner and consistent with applicable Federal and State regulations, KPMCP policies, the needs of Chiefs of Service, and required committees. This service is negotiated with Regional Pharmacy and the Richmond Chiefs of Service.

6. Service Provided: Provision of pharmaceuticals (pursuant to prescriptions and/or requisitions) and related supplies to outpatient Health Plan members and facility departments.

7. Hours of Service: Monday through Friday 9:00 a.m. to 5:30 p.m.

8. How Client Procures Service:
   8.01 By prescriptions which meet the requirement of State and Federal laws.
   8.02 By completed pharmacy requisitions.

9. Quality of Service Standards:
   9.01 All prescriptions will be labeled and filled correctly and have appropriate auxiliary labels attached.
   9.02 95% of all prescriptions will be processed within 20 minutes.
   9.03 All patients are treated with courtesy and respect.
   9.04 All prescriptions will be priced correctly.
   9.05 All pharmaceuticals dispensed will meet with high quality standards.
   9.06 Inventory control measures are taken such that all stocked pharmaceuticals and supplies are immediately available.
   9.07 All telephone calls will be answered within four rings.
   9.08 All State and Federal laws and regulations will be followed.
   9.09 Pharmacists will obtain clarification whenever necessary on prescriptions and orders.
   9.10 100% of clinic requisitions will be completed and delivered within 24 hours.
   9.11 Patient information handouts will be dispensed with all covered pharmaceuticals.
   9.12 Employees will be appropriately attired and wear name badges at all times.

10. Conflict Resolution:
    10.01 The pharmacist will contact the appropriate nurse or prescribing physician to resolve the problem.
    10.02 If no resolution the Assistant Chief/Chief Pharmacist shall contact the nurse or physician involved.
    10.03 If no resolution the Chief Pharmacist and the Chief of Service shall meet to resolve the issue.

11. Review and Update: The negotiated items in this document will be reviewed and updated annually or as required by the department or Chief of Service.

B. Specific Commitments to Nursing

Service Standards	Indications/Evidence of Success	Plan/Frequency/by Whom
The nurse can expect that a 24-hour supply of medications will be delivered to the patient's unit dose drawer, and that commonly used stock medications, emergency drugs, and diagnostic drugs on the agreed upon list (in Notebook in Nurses' Station) are in supply on the unit all shifts.	Is there a tray of Emergency drugs on the crash cart and on the shelf in the Medication Room? Is there a supply of stock medications on the agreed upon list on the unit when the nurse needs it for patient administration? Is the medication ordered for patient administration available in the unit dose drawer or refrigerator?	Will note if any complaints from nursing staff regarding supply of medications.
The nurse can expect that all outdated medications will be removed from the unit monthly.	No outdated medications can be found on the unit.	Pharmacist will do a monthly audit of all drugs on unit.

(Continued on next page)

Figure 17-3. (Continued)

Service Standards	Indications/Evidence of Success	Plan/Frequency/by Whom
When administering medications, the nurse is expected to complete a Communication slip and send it to the Pharmacy if the following occurs: —A medication dose is missed by the patient (e.g., with diagnostic tests, failure to give). —Medication borrowed from another patient's unit dose drawer. —Patient/nurse spoils dose.	When checking the patient unit dose drawer the Pharmacist has a Communication slip explaining missing or extra doses of medications.	Concurrent daily audits by the Pharmacist. Quarterly reports will be shared with the Assistant Director of Nursing Services.
When utilizing the stock medications, the nurse is expected to select the medication with the earliest expiration date.	Does the medication used by the nurse have the earliest outdate?	Two nurses will be observed administering medications by a staff nurse quarterly.
The nurse can expect a half-hour response for stat medications and one-hour response for routine medications from the Pharmacy upon receipt of the physician order.	Does Pharmacy deliver ordered medications to the unit within one hour of receipt of written physician order (excluding regular stock drugs)?	Will note if any complaints regarding delivery or requests from nursing staff.
The nurse/unit clerk is expected to pull newly written physician orders for medications from the medical record and place in the Pharmacy outbox within one hour after the order is written by the physician.	No yellow Pharmacy duplicates with written medication orders can be found in the patient's medical record one and one-half hour after the order is written by the physician.	Quarterly concurrent audit of 10 charts by the Unit Clerk.
The nurse/unit clerk is expected to complete a written requisition for all stock medication replacements. Twenty-four-hour turnaround time except for stat/emergency drugs.	Does the nurse/unit clerk have a written requisition when she/he requests replacement of stock medications? Are the drugs delivered in 24 hours of the requisition?	Will note if any complaints regarding delivery for requests.
The Pharmacist will premix IV medications daily, weekends, and on holidays.	Were the ordered IV medications delivered to the unit prior to the time of administration?	Will note if problems with regarding delivery.
On the day of discharge the patient's medication orders will be completed by the Pharmacist, with information regarding precautions in taking drugs and drug/food interactions included.	Patient expresses satisfaction regarding his or her instruction. Drug/food interaction and instructions checked off on the Patient Discharge Instruction form. Discharge medications are delivered to the unit as agreed.	Twenty-four hour audit by the Social Worker/QA Analyst.

NOTE: If the patient needs require service beyond this agreement, the patient will receive the needed service. If not able to, will negotiate what is possible with the client upon request.

Agreement Achieved:

_____   _____

Chief Hospital Pharmacist   Date

_____   _____

Asst. Dir., Nsg   Date

Reprinted, with permission, from Kaiser Medical Center, Redwood City, California.

Figure 17-4. Nursing Charter for the 5-South Ambassador Program: "People Caring about People"

Members of the 5 South staff to be appointed as Ambassadors to other departments within the hospital to serve as our diplomats, representatives, and negotiators for mutual problem solving.

Desired Outcomes:

- To demonstrate our support to other departments
- To demonstrate our values and philosophy of patient care
- To increase awareness of operations across department lines
- To identify and establish realistic expectations of departments supporting delivery of patient for care and the nurse's role in delivery of that care
- To facilitate the delivery of quality patient care on 5 South through networking with staff from other departments

Membership:

- Program Coordinator
  Bess Nuzzo, R.N.
  Charge Nurse, 5 South
- Ambassadors (one for each target department) appointed for one-year tenure
- 5 South Nurse Manager as Consultant to program

Role of Ambassador:

- Implement a planned visit to identified departments
- Observe operations of department, noting interactions with patient care areas, workloads, and problem-solving techniques of department
- Return to 5 South to debrief project coordinator and Nursing Leadership (Nurse Manager and charge nurses)
- Present brief written report for communication book and brief oral report to staff meetings
- Ambassador may be asked to participate in future problem solving with department *if* issues arise

Others Involved:

- Department Managers of the Transport, Pharmacy, Laboratory and Imaging Departments
- Staff ambassadors from each of the departments listed

Reprinted, with permission, from Pacific Medical Center, San Francisco, California.

What helps? Explicit behavioral norms and accountability, attention to building respect for diversity, and concrete experiences that build understanding between coworkers. Following are two strategies hospitals have used to accomplish these ends:

- Define and enforce behavioral norms for coworker relationships
- Create programs that build respect for diversity

Behavioral Norms for Coworker Relationships

Supportive behavior among coworkers can and should be an expectation of the job. Too often managers, supervisors, and executives let personality differences and frictions drive the quality of staff interactions instead of instituting a code of coworker behavior defined as appropriate and professional for the workplace.

It's important to make behavioral expectations explicit because some people don't instinctively or consciously know what constitutes constructive coworker behavior. If you don't institute explicit norms you will see a normal curve of behavior, with some employees being "awful" and a similar few being "wonderful." By developing an explicit code of behavior, you can raise the standard (the mean level of behavior) *and* reduce variation around this standard. Also, until such norms are conscious, managers have no right to enforce standards.

Some organizations develop coworker norms for the entire organization. Others use a decentralized approach in which work groups develop a code of conduct tailored to them. Following is one model that you can adapt to either approach. It has been used successfully to achieve this purpose.

Step 1: Conduct a staff meeting, as follows:

- Make a personal statement about why you think it's important to take steps to improve coworker relationships and outline the purpose of this meeting and the steps that follow.
- Warm people to the topic by asking them to brainstorm the consequences of positive versus negative relationships with coworkers (consequences for self, the organization, the department's external customers, and patients).
- Ask staff to consider coworker behaviors that make them feel valued, supported, and productive in their work and ask them to identify the coworker behaviors that have the opposite effect, depleting their energy and motivation to serve their customers well.
- Break into smaller groups or pairs, asking each group to share its lists and identify the "Big Five" dos and don'ts that, if adhered to, would have the most powerful positive effect on coworker relationships within this work group or organization.
- Reconvene the large group and make a grand list, streamlining it with the group's help by eliminating redundancy.
- After developing a manageably sized list, assert that you want these behaviors to become the code of conduct for coworker relationships.

Step 2: Institute a feedback device that periodically invites people's perceptions of the degree of conformance of self and others with the code.

Step 3: Present the results to the group. Then identify and pursue improvement opportunities.

Figure 17-5 provides an example of the code of conduct that resulted when The Einstein Consulting Group followed this process. *Positive Coworker Relationships in Health Care* by Wendy Leebov offers additional activities managers can use with staff to help coworkers improve their relationships.[4]

Figure 17-5. Code of Conduct (House Rules)

1. *Recognize every individual.* There's always a person behind the position. Break the ice. Say hello. Make eye contact. Express a few words of concern.
2. *Keep coworkers informed.* Educate. Help others fill their need to know.
3. *Make complaints and frustrations constructive.* Speak to the people involved in the problem; confront and work together to make things right.
4. *Appreciate.* Say a genuine thanks. Recognition sparks and inspires.
5. *Pitch in.* Accept and do with energy. Even if it's not your job, help or find someone who can. Take that call. Pack that box. Help each other and you help our customers.
6. *Be productive.* Concentrate on your work and produce results. Enable coworkers to do the same.
7. *Attend to the details.* Quality and accuracy in our individual work reflects on all of us.
8. *Listen.* When someone complains, speaks, up or confronts, listen and don't be defensive.
9. *Act and look professional.* You have a public importance and shape our image.
10. *Follow through.* Live up to your end of the job. Meet deadlines; keep promises. Everything you do or don't do, every deadline you meet or miss affects someone else. Earn people's trust and confidence.
11. *Take responsibility for making our company work better.* Initiate improvements. Make suggestions. Identify problems and implement solutions. Make waves for the good of the company. Good enough never is.
12. *Show respect.* Treat coworkers with dignity, empathy, and professionalism, no matter what their job. None of us is better than any one else.
13. *Be a telephone pro.* Take that call. Handle the caller with care. Return calls quickly. The phone is our lifeline.
14. *Stretch to serve our customer.* Go the extra mile. Without customers, there is no company.
15. *You are ECG.* Think "organization." Express optimism. Make your energy and attitude contagious.

Reprinted, with permission, from The Einstein Consulting Group, Philadelphia, Pennsylvania.

Programs That Build Respect for Diversity

There are no organizations more diverse than hospitals, and health care jobs are among the most stressful. Although some strains in coworker relationships are attributable to personality clashes, others stem from diversity—race, ethnic background, gender, or sexual orientation. Forward-looking hospitals are devoting time and attention to bringing diversity to the forefront and expecting and building respect for diversity among all staff.

For example, Grady Memorial Hospital in Atlanta integrated work on diversity into their service excellence strategy from the outset. Groundwork data collection included not only audits of service strengths and weaknesses, but also "think tanks" that invited employees to identify diversity issues that interfered with service provision. The issues raised were built into their awareness and training programs. Says Dewey Hickman, director of planning at Grady and the administrative overseer of their service excellence strategy, "You can't achieve excellent service and work well with other service providers unless staff respect each other; the diversity within our ranks creates barriers to this respect. That's why we decided to make diversity issues a focus within our service strategy."

A typical approach includes workshops that build a shared commitment to work-force diversity, based on a thorough understanding of its benefits:

- Educational sessions for all levels of management designed to engender a shared positive outlook on diversity, foster awareness of the problematic dynamics that take place in their organization, and build shared, concrete expectations for all staff delineating behaviors that communicate respect for and encourage the benefits of differences among staff.
- Educational sessions for all staff; and ideally physicians too, that sensitize people to differences, allow a safe environment for examining these differences and their consequences for the workplace, and identify friction points or problems that merit discussion and resolution (perhaps through development of teams).
- Intermittent programs (for example, forums, panels, news articles) that spotlight people from various cultures and sensitize others to their views, cultural patterns, and style preferences.

There are a multitude of consultants and curricula available to help you. Consider many until you find or develop the approach that fits best for your organization.

☐ Relationship Building and Skill Building

Coworkers and staff need to work together as partners, with teamwork and mutual support as the keys to smooth and productive relationships. Service improvement strategies don't work unless *relationships* (like work processes) are reexamined, redesigned, and continuously improved. Executive team members have to work hard on their own relationships so that they "sing one tune," speak the truth, give each other frank feedback, take risks in an environment of group support, and be vulnerable in the way continuous learners need to be. Administrators and physicians, physicians and nurses, nursing directors and pharmacy chiefs, and people from laboratories and nursing (to name just a few) all need to work on their relationships in order to make them work.

Relationships Don't Happen by Accident

The science of building relationships isn't as developed as, say, the science of cardiology. And health care leaders aren't necessarily trained or even interested in the relationship side of things. Some executives don't think it's necessary! Money, bottom line—that's what matters. To such people, relationships are "soft" and elusive. Also conscious attention to improving relationships doesn't fit with the natural or most comfortable style of certain executives. It goes against their grain. Some people are "process types" who like working on relationships; and others are more *task*-oriented, experiencing discomfort in the relationship arena.

Yet, when relationships are ignored or dealt with impatiently, the results are serious. You pay a steep price. Consider these familiar scenarios:

- The administrative team of Community General has high turnover. They did a climate survey that showed employees have little faith in leadership. Only 8 percent say top management functions as a unified team. Sixteen percent think top management is attuned to employee needs. When the top team sees the results
  - The CEO yells at the group.
  - The CFO says employees are *always* complaining, and, given the financial climate, they should be grateful to have their jobs.
  - The vice-president of patient services dismisses the results as unduly influenced by disgruntled nurses annoyed with the changes going on in nursing.
  - The vice-president of human resources suggests a shift to management by wandering around.
  - The vice-president for support services is absent.
  - The vice-president of marketing is away at a press conference.

  Nothing changes. People don't want to face the fact that their team is dysfunctional. The results continue to be high turnover, morale problems, and a very disaffected staff.
- Physicians and administrators are at odds. The administrators want to be all things to all people. Physicians, in the absence of a clear vision, engage in petty politics and power seeking more than ever.
- Members of the food and nutrition services staff get off the elevator with patient trays. Residents don't move out of the way. Staff think, "Don't we count?" The pecking order plays out in a kneejerk fashion that interferes with staff morale and ability to do jobs.
- At a management development workshop, department heads talk about a wheelchair shortage and, wanting to be constructive, map out a carefully sequenced process for addressing the problem. After working out proposed solutions in detail, one brave department head says (and others nod in agreement), "Let's face it. We're not going to go through with this because, even if we came up with a solution, we don't trust each other enough to follow through on our agreements. We'll still hoard the wheelchairs."

In every one of these scenarios, the parties involved remain at odds. The strain in their relationships is palpable. And their patients and other customers suffer. Why do such scenarios occur? Because great relationships don't happen by accident.

Relationship Building by Design

To build the trusting, productive teams or relationships that form the core of service delivery, people in groups need to address these questions with one another:

- Why am I here?
- Why are you here?
- What do we want to do together?
- How will we do it?

If teams don't address these questions; people are not united in their commitment and they do not move in an aligned fashion. By taking the time to address these questions, people become oriented to their common purpose, they develop trust, they clarify their roles in relation to each other, and they develop shared commitment.

A lot is happening on the relationship-building front. Consider for instance the burgeoning of process improvement teams that are the cornerstone of hospitals' quality improvement strategies. Instead of blaming and living with problems, teams from interdependent departments chart, study, and repair a problematic process. They also learn to hold more efficient, effective, and purposeful meetings.

At St. Rita's Medical Center in Lima, Ohio, 20 department heads convened to help each other pilot a systematic Customer-Driven Management process in their departments. The group divided into miniteams of five people who helped each other through an ambitious, staged change process. They combined learning with relationship building, naming their teams, mapping their experience, and regularly reviewing *how* they were working together and *how* they could work together better.

At one medical center, an administrator frustrated with two warring secretaries created a "Lunch Fund" for coworkers whose relationships were interfering with service delivery. The requirement: "You two must go *out* to lunch with one another three times over a two-week period!" At Rutland Regional Medical Center in Vermont, the executive team engaged in outdoor survival experiences to solidify their team and push their teamwork to new heights of support and courage.

In a long-term relationship-building process at the Albert Einstein Healthcare Foundation in Philadelphia, executives use red flags in their meetings to call the group's attention to a meeting gone awry so that they can take steps to bring the meeting back on course.

Many management teams nationwide are recognizing the necessity of holding retreats (or "advances") to build and periodically refresh their relationships, clear the air, and achieve a united and trusting leadership team. With initiatives like these, people recognize that relationships have to be strong for an organization to serve its multiple and diverse customers and staff effectively. Those focused on service improvement recognize the need to shift from a provider-driven to a customer-driven organization. To make this shift, a new style of relationship is required that reflects the following shifts:

- *From me to we:* Staff at all levels need a team orientation, not an individual one.
- *From parent–child to adult–adult:* We don't just want *healthy* parent–child or boss–subordinate relationships. We want adult–adult relationships in which everyone is respected and uses his or her own abilities fully to meet customer needs.
- *From competition to partnership:* We need to shift from a competitive model (competition for status and resources) to a partnership model.
- *From pecking order to parity:* We need to take steps to reduce the destructive and overblown pecking order in our organizations, because this pecking order *interferes* with the kind of massive team effort needed to meet and exceed customer expectations consistently, despite fluctuations in service volume and pressure. The residents who don't move out of the way of dietary workers pushing a rack of trays because they are *doctors* interferes with service to patients. A physician who addresses a nurse by first name but is miffed when the nurse does the same is refusing to see the nurse as a full partner.
- *From hired hands to hired heads:* We need to treat each other and our staff not as hired hands, but as hired heads fully activated and *trusted* to act in the best interests of the organization's service mission.

What can you do? Build relationship building into your strategy. Identify the source of conflict and the dysfunctional relationship that need deliberate team building. Is it the corporate and divisional staff? Is it physicians and nurses? Is it attending physicians and faculty in a teaching hospital? Is it residents and nurses in the emergency department? Set new norms and take new steps to reduce the issues that have become unmentionable because of distrust between people. Encourage others to point out when relationships interfere with desired results. Organizational consultant Charles Seashore tells the story of going to a glitzy gala where several hundred people convened—all decked out in their finery. As people arrived at the party, they were directed into the festive ballroom where they couldn't help but see on a large table in the center of the room an enormous dead moose. The evening wore on, with people dancing and enjoying themselves. But all evening no one said anything about the dead moose.

Our organizations have "dead moose" lying all around and people are afraid to talk about them. Until we talk about these dead moose, we will never have the quality of trust and teamwork we need to work together in our atmosphere of changing expectations and life-and-death ranges of feeling. Talking about the dead moose is partly an individual responsibility, but in many organizations it merits creation of structured settings for team building with skilled facilitators and time apart from the everyday routine. Relationships need special nurturing, time and attention, and a belief shared by all that we can improve them incrementally and substantially through deliberate effort.

Feedback Skills

No systems work unless communication with internal customers opens up. In addition to instituting structured vehicles to help, it's also important to strengthen the interpersonal skills of executives, managers, physicians, and *all* staff. If people resist giving each other feedback, keep important information to themselves, or avoid confronting problems in a constructive fashion, all structures fail.

The language of constructive feedback is very difficult. It needs to be learned and modeled—especially by managers. Too often managers harangue people into getting along better with one another, but neither they nor the organization spends the time or money to build the skills. Helping people embrace and use a simple model like the following can have a profound effect on the quality of internal customer relations across department lines and among coworkers.

Confrontation Model

- Your Intention: "I want to _____."
- Your Behavior: "When you _____."
- Consequences: "The consequences as I saw them were _____ (for me, the organization, our customers).
- Pinch of Empathy: "Now I realize it isn't easy to _____, because _____."
- What I want or expect in the future: "Still, from now on, I would like you to _____."

For example:

- Intention: "I want to have a better, more cooperative relationship with you."
- Behavior: "When you ask me to cover for you for a couple of minutes and then you leave your desk for an hour . . . ."
- Consequences: "I feel annoyed, because I don't want to abandon your area and my promise to you, but I have my own work to do."
- Pinch of Empathy: "Now I know some errands can take longer than you expect . . . ."
- What I want: "In the future, I want you to return when you say you will or I'll leave your area uncovered."

Staff also need to learn a similar model for giving each other *positive* feedback and appreciation. The above model, adapted to positive instances, reads like this:

Appreciation Model

- Your Intention: "I value our relationship and want it to be mutually supportive."
- Your Behavior: "When you offered to finish my report the time I had to leave suddenly because of the call from my son's day care center . . . ."

- Consequences: "It took a load of pressure off me, so I could focus on my family emergency."
- Pinch of Empathy: "I realize you have a tremendous workload of your own, and leaving your work aside had to be really inconvenient."
- Thanks: "I just want you to know how much I appreciate what you did. Thanks."

Imagine if these kinds of messages were frequent! The fact is that feedback drives improvement. Most colleagues want to do right for their customers and each other. If you can create an atmosphere in which skillful feedback flows from person to person across and within department lines, you will see people, of their own volition, make dramatic improvements.

Many executives, managers, and staff need training in the interpersonal skills that contribute to development of trusting relationships, such as constructive feedback, non-defensive listening, and win–win negotiation. By investing in the development of important staff skills such as these, you will reduce the strain in internal customer relationships and help everyone contribute to effective agreements and harmony.

☐ The Bottom Line

More than ever, effective service delivery relies on harmonious, cooperative "service partnerships" across department lines and between coworkers. Yet it's easy to become complacent, and in too many cases people settle for mediocrity in these relationships. The manager doesn't pay attention unless there are offensive things happening, and even then he or she might attribute problems to "human nature."

If you believe the competitive edge is excellent service to external customers and that internal customer relationships are key, then excellence in internal customer relationships is the competitive edge as well. The challenge remains to raise your standards, to actively seek missed opportunities, and to experiment with new ways to improve these relationships for the good of efficiency, quality of work life, and external customer satisfaction.

☐ Final Suggestions

- Remember that internal customer relationships affect external customer relationships and that every employee has internal customers.
- Devote time and attention to making these relationships strong—by design. Don't write them off as functions of different personalities or idiosyncrasies.
- Ground your strategies in a vision of partnership, in which all parties share responsibility for the quality of outputs.
- Install measures to monitor internal, not just external, customer satisfaction.
- Don't tolerate poor internal customer relationships endlessly. After working to improve these relationships, hold all managers and staff accountable for quality relationships. A service chain that affects patients is only as strong as its weakest link.

References

1. Bracey, H. Speech in CQI workshop, Philadelphia, PA, June 26, 1992.

2. Rawls, J., and Mulgrew, S. Service contracting. *Service Excellence in Practice* 2(2), Nov.–Dec. 1989.

3. Rawls, J. Speech on service contracting. Service/Quality Connection Conference, Chicago, May 16–18, 1991. Jointly sponsored by The Einstein Consulting Group and the National Society for Patient Representation and Consumer Affairs.

4. Leebov, W. *Positive Coworker Relationships in Health Care.* Chicago: American Hospital Publishing, 1990.

Chapter 18

Resistance to Service Excellence

S ome administrators feel angry at managers, physicians, and others who resist service improvement efforts, whereas others see resistance as an indicator that they have done something wrong strategically to cause it. The fact is, resistance to service quality improvement strategies is inevitable, even in the best organizations, because striving for service excellence requires significant change and change breeds resistance.

To develop a helpful mind-set in dealing with inevitable resistance, consider the following thought-provoking fable:[1]

Lee spent many years developing a vision. He finally has his vision clearly in focus. He begins a long trek—walking toward his vision, which is far off in the distance. As he walks in the direction of his vision, he sees another man approaching who looks like a mirror image of himself except that this other man has a long rope wrapped around his waist. As the two approach each other, Lee sees a chasm stretching between the two of them. As the other man approaches the chasm he tosses the end of the rope to Lee and yells, "Here, grab this!" Lee reflexively grabs the rope just as the man jumps into the chasm, hanging onto the other end. Now Lee is holding onto the rope with the other man hanging dangerously hundreds of feet below.

Lee yells into the chasm, "How could you do that?! I was approaching my vision and now look what you've done!" The man yells back from the depths, "Yes, and now my life is in your hands. Don't drop me!"

Lee yells, "Help me pull you up. Wrap the rope around your waist and it will gradually shorten and I'll pull you up." The man at the end of the rope yells, "No, and my life is in your hands!"

Lee becomes aggravated and shrieks, "Look, you can help save yourself. I'll anchor myself against a rock up here and you slowly climb the rope." The man yells from below, "No, and my life is in your hands, so don't let go."

Becoming even more frustrated and frightened, Lee asks, "Do you have any ideas how you can help save yourself? I'll help you in any way I can!" And the man at the end of the rope yells, "No, and don't let go. If you drop me, I'll die!"

Lee becomes even more disturbed. After all, he's exhausted from holding the rope with the man's weight on it; and Lee is making no progress toward his vision.

And the man hanging from the rope won't do anything to help. Lee yells, "Look, I've had it with you! You don't seem interested in saving yourself. I've done all I can. I am going to hold on to you for 30 more minutes. If you don't do something by then to climb up here, I am going to let go of the rope."

The man replied, "You can't. I'll die. My life is in your hands." And he did nothing to save himself.

Lee waited 30 minutes and then let go of the rope.

This fable is instructive about resistance. It raises the critical question, "Who's responsible for overcoming resistance?" According to the fable, this responsibility begins with the people with the vision, becomes shared, but ultimately rests on the resister. Leaders need to take proactive and reactive steps to handle resistance and provide extensive support. But ultimately they need to be ready and willing to let go of the rope if the resistant people persist in paralyzing other people's efforts to achieve your vision.

☐ Resistance Takes Many Forms

Resistance takes many forms, as seen in the following examples:

- An executive gives lip service to the concept of service excellence. He's a hard-line manager who lives by "do as I say, not as I do." He expects employees to conform to rules and engage enthusiastically in the service strategy upon demand, with minimum concrete training or support.
- Helene always has an excuse. The other patient, the other tech, the other department is always the cause of whatever problem is at hand. She is quick to point the finger at everyone but herself. She reacts the same way with regard to service excellence. She's exemplary. She thinks that other people cause the problem.
- Mark works as a nurse, but you'd think he complained for a living. He is usually annoyed, usually griping, and usually lowering the morale of his colleagues. He is quick to say, "This will never work; we're too short-staffed," or "Administration doesn't care anyway." The glass is always half empty, never half full. Mark sees only the pitfalls in formal efforts to improve service and the burden of more pressure to perform.
- What does Leslie think about service excellence? You can't be sure. She's late for improvement team meetings. She sits quietly with raised eyebrows. She always has an excuse for why she didn't do what she promised to do.
- Sandy still feels insulted by the concept of service excellence no matter what you do or say. She's seen herself as a superstar for years.
- Larry works in engineering. He doesn't see the point of his being involved in service improvement because he doesn't serve patients and he's busy.
- Your whole emphasis on service excellence passes Mary by. She thinks your hospital is fine the way it is, especially compared with other hospitals. She also thinks that courtesy is learned in childhood, that the employee who is rude now cannot be changed.
- Joan is angry about the emphasis on service. She thinks it's the administration's way of haranguing nurses to be a doormat for patients, their families, and physicians. Joan mistakes "service" for "servitude" and sees the focus on service as a threat to her self-esteem.
- Tom has been schooled in the philosophy that employees are tools of production, not competent people capable of good judgment in customer interactions. He is unwilling to give up some control to enable frontline people to act quickly, responsibly, and creatively in the customer's behalf. He thinks it's his role to develop service rules (since he knows best) and then police people for service violations. Also,

he disparages the people who claim that faulty work processes create service problems.

☐ What Drives Resistance?

According to experts on resistance, *individuals'* reasons for resistance to change fall into six categories:[2,3]

1. *Habit:* Doing things the way you always did means merely responding to stimuli without thinking. That's easier than deciding to act in new ways.
2. *Selective attention and retention:* People tend to notice and absorb only those things that fit their own ways of thinking and acting. They reject what's not congruent.
3. *Dependence:* People with low self-esteem or little confidence resist change until the people they depend on embrace the changes.
4. *Fear of the unknown:* People get nervous with the uncertainty that accompanies unknowns. "The devil you know is better than the devil you don't."
5. *Economics:* People fear that changes might somehow upset the apple cart with the consequence of threatening their jobs.
6. *Security:* Change challenges people's sense of security. People find comfort in doing things the same way as always, even if it doesn't serve the organization. They may be in a "fur-lined rut."

At the *organizational* level, not the individual level, there are five kinds of resistance:[4]

1. *Power and territory:* Some people resist because they think the changes will rearrange or encroach upon their territory. For instance, some managers are threatened by cross-functional process improvement teams because problems and the approach to work within their departments become public.
2. *Organizational structure:* Job descriptions, departments, and lines of authority tend to be resistant to change. They become self-perpetuating. Because of their complexity and interconnectedness, no one wants to take on what seems like the gargantuan task of changing them.
3. *Resource limitations:* Health care organizations have constraints on how much they can invest in service improvement. Some people resist service strategies because they know that the organization lacks the resources to implement everyone's favorite proposed service improvement.
4. *Sunk costs:* Past decisions about buildings, work processes, and people feel like investments that executives don't want to throw away. The result is resistance to making changes that upset these past decisions. This applies even at the level of retaining the 25-year loyal employee who is a thorn in the organization's service image.
5. *Interorganizational agreements:* People might want change but be (or feel) locked into agreements that don't serve their service goals, such as agreements with suppliers, other organizations, physician corporations, and the like.

Beyond these classic reasons for individual and organizational resistance to change, employees demonstrate three patterns of resistance to service improvement strategies in particular. Some employees and physicians are insulted by the notion of a designed strategy for service excellence. They already think of themselves as professional when it comes to extending themselves to patients. Others are cynics who doubt the effectiveness of their organization's long-term commitment to service excellence: "This is just another flash in the pan," or "You must be joking, you can't change people." And still others are so full of resentment toward the organization that they refuse to cooperate.

329

They will get better only when they are treated better by the organization: "If you muck-amucks give me the respect I deserve and solve the problems that make my life miserable, then I'll bend over backward for our patients; but until then, get off my back!"

The insulted are insulted for a reason. The cynics are cynical for a reason. The resentful are resentful for a reason. Arguing against their reasons or attempting to squelch them doesn't help. Their reasons are real and contain at least a grain of truth. Still, you have to be so committed to your vision of service excellence that you don't allow these reasons to push you off course.

☐ Resistance Is Normal, Even Healthy!

Resistance to change serves a function—to maintain the status quo or the organization's perceived state of equilibrium. If resistance to change never occurred, organizations would no doubt be entirely unstable; they would lack focus and integrity. Resistance serves to maintain equilibrium in organizations until the reasons for change are both conscious and compelling.

Behavioral scientist Kurt Lewin described organizational change as a three-step sequential process:[5]

- Step 1: Unfreezing or thawing out established patterns
- Step 2: Changing or moving to a new pattern
- Step 3: Refreezing or maintaining the new pattern

Resistance is especially inherent in the first step, unfreezing. Unfreezing is inevitably unsettling, because it stems from tension that drives people to search for new ways to do things. Such tension is typically generated by an awareness of competitive pressures, falling standards, image problems, a financial downturn, and the like. If your people don't feel this tension, you have to take explicit steps to create mild states of anxiety, or they will not be motivated to change. No wonder the concept of service excellence meets resistance. Who wants to feel anxiety and pressure to abandon old ways that seemed to work fine for years?

☐ Resistance Tactics for Service Strategies

According to O.D.R., Inc., resistance is increased under specific circumstances. The following lists some of these circumstances:[6]

- The purpose of change is not clear.
- People don't believe the change is needed.
- People are not involved in planning the change.
- Communication regarding the change is not clear.
- The change has a relatively high tangible, intellectual, or emotional cost.
- Rewards for accomplishing the change are inadequate.
- The change represents certain values that are in direct conflict with the organization's values.
- There is weak political support for the change.
- The change affects the way people relate to others in the organization who are important to them.
- People don't feel confident that organizational resources required for the change will be made available.
- People expect the change to have a negative impact on their area's budget.
- An inappropriate amount of time is allowed between the first announcement of the change and its implementation.

- Daily work patterns are not adequately considered when the planning is done for the change.
- People believe there is a negative effect on key aspects of their jobs.
- The change is not seen as meaningful.
- People are punished inappropriately for making errors while implementing the change.
- People don't feel secure about the way they will be doing their work because of the change.
- People don't think they have the skills and knowledge necessary to implement the change.
- People have a low level of respect and trust for the sponsor of the change.
- People have a low level of respect and trust for those responsible for implementing the change.
- People are overly stressed and burdened by their current work loads.
- A change represents a threat to personal interests such as salary or prestige.
- The objectives of the change are incompatible with personal or career goals.
- There are many permanent consequences that would make it difficult to reverse a change.
- A change requires people to acknowledge past failures, or it generates doubts about their judgment in past decisions and actions.

So what can you do? In the long run, resistance will fade as, through successive approximations, you align your organizational practices with your service mission. The more your practices related to accountability, measurement, communication, reward and recognition, training, and other pillars advance continuous service improvement, the less resistance you will see, because your culture will create a "current" that will carry people along if they choose to swim in your organization.

In the short run, however, there are many things you can do. We suggest the following 16 components to confronting resistance.

Unite in Your Commitment

Decide firmly what you really want to achieve with your service improvement strategy. Work on your vision until it is solid and has been embraced by a critical mass of your organization's leaders. Commit to hanging onto this vision together despite bouts of inevitable resistance. Don't permit yourself or colleagues to be distracted from your course.

Be Sure the People at the Top Are Personally Aligned with Your Service Mission

Eliminate double standards. Double standards breed resistance. One of the most effective ways to soften resistance is through positive role modeling by executives and middle managers. Managers must demonstrate excellent service habits visibly as they interact with employees and physicians. When resistant employees see this behavior, they feel much less righteous in their resistance. When managers do not practice what they preach, the seeds of resistance blossom.

Do the hard work involved in bringing leaders' individual behavior and decisions about time and resource allocation into alignment with your service focus.

Create Hope and Possibility through Benchmarking

Make sure people see positive change as achievable. Early on, assemble groups of managers to visit organizations that have exemplary service strategies and results to show for it. In the same vein, circulate articles about other health care organizations with exciting

331

strategies. Managers will learn vicariously about what's involved and become more comfortable with it. Also that motivation to "keep up with the Joneses" will get them interested or constructively competitive with other like organizations. Show managers that *not* working on service is obsolete. Most managers don't want to feel or be obsolete.

Be Sure All Organizational Leaders Can Articulate the Rationale for Your Strategy and Their Personal Commitment to It

Anticipate the concerns people are likely to voice and prepare to handle them persuasively. For instance, how would you respond to employees or physicians who ask or assert:

- Why are we doing this?
- We've been successful before, so why do we need to abandon our ways of the past?
- We're succeeding now and we're satisfied with it.
- Isn't this just a flash in the pan like everything we do here?
- Now whose bright idea is this and what is he or she trying to prove?
- How can you be sure we'll be more successful as a result of this strategy?
- Whose responsible if it fails?
- We're already swamped. How can we do this too?
- It's a waste of time.
- We're unique. This has been done elsewhere, but it won't work here.
- We're already strapped financially. We don't have the money to do this right.
- It sounds great to me, but others here won't buy this.

Consider practice sessions in which your strategy leaders and eventually *all* managers and supervisors help each other address these questions and give each other feedback on content and style until everyone sings in harmony. Invite your training professionals to help by briefing people on the helpful skills of active listening, fogging, personal ownership, and the "broken record" technique.

Enlist the Help of Already Credible People

Joiner Associates Inc. describes the "demography of change" with the normal curve in figure 18-1. The figure shows that most people tend toward neutrality in relation to impending change with a minority at the extremes of resistance and support. The firm

Figure 18-1. The Demography of Change

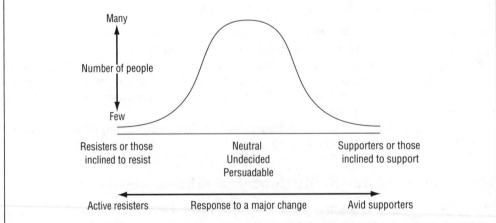

then juxtaposes degree of support against extent of influence over others, as shown in figure 18-2, pointing out that strategy planners need to plan tactics for each specific group (member)—champions, neutrals, and adversaries—in order to minimize resistance and maximize support for the proposed change. These steps toward converting resisters are suggested:

- Identify movers and shakers (groups 1, 2, and 3).
- Work with the neutrals (this means listen, listen, listen) (groups 8, 5, and 2).
- Get the help of the 1s and 4s to convince the 2s and 5s and neutralize the 3s and 6s.

The firm's recommendations support our experience. It's important early on to engage the organization's informal "opinion leaders" (including malcontents if they are opinion leaders). Trendsetters on your side will enlist others in droves. Feature the opinion leaders, engage them in needs assessment and strategy planning, make them facilitators, and recognize their power to help the organization change, no matter where they appear in your organization's pecking order. If this group includes malcontents, be sure to:

- Directly and constructively solicit their criticism and use it in forming your strategy, because they speak for others as well. No institution is perfect, and employee complaints are usually at least partially legitimate. For example, redressing complaints about equipment or cumbersome procedures often enables employees to deliver better service to customers.
- Solicit people's advice about strategy questions. Such action causes potential resisters to have an investment and stake in the eventual strategy.
- By involving a wide variety of people up front, you are inviting them to bring their feelings out in the open where you can handle them. If you let these feelings stay hidden, they'll erode your best efforts later.

Figure 18-2. Subgroups That Merit Special Planning

	No Influence	Moderate Influence	Movers and Shakers	
Very high	7	4	1	Champions
Degree of support for this change	8	5	2	Neutrals
Very low	9	6	3	Adversaries

Very low ←————————————→ Very high

Extent of influence over others

Plan and Prepare Formal Components of Your Strategy with Anticipated Resistance in Mind

Consciously build in rationales and approaches designed to minimize the anticipated resistance instead of fueling it. Taking measures to prevent resistance is more efficient than trying to cure it. For instance, hold employee focus groups in which you summarize all known components of your forthcoming strategy and urge participants to play the role of "skeptics," asking every possible skeptical or cynical question that comes to mind. Then join with your strategy planning team and see if you can amend your strategy to prevent any of the skeptics' questions or at least prepare everyone to answer them before they are asked.

Take into Account and Plan for the Range of Employee Feelings That Are Likely to Arise

Once again, the three groups most likely to show resistance are the insulted, the cynical, and the resentful. These groups are summerized below:

- *The insulted:* Acknowledge that people are already good at service but that being "good" isn't enough in today's environment. Focus on shifting the norm from satisfaction with the status quo to a powerful value on continuous improvement. Then concentrate your efforts on raising awareness, not on training, and emphasize moving from "good" to "great." This action sends a motivating, nonpunitive message. Emphasize the new economic challenges hospitals face and the need "to pull out all the stops" to compete effectively. Tell the truth and avoid rhetoric. Workshops shouldn't be pep talks. Employees need to know that excellent service on their parts and continuous service improvement aren't grounded in lofty rhetoric but are consistent with their personal goals and the organization's goals as well as wise competitive responses to the increasingly fierce health care market. When employees see the organization relying on them to be the "excellence factor," a driving focus on service excellence becomes flattering, not insulting.
- *The cynics:* Donald Kanter and Philip Mirvis of Boston University find an "us against them" syndrome surfacing in the United States. They claim that handling hostile, cynical staff members who have a high opinion of themselves is becoming a significant management problem, let alone the challenge to create change in our human resources.

  The new generation of cynics requires thoughtful approaches to corporate culture and therefore to service improvement. According to Kanter and Mirvis, cynics believe that corporate communications are designed to deceive and manipulate them. They suggest that communicating with cynics requires a special approach including the following features:[7]
  - When presenting information, allow all sides to be heard. Even antimanagement positions should be heard so that cynics cannot claim a cover-up.
  - Communications should be phrased so that people have a chance to make up their own minds; communications should not be simply direct transmissions of management policy.
  - Communications should not raise employee expectations unduly.
  - Management presentations should be factual and detached. Information, not propaganda, should be offered.
  - Communications should come from senior management known to the work force.
  - If the message is important, its initial presentation should be followed up by informal meetings of small groups at which the message is reinforced and fence sitters are encouraged to consider all sides.

Confronted with your ambitious service excellence strategy, cynics become skeptical. Perhaps they had embraced similar programs in the past, only to see them fade away because of waning administrative support or lack of follow-up. The cynics need to know that this strategy isn't just another flash in the pan. All communications (workshops, memos, and the like) should emphasize that the administration has made a serious, ongoing commitment to service excellence and that a long-term plan is in place. Challenge the cynics to suspend their disbelief and become part of the solution. Dare them to excel, and convince them that their efforts will be continuously augmented by the entire organization.

- *The resentful:* Develop with executive management a clearly defined mechanism for employee participation in problem identification and process improvement, for prompt action on employee suggestions, and for prompt feedback so that employees know the results of their complaints and their everyday efforts to contribute to customer satisfaction. Resentful employees need to be aware that your organization recognizes the need for extensive, ongoing "body work" (process improvement) and not just a glossy "paint job" to make service improvement real.

Good faith has to be developed between the administration and employees who resent the service focus and increased pressure to contribute. Workshops can help by offering employees the chance to vent their frustrations, frustrations that should be seriously listened to, recorded, and turned over to the right people for action. Dialogue is essential to decrease resentment and create new openness to change on the part of resentful people.

See Resistance as Feedback

Don't keel over or get angry when resistance strikes. Adjust your mind-set so that you see resistance as feedback—and as useful feedback at that. Listen to it and act on it.

When asked questions you can't answer, admit it. If you fudge, the resister sees your pretense and loses trust in you. Better to say, "That's a good question; let me think about it," or "That's a tough question; let me see if I can get an answer for you." Then regain the initiative by asking, for example, how detailed an answer the resister thinks is necessary, how soon the resister wants an answer, and so forth. Take notes on everything the person says to show that you're taking the questions seriously and, in fact, are already working on it.

Don't Move Forward without Getting Middle Managers on Board

If it takes a long time, spend it. At the management level, create discussion opportunities that build service commitment, training opportunities that build skill, and support systems that reinforce attention and effort toward service improvement. Help managers and frontline supervisors recognize and handle resistance first in themselves and then in others. Don't skirt it; caringly confront it and help managers and supervisors work it through. Suspend using executive orders and fear to motivate until you have provided patient, persistent, and extensive supports to managers and supervisors to help them make necessary changes and embrace your strategy as theirs.

Start Slow and Small

If you haven't started yet, move carefully. Develop small wins that create positive expectations about change and that build the skills and comfort of some people, then other people, then other people. Value incremental change and accept the fact that aligning your organization with your service commitment takes most organizations 5 to 10 years of *major* effort and then a forever process of continuous improvement and course corrections.

Use Data, Not Harangues, to Drive Improvement

Don't skip over installation of meaningful measures of service performance, because the data that these measures yield drive improvement more than urgent appeals by the organization's leaders. In some organizations, leaders lecture staff about what staff need to do to improve service. Their words smack of rhetoric and breed accusations that the leaders don't practice what they preach. It is much more effective to use customer feedback data to focus staff on the need for improvement than it is to preach about the importance of improving customer service.

Take Steps to Engage Employees as Owners, Not Only as Participants

Help people connect their vision to the vision and goals of your strategy. Help employees and physicians to align personally with your service commitment by articulating their own personal vision and values and then connecting them to the vision and values that drive your service strategy.

For example, in workshops or in staff meetings designed to achieve "personal alignment" with your strategy, ask employees or physicians to address these six groups of questions with one another:

1. What do I want to accomplish in my career? Years from now, what do I want my coworkers and customers to say about me? What will be my legacy? What values, ethics, and behaviors do I want to reflect in my daily work?
2. If I live my vision and values, how will others benefit?
3. What thoughts, actions, and attitudes on my part will help me live my vision and values?
4. How do my vision and values for myself fit with the vision and values for this organization's service strategy? How do my vision and values not fit with this organization's service strategy?
5. How can I move toward my personal vision and live my values in the context of our service strategy?
6. What's in it for me?

Provide Growth Opportunities to Help People Change

Some people resist change, claiming it's a bad idea, because they are afraid they won't be able to do what's expected of them. New expectations lead to a confidence crisis and indeed some people may not have the skills to meet the newly raised standards. That's why you need to go beyond communicating clear expectations and provide training, mentoring, coaching, and practice in an atmosphere of mutual learning and support, not fear, so that people have the chance they deserve to develop new muscles.

Help People Build Skill at Resistance Comebacks

What about those annoying one-liners that catch you off guard in the hallways and elevators?

- "How's your sweet little service excellence program going?"
- "Marge, you're not smiling!"
- "Service excellence—the farce of the year. When's the next showing?"
- "How did a sharp person like you get suckered into this service improvement bit?"

The Einstein Consulting Group has developed a toolkit of the following skills for responding to sarcastic cracks, loaded innuendos, or straightforward resistant comments:

- *Be a sounding board:* Find out why. Ask open-ended questions. Let employees vent their frustrations. Express concern and empathy.
- *Enlist support:* Don't be afraid to ask for help. Be clear about your own identification with the service mission.
- *Stand firm:* Let resisters know that service excellence goes with the territory. Keep emphasizing that service is everyone's job.
- *Show humor:* "What have we got to lose?" "Why not try it; things can't get much worse."
- *Share benefits:* Point out to the resisters what's in it for them. Give good logical reasons why service improvement is really good for employees and physicians: for example, less stress and a more pleasant, cooperative environment.
- *Meet resisters halfway:* Rearrange schedules, solve problems, offer alternatives, and use their input.
- *Charm and disarm:* Make resisters feel special. Let them see that they are valued but that, of course, everyone "has room for fine-tuning."
- *Tell a tale:* Sometimes people need to hear other people's service successes, improvement, and recovery success stories.
- *Command respect:* Don't tolerate abusive resistance. Remind the abusive resister that you're a person, deserving of respect.
- *Give logical explanations:* Describe why service excellence is good for the organization, for patients, and for the resisters to the strategy. Share the realities of the economic picture. Point to competition and market research, for example.
- *Switch the focus:* Ask the resisters questions. Put *them* on the defensive. Listen to their rationales and address their concerns.
- *Change the environment:* Surprise resisters. Make quick improvement so they see that something is actually happening. Communicate about progress constantly.
- *Get their opinions:* Engage resisters as opinion leaders. Involve them in think tanks, focus groups, and advisory committees.
- *Hold up a mirror:* Show resisters how their resistance sounds and what it looks like. Some people don't even know they're being negative.
- *Provide an experience:* Let the resisters talk to patients and view a positive interaction. A good role model helps.
- *Take a strong personal stand:* Stick your neck out if you believe in what you're doing: "You might think I'm crazy but I really believe that a focus on continuous service improvement is good for us, and I'm going to do what I can to make it work."

Be Patient but *Expect* Alignment

Develop exquisitely clear performance expectations and put teeth into your strategy. Make the expectations clear to your employees before you enforce them so that people have a chance to *choose* to perform. Ambiguity about performance expectations breeds testing of limits on the part of a small but visible number of employees. The antidote is clarity, unequivocal and explicit job expectations backed up by enforced consequences, both positive and negative, for employee actions.

Some people resist or rebel in hopes of being let off the hook. If their resistance reaps these benefits for them, expect an epidemic of resistance. An employee who does not meet your service standards cannot be allowed to get by. You put teeth in your service expectations by developing policies, job description statements, behavioral expectations, a performance appraisal system, and so forth. Now you must follow through. Without enforcement, excellence crumbles; and the same few people who drag down morale and the organization's image continue to do so, dragging good people down with them. Confronting problem service performance by an employee is something no supervisor (or executive) likes to do, but tolerating poor or mediocre performance compromises your service commitment.

Recognize Ambivalence in Yourself and Others and Resolve It

Although everyone knows that health care delivery is in the midst of hard times, employees and physicians understandably are resisting this reality and wishing for the good old days. What should change agents do in this atmosphere? First of all, examine your own beliefs and feelings. Do you feel guilty pushing for change when people keep reminding you of all the ground they feel they've lost—all the ways they're being victimized and oppressed by the new realities? Or do you understand the feelings but refuse to accept them as excuses for inaction or refusal to change?

It's important to empathize with these feelings, but then move quickly to insist on the need to improve service anyway. Push for what you know needs to happen in the face of today's harsh realities. Change agents need to show bravado in the face of resistance and tenaciously resist submitting to pressure to "be understanding and back off." Otherwise, you join the ranks of the demoralized. Our careful message that mixes empathy with determination to press forward might sound like this:

> I can understand that you're exhausted from taking care of so many patients. *Still,* I believe attention to service quality is essential! I realize the belt tightening around here has been very painful as we stretch to make do with fewer resources. *Still,* this is no excuse for inattention to meeting our customers' needs with care and sensitivity in the time we do have with them.

The fact is, individuals have vast room for improvement in every minute they spend in a service interaction. The following excerpt from a letter written by a patient to a hospital administrator about the treatment she received in radiology is testimony to this fact:

> I had some X rays and a CAT scan last week. After putting on a gown, I appeared in the waiting area. The tech, looking at the floor, said mechanically, "This way." She walked me to the procedure table and said mechanically, "Lie down on your back."
>
> In the same amount of time, she could have said, "Hello, Ms. Smith. My name is Cindy. Follow me, please." And then as we approached the table, she could have said, "You'll need to lie down on your back on this table. I realize your back is hurting you, so may I help you up?" This second way would not have taken *one second* more of Cindy's time and I would have felt more welcome, less fearful of jarring my already aching back, and more confident that I was in good hands.
>
> I ask you, is high acuity, busy-ness, and short staffing an excuse for mediocre treatment? How can health care professionals feel proud of this? And how can managers feel so unambitious as to let this remain the standard of service in your organization?

Change agents, including managers, need to resolve their ambivalence about raising service standards, to confront resistance head on and challenge people whose actions or words say "I refuse to examine my own behavior; I refuse to take any responsibility whatsoever for making improvements here." Beyond that, such agents can be role models of people who see change as an adventure instead of a threat, as a learning opportunity and pathway to personal renewal, rather than as yet another burden.

Ideally, these resistance-prevention approaches should be implemented at the beginning of a service strategy. However, these same techniques are useful at many points in an ongoing service improvement strategy.

☐ Final Suggestions

Some resistance to essential changes is inevitable in an organization that is committed to continuous service improvement as a modus operandi. As you encounter this resistance, consider these suggestions:

- *Don't label resistance a negative trait:* As an expected stage in a change process, read it as an opportunity for progress in making people aware of new, more ambitious expectations. Then, with empathy, help them focus on the future and the benefits change can bring if everyone contributes to your service mission.
- *Don't harbor grudges against resisters:* So often, people spearheading service strategies have turned initially resistant people into believers and supporters. Remember the power of your own expectations and *expect* resisters to become your strategy's success stories and best advocates.

Resistance to change is more than just inevitable; it's also a natural reaction to unsettling shifts in the status quo. Remember that everyone, even the most forward-thinking individual, has some difficulty handling change. Consequently, resistance to change is a force that must be planned for as you develop and deepen your strategy and a source of energy that you can use to grow and cultivate support and action. Because resistance is natural and is to be expected, don't be intimidated by it. Provide clarity, time, support, and the stability of a persistent message. Then, if people make the choice of refusing to move with you toward your vision, remember the fable at the beginning of this chapter, and let go of the rope.

References

1. Adapted from: Friedman, E. H. *Friedman's Fables.* New York City: Guilford Press, 1990.

2. Hellriegel, D., Slocum, J., and Woodman, R. *Organizational Behavior.* St. Paul, MN: West Publishing Co., 1983.

3. Zaltman, G., and Duncan, R. *Strategies for Planned Change.* New York City: Wiley Interscience, 1977.

4. Hellriegel, Slocum, and Woodman.

5. Lewin, K. Frontiers in group dynamics. *Human Relations* 1:5–41, June 1947.

6. ODR, Inc. *Change Resistance Scale.* Atlanta, GA: O.D.R., Inc., 1991.

7. Kanter, D., and Mirvis, P. Managing jaundiced workers. *New Management* 3(4):50–54, Spring 1986.

Chapter 19

Innovations in Service Quality

Many health care organizations that have methodically built a customer orientation into their everyday culture become frustrated with constraints posed by traditional operating structures. Feeling that incremental service improvement is no longer enough, they enter the "land of innovation," instituting structural and operational changes in health care delivery protocols that dramatically improve service quality and heighten customer satisfaction.

In *Busting Bureaucracy,* Kenneth Johnston describes three goals for service improvement efforts:[1]

1. The "customer-*sensitive*" organization maintains its current organizational form while working to bring service quality up to and beyond customer expectations. The degree of bureaucracy that customers and staff experience might lessen as a result.
2. The "customer-*focused*" organization incorporates an explicit customer focus into its mission statement. It aims to achieve extraordinary customer relations, but it maintains its present form of organization, including hierarchy, rules, detachment, functional lines of organization, and an emphasis in hiring based on technical qualifications.
3. The "customer-*driven*" organization willingly, even eagerly, alters its organizational forms in order to achieve extraordinary customer satisfaction and an extraordinary organization.

Few organizations have gone as far as becoming truly *customer-driven*. Following is a description of three structural innovations by hospitals experimenting to achieve breakthroughs in customer satisfaction—structural innovations that we believe reflect the highest level of effort in service improvement—thus becoming customer-driven organizations:

- Patient-focused care
- The Planetree model
- The Cooperative Care program

☐ Patient-Focused Care

In an article in *Healthcare Forum Journal*, Janet Henderson and James Williams provided the following typical scenario:[2]

> As his wait for the physical therapist approaches 30 minutes, the patient at Pigeon-hope Hospital is becoming increasingly frustrated. While he is pleased that his surgery two days ago was a success, he is anxious about the recovery process. And he is getting irritated at the amount of time he has spent waiting throughout his stay—not to mention being fed and transported at times that have seemed more convenient for the hospital than for him.
>
> Not being the reticent sort, he has begun to air his complaints to several of the staff. But he senses that few really have time to care about him—only about efficiently performing their tasks. While most are pleasant and seemingly professional people, he doesn't feel that anyone in the hospital has the "total picture" of his treatment and concerns.
>
> He begins to count how many different people in the hospital he has come in contact with during his two and one half day stay. When his count reaches the mid-thirties, he is interrupted by the physical therapist. She is ready to see him now.

This is a typical situation in the hospital of the past and in many of today's hospitals. But the wave of the future is the innovative care delivery system of the patient-focused hospital. The *patient-focused hospital* (a term coined by J. Philip Lathrop, vice-president of health care practice with Booz-Allen and Hamilton) has been shown to achieve significant gains in service quantity, quality, and customer satisfaction through *structural* change in how health care is delivered.

According to Lathrop in an article titled "The Patient-Focused Hospital," today's hospitals are in fact sadly *un*–patient-focused. For example:[3]

- Direct care for patients counts for less than 25 percent of hospital personnel expenditures.
- A typical patient interacts with about 60 different employees during a four-day stay.
- Most hospitals have 100 to 150 activity centers and more than 350 different job classifications (nearly half of which have only one incumbent).

Lathrop identifies some painful symptoms that cost patients dearly in terms of confusion, lack of continuity, impersonal care, and cost. For example:[4,5]

- A one- or two-hour odyssey for a routine X-ray exam is considered "good service."
- More than half of all basic lab tests are ordered "stat."
- Five-minute EKGs require nearly an hour's worth of scheduling, documentation, and transportation—all to "optimize" the time of a high school graduate with two weeks of in-service education.
- The presence of specialists and technicians whom we wouldn't dream of asking to do anything but their own narrow, and often self-defined, duties—even if it means they are idle much of the time—must be tolerated.
- Separate job classifications for housekeepers who clean tiles and housekeepers who clean carpets are somehow justified.
- An outpatient processing system that thinks nothing of charging premium prices for a half-day's ordeal just to get a chest film, an EKG, and a specimen drawn is considered efficient.
- An infrastructure nightmare allows clerks and secretaries to outnumber the inpatients in a large hospital.
- Multiple entries in every patient's record every day document a hand-off approach in the process of care (for example, "The patient was alive when I handed him/her off.").

- A nurse pokes her head into the patient's room *often* to ask, "Has _____ been in to see you yet?" (Thus the patient gets the impression that nobody knows what's going on.)
- The nearly pandemic "I'll get someone" syndrome, which follows the "You mean they haven't done that yet!" syndrome, is contagious.
- Physicians arrive on nursing units only to find their patients away at X-ray, physical therapy, or some other ancillary service.
- Caregivers deserve frequent flyer status, for they travel many miles daily through hallways; up and down stairs; and on elevators to find, transport, and serve patients.
- An average of fewer than five incumbents per job classification (excluding nursing) leads to extremely high levels of structured idle time.
- Forty to 70 minutes are devoted to busywork (transportation, scheduling, documentation) and patient interactions with three or four different staff members (two transporters, a nurse, and a technician) just to perform a centralized EKG, an inexpensive procedure requiring an inexpensive machine and an in-service-trained paraprofessional.

Most of these symptoms are the result of a structure that is compartmentalized and fragmented. Such a structure makes continuity of care impossible, it wastes money, it frustrates and bores caregivers, and it interferes profoundly with patient satisfaction. In a patient-focused hospital however, hospital operations are driven by a concentration on patients as the highest priority. Translated into many forms, the patient-focused hospital has shown its potential to heighten patient satisfaction dramatically while increasing the direct care provided to patients by 60 percent, increasing staff satisfaction, and reducing personnel-related costs by as much as 40 percent.[6] The main assumption on which experiments in patient-focused care rest is that a hospital's organizational structure must be changed in ways that reduce specialization, complexity, wasted personnel time, and bureaucracy. Typically, such experiments restructure patient care in two key areas: (1) in nursing jobs especially, so that there's a better fit between the individual's training and expectations, and (2) in the patient care delivery system so that fewer health care specialists do more for the patient and do it closer to the patient's bedside. Key tactics for achieving these changes include:

- *Cross-training:* To decrease the myriad of staff who interact with the patient, fewer staff are trained to perform more functions, thus becoming more versatile and less specialized. As a result, they have less downtime and can do more for the patient without having to communicate with or seek approval from other service providers.
- *Redeployment of ancillaries:* Ancillary care providers are also cross-trained. Medical, laboratory, and respiratory technicians, in addition to nurses, provide routine care. These services are provided at the patient's bedside, which reduces the handoffs and transportation nightmares described above.
- *Care teams "own" their patients:* Two or three multiskilled professionals work together in teams to serve an assigned group of patients. These teams maintain continuity across shifts and days of stay. They also admit their own patients and do medical record coding and abstracting. Because these teams take on routine chores such as linen changing, tray delivery, and blood drawing, patients and their families know who their caregivers are and see them often. Thus, patients do not feel anonymous, dehumanized, or lost in a complex system of people and services. Patients who stay for three days are likely to interact with fewer than 15 employees, not the 50 or 60 they interact with in a traditionally structured system.
- *Care close to the patient:* The goal is to decentralize care, bringing care and service to patients, instead of making sick patients search out needed services. The result is less patient discomfort, reduced waits and turnaround times, and more personalized service, because patients know their handful of caregivers.

343

- *Increased consistency, quality, and efficiency through use of protocols:* Most care is driven by protocols, and caregivers would need to engage in the unpopular task of charting only when care departs from the protocol. This reduction in paperwork produces more time for patient care.
- *Greater staff gratification and reduced turnover:* With this model, staff do more things for fewer people and gain more gratification from getting to know their patients and families better. Their more versatile use of skills is more stimulating than doing the same specialized function day after day, patient after patient. The interactions between staff and patients are more vibrant and staff are less likely to jump ship due to burnout.

According to David Weber in his article "Six Models of Patient-Focused Care," there is an "urgent need for radical surgery to cure a syndrome in which record keeping, scheduling, transporting, supervising, attending meetings, tidying up, serving meals, and simply standing around idle now consume fully 84 percent of the typical hospital's value-added personnel activity."[7] Lathrop adds, "For every dollar spent on direct care, we spend $3 to $4 waiting for it to happen, arranging to do it, and writing it down. This can't be fixed by working harder and faster."[8] Both believe that it is only through structural change that leverage in quality can be found.

Many hospitals are experimenting with patient-focused care, and Weber describes six such models.[9] These models were developed by pioneering hospitals with leaders eager to experiment with structural change that would both decrease cost and improve service quality. The hospitals are Lakeland Regional Medical Center, St. Vincent Hospital and Health Care Center, Vanderbilt University Medical Center, Bishop Clarkson Memorial Hospital, Lee Memorial Hospital, and Robert Wood Johnson University Hospital. With the permission of *Healthcare Forum Journal*, excerpts from the descriptions of four of these pilot efforts are reprinted in the following subsections.

Notice that not only does patient and family satisfaction improve in an atmosphere of patient-focused care, but the quality of life for physicians and staff also improves. Early data also indicate that the improved flow of services to the patient and the increased contact with a smaller number of caregivers results in decreased cost.[10]

Lakeland Regional Medical Center (Lakeland, Florida)

The Lakeland Regional Medical Center (LRMC) was where Booz-Allen's model of hospital decompartmentalization was first elaborated. Located in the geographic center of Florida, the 897-bed LRMC is the sole acute care/surgical provider to the 180,000 residents of Lakeland and its surrounding county populace of 410,000. The hospital performs some 15,500 surgical procedures annually, including about 500 open-heart surgeries.

With an operating margin of 6.5 to 7.5 percent over the past two years, "our financial situation has been stable, not deteriorating," observed Senior Vice-President for Patient-Focused Development David Jones. Nevertheless, by the end of 1987, LRMC management had become convinced that, as CEO Jack Stephens emphasized, "preservation of the status quo was clearly going to lead us into a tragic, crisis situation." Although the work with Booz-Allen "began as a cost-saving effort," he said, it soon became apparent, he said, that "many quality pieces would have overriding impact."

By the beginning of 1989, operations research had been completed and planning for implementation of the pilot project begun. A 40-bed unit capable of expansion to 85 beds in a renovated wing of the hospital was selected to house the initial experiment. It would be a self-contained surgical service with its own minilab, diagnostic radiology rooms, supply stockrooms, and administrative records/clerical area.

Bedside care would be provided by teams of multiskilled practitioners made up of a care pair—a registered nurse and a cross-trained technician—backed by a unit-based pharmacist, a unit clerk, and a unit support aide to help with transport, restocking, upkeep, and maintenance. The aim was to enable each care pair on each shift to meet up to 90 percent of the pre- and postsurgical needs of four to seven specific patients admitted by 29 physicians specializing in general, vascular, ENT, plastic/oral surgery, and neurosurgery. Unit management would be handled by a master scheduler, a clinical manager coordinating day-to-day activities of six or seven care teams, and an administrative director with overall unit human resources, planning, and budgeting responsibility.

In July 1989, cross-training for the Patient-Focused Surgical Services (PFSS) nurses and technologists began. The latter included licensed vocational or practical nurses (LVNs or LPNs), patient care assistants (PCAs), respiratory therapists, and radiologic technologists. Six-week, full-time classes based on materials prepared by LRMC staff followed by competency-based testing in each area were offered in routine phlebotomy, EKG, respiratory and physical therapy, laboratory testing, and diagnostic radiology procedures.

Between them, the care-pair team would be competent to shoulder the full range of direct patient care, records processing, and "hotel" functions—from admitting, charting, charging, tray passing, transportation, and room cleanup to care planning, assessment, therapeutic intervention, diagnostic test administration, and outcome evaluation.

"One of our functional models is 'never pass over something you can do yourself,'" declared Phyllis Watson, LRMC vice-president of nursing. "We're going counter to the trend in the industry, which is to do fewer things for more people. We say we're going to do more and more things for fewer people."

"In the beginning," admitted Watson, "all 2,300 employees expressed fear and trepidation." High on the list of concerns, of course, was the blurring of professional and nonprofessional roles. But the consensus among PFSS nurses today, she maintained, is that "there are no demeaning tasks when it comes to taking care of patients. Besides, they say they'd rather pass trays than spend an hour on the phone." Other benefits—gains in terms of decentralized and simplified services (among others), as well as charting by exception—are described in the following sections.

Huge Gains
By decentralizing lab services, turnaround time for routine tests in the patient-focused unit plummeted from an average of 157 minutes under the old regimen to an average of 48 minutes—a 70 percent improvement in responsiveness. Diagnostic radiology procedures were simplified from 40 steps consuming 140 minutes on average to 8 steps taking 28 minutes—an 80 percent reduction in turnaround time.

Compared with traditional nursing service, care pairs were able to double the time they spent actually ministering to patients' medical, technical, and clinical needs. Not surprisingly, perhaps, errors have been greatly reduced. Fewer patient falls were recorded in the patient-focused surgical unit than in any other comparable conventional LRMC service except surgical intensive care and gynecology. Medication errors were the fewest in the hospital.

Staff, physician, and patient satisfaction levels all soared too, according to surveys. Patient-Focused Surgical Services RN turnover was the lowest in the institution—3 percent for fiscal year 1989–90. Physicians unanimously hailed the improvements in test result turnaround time, reduced paperwork, and efficiency in making rounds. Perceptions of quality, responsiveness, and caregiver concern were 13 to 17 percent higher among PFSS patients than those treated elsewhere in the institution.

Moreover, the lengths and variability of patient stays were sliced appreciably—by 1.3 days on average for a colonectomy, for example. More than 60 percent of PFSS patients were seen exclusively by their primary physician throughout their hospitalization. The average number of different hospital personnel who interacted with PFSS patients during a stay was just 13, 10 of them care pairs. That was 75 percent fewer than the 27 nurses, 10 dietary, 6 ancillary services, 5 central transport, 3 environmental services, and 2 "other support" employees who used to bustle in and out of rooms during an average LRMC stay.

Chief executive officer Stephens estimates that his institution has spent some $5 million on the enterprise so far. Capital costs were the least of the bill—$100,000 for X-ray equipment, $150,000 for laboratory decompartmentalization, and $100,000 for patient room computer terminals. Direct bedside care costs in PFSS compared to a traditional unit, however, were 9.2 percent lower—$12,034 per occupied bed versus $13,256 elsewhere in the institution.

"We don't know that this is sustainable, but we think it is," he said. "In fact, we think it will increase and create a critical mass that will allow us to reduce the infrastructure even further. But if it just doesn't cost us any more, we think that's enough to go forward."

Charting by Exception

Among critical "enablers" underlying the success of the project, according to Watson, was the painstaking and resource-intensive development of problem-specific care protocols organized by day and phase of stay, delineating caregiver activities as well as some physician orders.

These were the underpinnings of another key enabler, a system of charting by exception. Whereas LRMC nurses once spent 29 percent of their precious time and energy scribbling down observations (including such vapidities as "skin warm and dry; patient slept well"), they now consult five-day flow sheets based on the patient-specific protocols. Only variations from the expected course of treatment and recovery are noted. As a result, medical documentation in PFSS occupies an infinitesimal 2 percent of nurses' working hours.

Computer terminals in each PFSS room linked to the hospital mainframe support decentralized admitting, charging, discharging, and bed control. To arrange for an admission and an operating room, a surgeon's office calls the master scheduler, who triangulates a conference call with PFSS to specify the care team the physician wants and to pinpoint the anticipated length of stay, based, said Watson, on "a few smart questions." Assisted by specially developed software called "Carelink," the master scheduler has been able to hit the target work load for care pairs 87 percent of the time.

To simplify communications and reduce noise and distractions, a single telephone number for the unit is attended by a single receptionist. Care providers wear silent, vibrating alphanumeric beepers that deliver specific messages such as "go prep Mr. Lathrop for surgery." For situations in which beepers would be impractical, care team members can be reached by zone phones covering their own clusters of rooms. Patients wear the appropriate number on their wristbands. Care providers spend virtually all their time in one or another of the patients' rooms; they are never summoned to a central area to answer the telephone.

Designing a compensation and career advancement program that will suitably reward and motivate multiskilled practitioners has been a challenge, Watson acknowledged. With Management Science Associates, Lakeland has devised a two-part pay scale in which range is based on skills (up to 600 points determined by competency testing) and education (400 points), with differentials awarded according to an annual assessment of the year's achievements in leadership (counting for 45 percent), cross-training (35 percent), and professional development (20 percent).

Convinced by the pilot experience that the patient-focused structure enhances service, increases satisfaction, improves quality, and reduces expenses, LRMC plans to expand the PFSS to 235 beds within the next two years, incorporating the operating room and postanesthesia care units. From there, says Stephens, the development team and Booz-Allen will work on rolling out four additional patient-focused "hospitals" grouped around cardiovascular/trauma/critical care, outpatient/inpatient diagnostic, general medical, and family care.

Vanderbilt University Hospital and Clinic (Nashville, Tennessee)

A 630-bed facility, Vanderbilt is an academic medical center that treats some 26,500 inpatients each year. A renovated orthopedic unit of 31 private rooms on two levels was selected as the patient-focused pilot. Three classes of multiskilled personnel—clinical associates, administrative associates, and service associates—work collaboratively under an operating philosophy that dictates, "Never hand off what you can do yourself."

Clinical associates, according to CEO Norman Urmy, share duties from emptying wastebaskets to taking X-ray films, but they are forbidden by state law from assuming laboratory functions. Patient financial counseling is the only other routine activity dispatched off-unit.

"Some people estimated it would take nine to 14 weeks of one-on-one training to impart a skill," explained executive director of nursing services Judy Spinella. "At that rate, the necessary cross-training could have taken years. So we decided that some 'nice-to-know' would have to go. A lot of 'need-to-know' had to stay."

Urmy calculates that cross-training alone cost about $70,000, "but we don't think that's too much to pay for this good a show." Projected across the institution, patient-focused restructuring can support a 9 percent reduction in staff, he said.

As elsewhere, the development of protocols and their incorporation in a customized "critical path" detailing "milestones" for each day of each patient's stay has been a critical ingredient in the success of the project, Spinella emphasized. "The plan is only changed where necessary, and it allows documentation by exception."

In pre-pilot attitude surveys, literally zero percent of the hospital staff expressed satisfaction with the amount of paperwork they were burdened with, she reported. But in the patient-focused orthopedic unit, an astonishing 80 percent declared themselves satisfied with documentation requirements.

"It used to take four hours to turn over a bed between patients," she continued. "Recently I overheard two service associates complaining because it had taken 15 minutes!"

Bishop Clarkson Memorial Hospital (Omaha, Nebraska)

More than $1 million in construction costs and $236,000 in equipment purchases underlie Bishop Clarkson's pilot patient-focused project, a 35-room oncology unit staffed by 40.7 FTEs, 28 of them multiskilled "care partners." Each room in the pilot unit, which opened July 31, 1990, is equipped with a "patient server" housing a computer terminal for order entry, care planning, and online reporting to radiology, laboratory, and pulmonary services; a telephone; and supplies sufficient to meet 90 percent of the care partners' needs.

A radiology suite supports on-unit test procedures except those involving MRI, CAT scan, fluoroscopy, and ultrasound. A satellite pharmacy fills all chemotherapy and first-dose oral, injectable, and topical prescriptions.

Patient-focused care at Bishop Clarkson, according to neurosensory administrative manager Kevin Moffitt, unit manager Lisa Tracey, and medical director Tom Tinstman, MD, has yielded signal advantages. Ten steps have been sliced from the admitting process, whittling the average time from patient check-in to order entry and the actual paging of the physician from almost eight hours to 23 minutes. Patients receive an antibiotic ordered by the physician in 5 steps instead of 12.

The very appearance of the unit to someone "looking down the hall" is vastly different from the rest of the 523-bed hospital, Tracey pointed out. On conventional floors, a central nursing station is the focus of activity, with charge nurses, team leaders, nursing assistants, housekeepers, patient transporters, phlebotomists, EKG technicians, physical therapists, and respiratory therapists milling about this hub.

In the patient-focused unit, multiskilled care pairs and support generalists appear only occasionally as they move from room to room. All charting, care, and conversations between physicians, nurses, patients, and their families take place at the bedside.

Based on operational gains and the accompanying boosts in physician, patient, and staff satisfaction levels, Bishop Clarkson opened a patient-focused kidney center with 37 inpatient beds, outpatient dialysis, transplant, and home dialysis services. Unlike the

347

oncology unit, whose restructuring was implemented from the administration down, the kidney center was redesigned by its own team, Moffitt said.

Planning is also under way to convert a two-floor critical care unit including 48 ICU and 22 intermediary care beds to patient-focused operations. Orthopedics, neurology, and maternity care stand next in line—and after that, said Moffitt, even those hospital activities that have so far been "out of play."

Robert Wood Johnson University Hospital (New Brunswick, New Jersey)

For the past three years, an alternative patient care delivery model embodying many of the concepts underpinning other patient-focused restructuring efforts has been in operation at 416-bed Robert Wood Johnson. Beginning in a 32-bed surgical orthopedic unit, the model has been expanded into eight other departments, including critical care.

Key elements of the program include the management and coordination of individual patient care by an RN clinical care manager (an exempt rather than hourly position), who ensures that anticipated outcomes for a caseload of about a dozen patients are achieved within established protocol time frames.

Assessment, planning, and provision of direct and indirect care for patients are the jobs of the primary nurses, about six of whom are overseen by each clinical case manager, with one or two associate nurses—LPNs—providing assistance. Task such as making unoccupied beds, preparing patients for meals, and distributing water and linen, though, are handled by "support services hosts," who are assigned to specific groups of patients. Each unit is also staffed by a pharmacy technician who prepares all medications and intravenous solutions according to each patient's dose administration schedule. "We're trying to hone down what we see as the professional work of the RN," emphasized Mary Tonges, vice-president of nursing. "This does not involve cross-training."

In the restructured critical care unit, however, some functions like glucose scans, CPR, and patient bathing have been delegated to critical care technicians, a newly created position. "We've also decentralized a number of systems to the bedside," she said, including a telephone for each, a large tool chest adapted to contain all medications and supplies for the patient—stocked by the support services host and pharmacy technician—and a split-screen TV monitor so nurses in one room can observe a patient in another.

Quality of care, worker satisfaction, and patient satisfaction indexes have all been positive, Tonges reported. Lengths of stay have been sliced by 26 percent in the units where the system has been in operation longest.

For additional references on patient-focused care, see "Operational Restructuring: 19 Pioneering Models" in *Healthcare Forum Journal*, 830 Market Street, San Francisco, CA 94102, 1992.

☐ The Planetree Model

Research on human responses to stress and their impact on the immune system emphasizes the powerful influence of environment on health. Some organizations are designing "healing environments" to enhance therapeutic outcomes and patient and family satisfaction. *Healthcare Forum Journal's* "Healing Environment Compendium" focused an entire issue on healing environments and alternative delivery systems that emphasize patient comfort, satisfaction, and responsibility.[11]

The Planetree model, a pioneer in the quest to humanize health care in our high-tech age, originated in 1981 on the campus of what was then the Pacific Presbyterian Medical Center (and is now part of San Francisco's California Pacific Medical Center). It began as a resource center for patients, their families, and the public, including a library of medical texts, news clippings, and health material available for study at no charge.

Four years later, Planetree expanded to include an inpatient unit that has become a widely respected prototype for a humane or "healing" hospital environment.[12]

Named after the tree in whose shade Hippocrates is said to have taught the healing arts in ancient Greece, Planetree was developed by Argentine-born Angelica Thieriot, a member of a prominent San Francisco family. After experiencing several hospital experiences that she perceived as depersonalizing, alienating, and confusing, Thieriot set out to develop a health care alternative that would integrate the technological capabilities of western medicine with the spiritual dimensions acknowledged by the healing arts as Hippocrates understood them, specifically compassion, comfort, aesthetic beauty, dignity, shared knowledge, and the freedom of informed choice.

The Planetree unit was painstakingly designed and redesigned to comfort and cater to acutely ill people. It includes facilities that make the atmosphere homelike and comfortable, including the following:

- A kitchenette where patients and their families can cook at all hours and learn to cook healthy meals under the guidance of Planetree's nutritionist
- A corridor that invites walking around because it is spacious, carpeted, equipped with incandescent track lighting, and trimmed in wood with sound-dampening wallpaper
- Colorful patient rooms, including beds made with floral sheets and colorful spreads; pastel, not white, privacy curtains; and a bookshelf and bulletin board for personalizing the environment
- A lounge with VCR and big-screen TV, equipped with light-hearted movies

Its people, policies, and procedures encourage patients and their families to become knowledgeable, participate actively, and take responsibility for the regimen in the hospital and after discharge. For instance:

- Patients and families are encouraged to read all about the patient's illness in the Resource Center.
- The patient is a key participant in considering treatment options and making decisions about them.
- The nurses station is open, accessible, and inviting to patients.
- Patients are encouraged to read their charts and to write their own observations or progress notes in them.
- Medication is under the control of the patient and family; they are coached to develop and control a medication schedule suited to the patient's sleeping hours and mealtimes.
- Family and friends, including children, are welcome to visit at any time or to stay overnight and to participate in patient care as "care partners."

Other features include:

- Primary nursing, in which one RN coordinates the patient's care plan throughout the patient's stay
- Access to alternative techniques, such as therapeutic touch, homeopathy, stress reduction, resident storytellers, and much more

With leadership from Robin Orr, Planetree's national director of hospital projects, Planetree has been replanted in several parts of the country in widely divergent settings, including San Jose Medical Center, Beth Israel Medical Center in New York City, and Mid-Columbia Medical Center (a 49-bed rural hospital in The Dalles, Oregon). Other experiments in healing environments extend beyond hospital walls. For instance, Vidark-liniken (a house of healing) in Sweden and Dr. Patch Adams's Gesundheit Institute in

Arlington, Virginia, are two examples in which the environment is carefully designed with the patient at its center, and alternative (holistic) healing methods are the mainstay, not the periphery, of patient care.[13,14] It can be expected that many more models and experiments will create the capability to achieve breakthroughs in patient responsibility, health outcomes, and satisfaction.

☐ The NYU Medical Center Cooperative Care Program

The NYU Medical Center Cooperative Care program is an innovative model of a delivery system of acute inpatient hospital care.[15] Its special feature is that a live-in family member or friend acts as the patient's "care partner." This model emphasizes education in order to encourage full patient and family involvement in care during the acute hospitalization, thereby preparing both parties for management at home after discharge. The education-intensive experience of Cooperative Care provides an alternative to traditional inpatient hospital care. Specifically, it increases patient and family knowledge and satisfaction, adherence to the medical regimen, and appropriate self-management. The functioning ability of the patient-care partner team improves and their anxieties about self-care decrease upon discharge, which also results in decreased future use of high-cost health care resources, particularly rehospitalization.

Inclusion of the patient's family and support system into the period of hospitalization leads to more humanistic hospital care. Housed in a homelike setting (with doors that lock from the inside) without physicians, nurses, or nurse-aides on the patient-room floors, the Cooperative Care patients are brought to the centralized hospital services by the care partner for their clinical nursing and physician assessments and treatments, and for comprehensive individual and group education sessions. These two elements (the "Therapeutic Center" for clinical functions and the "Education Center" for instructional functions) are interdependent and enable the unit to provide a very high level of personal care for a broad spectrum of acutely ill patients.

The professionals in this partnership include the patients' physicians, the Therapeutic Center's Senior Nurse Clinicians (who carry out the diagnostic and therapeutic regimen while the patient is hospitalized), and the Education Center's multidisciplinary staff of nurse educators, nutritionists, social workers, pharmacists, and a movement therapist. This multidisciplinary team is responsible for:

- Orienting patients and care partners to Cooperative Care at the time of admission
- Performing an assessment of the appropriateness of the patient for Cooperative Care on entry
- Determining whether an adequate care partner is available and, if not, interceding to assist the patient in making arrangements for an adequate care partner
- Providing and evaluating education services for patients and care partners

This partnership of patients, families, and professionals provides the optimal approach to care during hospitalization and preparation for competent management at home after discharge.

☐ Final Thoughts

Health care providers are experimenting with a wide variety of structural and environmental changes that create new possibilities for the health care system and, specifically, create the potential for breakthroughs in patient and family satisfaction. The fact is, the current health care system, like any process, has limits—limits in this case on how well or consistently it can satisfy patients. If your organization is interested in breakthroughs in customer satisfaction, you will no doubt need to enter the land of structural change and experimentation. Fortunately, exciting models are springing up and can used as benchmarks (see discussion of benchmarking in chapter 7) that help you learn from the best of the best and avoid reinventing wheels.

Notes and References

1. Johnston, K. *Busting Bureaucracy.* Homewood, IL: Business One Irwin, 1992, p. 81.

2. Henderson, J., and Williams, J. The people side of patient care redesign. *Healthcare Forum Journal* 34(4):44, July–Aug. 1991.

3. Lathrop, J. P. The patient-focused hospital. *Healthcare Forum Journal* 35(3):76, May–June 1992.

4. Lathrop, J. P. The patient-focused hospital. *Healthcare Forum Journal* 34(4):17, July–Aug. 1991.

5. Lathrop, 1992.

6. Lathrop, 1992.

7. Weber, D. Six models of patient-focused care. *Healthcare Forum Journal* 34(4):24, July–Aug. 1991.

8. Lathrop, 1992.

9. Weber, pp. 23–31.

10. Weber, pp. 23–31.

11. Healing environment compendium. *Healthcare Forum Journal,* 35(5), Sept.–Oct. 1992.

12. Weber, D. Planetree transplanted. *Healthcare Forum Journal* 35(5):30–35, Sept.–Oct. 1992.

13. Coates, G., and Siepl-Coates, S. Vidarkliniken. *Healthcare Forum Journal* 35(5):27–29, Sept.–Oct. 1992.

14. Dr. Patch Adams's Gesundheit Institute, personal conversation, Arlington, Virginia, May 14, 1987.

15. Anthony Grieco, M.D., Medical Director; Kimberly Glassman, R.N., M.A., Clinical Assistant Director of Nursing; Shirley Garnett, R.N., M.S., Manager, Education Center, "Cooperative Care: Patients, Families and Professionals—Partners in Education and Care," NYU Medical Center, 530 First Avenue, New York City, NY 10016, 1991.

Chapter 20

Making Service Improvement an Ongoing Process

Since startup of a service improvement strategy takes extraordinary effort, time, and attention, many—in fact *most*—organizations slacken their efforts after what is really only the kickoff phase, even though the kind of culture change that is prerequisite to *continuous* service improvement is a complicated and long-term task. It takes three to five years to get a strategy going full steam ahead—and even then the effort can never ease up.

Long-term efforts are needed for three main reasons. First of all, *the scope of needed changes is enormous.* As shown in figure 20-1, Joiner Associates uses the iceberg analogy to describe the magnitude of effort needed to change organizational culture. Initially, change strategies address the more visible, surface forces that influence service performance. But enduring culture change requires digging deeper, beyond these apparent or surface forces, to align all formal, informal, and "below-the-surface" aspects of the organization with your service mission.

Second, *organizational habits change slowly.* Behavioral science research has shown that, while an individual can change behavior quickly, the change does not become habitual unless it is sustained for at least 21 days in a row. If it takes that much practice and repetition and persistence for an individual to change a simple behavior, imagine the difficulty of creating not only organizational change, but new organizational *habits* that endure without rigorous and sustained attention to them. In pursuit of continuous service improvement, organizations need to not only make changes but also develop new habits in customer focus, management behavior, measurement, feedback, approaches to problems, employee skills, and accountability practices. Continuous service improvement requires substantial policy change and implementation, prolonged behavior change on the part of staff, and substantial and sustained improvements in relationships within the organization. Development of this myriad of habits inevitably takes years of sustained attention, repetition, and reinforcement, not to mention incremental improvement until the changes sustain the effects that they were intended to produce.

Third, *individual differences affect the pace at which staff align with the service mission.* Joiner Associates uses the graphic in figure 20-2 to show the normal curve of reactions to the need for change among a diverse workforce. The explorers chart the path. The pioneers go first, preparing for the arrival of the settlers who follow after the changes are implemented. The stragglers drag their feet, and the urbanites dig in their heels, refusing to make the change. No wonder it takes time to bring staff in all of these categories up to speed with a service-oriented culture!

Given these reasons why long-term follow-through is inevitable, organizations that stop short not only fail to produce the results they seek, they also create a culture of learned apathy on the part of staff. Employees and physicians come to expect organizational change initiatives to start with a bang, peak, and then fizzle. They learn to ignore them or greet them with understandable cynicism. They must be helped, perhaps even taught, to help the strategy live through its slow times. And they need to see rejuvenated efforts not as new startups (thus fulfilling their expectation that programs come and go), but as continuations of the original strategy.

☐ Stallouts and Why They Happen

Some leaders are fully aware of the need for long-term follow-through, but their strategies stall anyway. Stallouts happen primarily for 10 reasons. Consider the extent to which these reasons apply to your organization. If you start by identifying the causes of your faltering strategy, you can develop tactics for follow-through.

1. *Impatience:* Often leaders have so much on their plates and are so accustomed to pushing for results *now* that they lose patience with the long-term work that needs doing. Also, many disregard the well-known fact about change: "It may get worse before it gets better."

Figure 20-1. Changing the Culture: The Organizational Iceberg

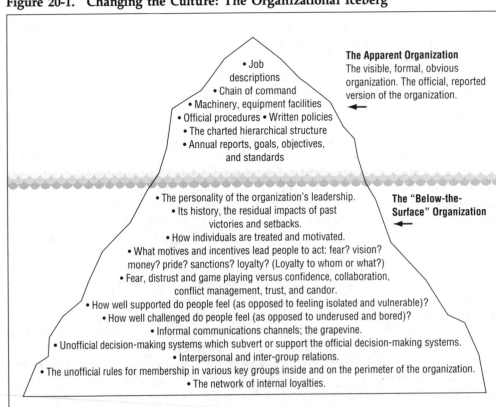

Figure 20-2. The Normal Curve of Reactions to Change

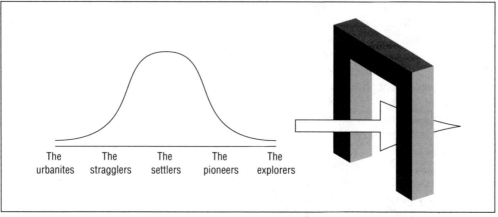

2. *Shortcuts:* Some leaders think they can skip some of the infrastructure building that other organizations seem to need. For instance, without adequate attention paid to building ongoing feedback systems into everyday operations, people have to pontificate about the need to make improvements, instead of having data to make the need for improvement both obvious and focused. Another example of a shortcut that creates downfalls is new employee orientation. Hospitals too eager to get new staff to the floors bypass adequate orientation and then have to spend inordinate time later rehabilitating employees who were inadequately prepared to begin with.

3. *Distraction:* In too many cases, organizations intend to follow through but divert their energy, focus, and resources because of growing economic problems that create additional pressure on the system. People then flip into a reactive mode, forgetting or considering it a luxury to pursue their service improvement strategy.

4. *Separation of strategy from everyday business:* Sometimes organizations feel they've hit a dead end in their efforts to improve service. In our view, this happens especially in those organizations that create a parallel structure, or shadow organization, to pursue service improvement without phasing in the integration of service management and service improvement activity into every department, every cross-functional effort, and the organization's strategic plan. The tactics remain above and beyond business as usual, instead of changing business as usual to incorporate ongoing service improvement.

5. *Status quo middle management:* Service improvement doesn't become routine behavior unless middle managers drive it. Yet many organizations fail to provide the expectations, training, support, and reinforcement middle department directors and supervisors need to change their mind-set and everyday practices to support ongoing service improvement. At best, ideas instituted by service strategists work, but habits don't change.

6. *Training that neglects one side of the brain:* People at all levels need training to help them become effective in service interactions and to become improvers of service quality. Some organizations focus training on building the analytical skills people need to make process improvements, but they neglect the soft skills that improve service relationships and make interactions harmonious and personally gratifying. Other organizations do the reverse, focusing on the soft skills, but failing to invest in teaching staff to solve tough service problems and introduce efficiencies that at the same time heighten customer satisfaction.

7. *Quickness to perceive failure:* Organizations may become disappointed with their results and conclude that the strategy was a bad idea, when really it was a good

idea poorly implemented. This premature conclusion is likely when results are slow in coming or when well-laid plans were poorly implemented. To guard against this, implementation steps need to be evaluated—first to make sure they happened and then to examine their effects.

8. *Leadership fade-out:* Some organizations have what appear to be sound plans but leaders fade out of the picture. Managers must actively lead—not delegate—service improvement efforts, even after an energetic startup and articulation of commitment. They have to get involved, stay involved, and get reinvolved when others' focus or energies appear to be fading.

9. *The problem obsession:* Some leaders are never satisfied and don't stop to celebrate improvements. Instead, they move immediately onto the next problem to be solved. Staff become demoralized, fatigued, and feel unappreciated because they live in an atmosphere of perpetual "never enough." These leaders see the half-empty glass, never the one that's half full.

10. *Heavy-handed top-down approach:* Frequently strategies stall because eventually resistance among staff overwhelms the energy for change. Usually such resistance happens because of inadequate opportunities for staff involvement. The fact is, people don't resist change; they resist being changed.

☐ What to Do with a Stallout

In the event of a stallout, the worst thing to do is ignore it. Doing so wastes every cent and every minute of precious time already invested in the effort. Furthermore, you can expect to see backsliding in the progress made to date. Once a strategy stalls, insiders may resist refreshing it, because in many ways it means starting over, doing what should have been done in the first place. What distinguishes a successful service improvement strategy from an unsuccessful one is not why it came into being in the first place and not what kind of plans you started with and whether these proved to be on target or not. *What distinguishes a successful service improvement strategy from an unsuccessful one is not its past, but its future.*

So how do you figure out which aspects of your approach are working and which are not? How do you plan your next steps? Start with an audit. Look at the data on the indicators you established to monitor service performance, customer satisfaction, and your strategy components themselves. Also consult employees and physicians. They have valuable insights about what's working, what isn't, and what's needed to move forward. The focus group plan described in figure 20-3 is one way to collect this kind of rich, qualitative information.

After you have consulted the service performance and customer data and have used a method such as the focus group described above to collect qualitative information from the people who play a role in implementing your strategy, bring together your planning team to review this information and set directions for the future. Specifically:

- Compare your results so far with your original goals and hopes.
- Consider what you have and have not done to strengthen your service culture by propping up the 10 pillars of continuous improvement. What policies and procedures have you installed to advance service quality? What changes have you made to align existing practices with your service mission?
- Identify and tackle issues related to the leadership and responsibility for your strategy.
- Determine some breakthrough objectives for strategy improvement. A "breakthrough objective" has a strong impact on many other objectives you want to achieve. For example:
  - Improve the timeliness of service hospitalwide; decrease service cycle time

—Improve communication hospitalwide—with patients and physicians

—Bring the maximum possible services *to the patient* (not the patient to the service)

If you tackle such an objective, you will see powerful ripple effects. Everyone in the organization can contribute to it in some ways. If everyone focuses energy on making even small, incremental contributions to one or two breakthrough objectives, it adds up to a breakthrough. After discussing the findings from your strategy assessment, consider using a process like the one described in figure 20-4 to identify one or two breakthrough objectives to guide your follow-through strategy.

Figure 20-3. Taking Your Strategy's Pulse

Set up various focus groups, some with managers, supervisors, frontline employees, and physicians—grouped homogeneously.

1. Welcome and introduction to the focus group's purpose and process. Make these key points:
   - The focus group process is similar to that used by the hospital's marketing department to invite consumer views about quality, service needs, and new programs.
   - "As people know, the organization introduced a service improvement strategy to improve customer satisfaction. This strategy can only work through YOU. That's why we're interested in learning what you think about what we've done so far and what you think needs to be done to make our strategy more effective. We value your opinions and want to know them, so we can make course corrections or continuous improvements in our strategy."
   - "There are no right or wrong answers. And we don't have to reach consensus. We want to know what everyone thinks."
   - Ask permission to tape record or take notes.
   - Promise confidentiality—that people will not be quoted by name in your report.
   - Promise a written summary of what groups tell you and about any strategy plans and actions taken as a result.

2. Pass out paper. Ask people to take five minutes to jot down—in a stream of consciousness way—their perceptions of your strategy so far (descriptive) and their reactions to it (evaluative). "How might you describe our strategy to a knowledgeable person you trust who has nothing to do with our hospital?" Then ask people to share highlights of what they wrote.

3. Find out the extent of people's awareness of the strategy: "What are the main facets of our strategy so far? What have we actually done that you are aware of?"

4. Post a list of components of the strategy that have already been implemented. For each component, ask people if they were aware of it and, if so, what they thought that step did and did not accomplish.

5. Ask people what they think the strategy is really about: "What would you say are the key concepts and changes that this strategy is trying to promote? What do you think we are trying to change here as a result of our strategy?"

6. Ask people about results/effects so far: "In your view, what if any results have you seen from our strategy so far?"

7. Ask people about highlights and strengths: "What comes to mind as highlights of our strategy so far? What have you liked or appreciated?"

8. Ask people about ineffective aspects: "What haven't you liked or appreciated about our strategy so far? What are your complaints? What are your disappointments? What is the number one complaint you hear from other people?"

9. Ask people for suggestions: "Imagine that it's your responsibility to further develop and improve our strategy over the next year. What would you want to do? What do we need to do to strengthen our strategy? What should we *start* doing and what should we *stop* doing?"

10. Invite other perceptions and comments that weren't triggered by any of the above questions.

11. What to do with the results:
    - Summarize them fully on paper and prepare to present them to your Service Quality Council/Steering Committee/Commission/Task Force—the team that will translate them into plans.
    - Communicate a straightforward unsanitized summary of the results of the focus groups to participants, thanking them for participating and reassuring them that their contributions will shape strategy improvements.
    - Communicate an unsanitized summary of the focus group process and findings to ALL employees and physicians, alerting them to the fact that you will be building a new plan based on the findings and inviting their recommendations.

Figure 20-4. Helping a Group Select Breakthrough Objectives

1. Brainstorm everything people want to accomplish in your follow-through plan. Write each idea on its own Post-It™ note in preparation for making an Affinity Chart.

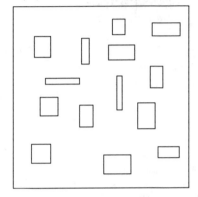

2. Engage the group in making an Affinity Chart, grouping related ideas and identifying "headers."

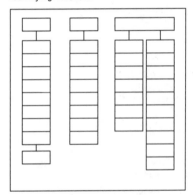

3. Do a "Relationship Diagram" in which you look at each pair of strategy alternatives and ask, "Which, if either, influences the other?" First, arrange all the strategy alternatives in a circle.

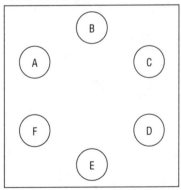

4. Now, looking at two alternatives at a time, decide which influences which and draw arrows indicating the direction of influence if there is one.

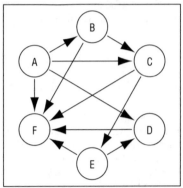

5. Then count up the "drivers" (the alternatives with the most arrows leading out of them to other alternatives). This will tell you which strategy alternatives have a ripple effect on the most other alternatives.

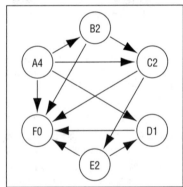

6. Draw conclusions. If one alternative drives several others, and if that alternative is amenable to change, it would be a logical focus for further strategy work. It has the power of a root cause, because positive change within it will in turn affect other change as well. In this example, alternative A drives four others and is a logical focus for follow-through because it has a great impact.

7. Develop a hospital wide plan for tackling the breakthrough objective.

☐ Key Roles in Follow-Through Planning

Unfortunately, no universal formula exists for effective follow-through. As is true with any challenging organizational priority, progress over the long haul takes periodic stock taking, planning, and implementation and then more stock taking, planning, and implementation in an endless cyclical process.

However, one thing is clear: The people involved in advancing your strategy need to be committed and visionary. They also need to fulfill four necessary roles throughout the life of your strategy. Borrowing the four hats of the creative person developed by Roger Von Oech in *A Kick in the Seat of the Pants*,[1] your service improvement team needs to serve as explorers, artists, judges, and warriors in order to press your strategy forward:

- *Be the explorer:* Your team needs to collect information and scrutinize results along the way with an eye to understanding the dynamics that cause success or disappointment. Look for relationships, breakdowns, barriers, dips, and swings. Look to other industries to see how they stay in touch with their customers and meet their needs. Look at how plumbers solve those difficult systems problems. Your follow-through plans will be most appropriate if they are grounded in a knowledge of the territory.
- *Be the artist:* Having gathered all this information and knowing your problems and weaknesses, your team needs to draw into your strategic process creative people who can help you craft solutions that create the textures, colors, and forms to suit your people, culture, and problems. The artist, remember, chips away at the sculpture to create the work of art. Remove the constraints to people's thinking and encourage the freewheeling creativity that just may help your people stride—or even leapfrog—forward.
- *Be the judge:* Your team needs to be discerning and strategic and to courageously acknowledge what works and what does not and choose what will enhance your strategy and its results. Letting problems slip by year after year, letting people who drag down your organization's image do so year after year, adopting strategy ideas that are weak or unjustifiably costly or difficult are actions that reveal an unwillingness to judge and take action for the sake of your vision of service excellence.
- *Be the warrior:* The warrior has stamina. The warrior may be obsessed with the objective and will ramrod through and over obstacles to get to that objective. Your team needs to be the warrior for service excellence. You need to lobby, advocate, and persistently pursue change.

Following through means becoming a "learning organization." Your organization needs to foster ongoing experimentation and learning, tapping into people's intrinsic motivation to learn from their experience and, as a result, do better and better. According to Peter Senge, the learning organization is a place where people continually expand their capacity to create the result they want, where innovative and expansive ways of thinking are encouraged, where collective hopes are liberated, where intelligent failure is rewarded, and where people are continuously learning how to learn together.[2]

☐ Final Thoughts

Eventually, health care organizations will have weathered the storm of conversion to a service-oriented, customer-driven culture. They will exude a strong service orientation that drives their behavior, systems, and decisions. When health care organizations reach this point, service improvement will require ongoing course corrections, but not the exhaustive energy needed to create a customer orientation in the first place. Service improvement will be an everyday management priority, a habit. It will be in every manager's bloodstream and it will be ingrained in every department's way of doing business daily.

However, until that utopia is realized, and to sustain it once it does, you have to do all you can to help your organization achieve the objective of service excellence for the sake of patients and their families and friends and for the sake of employees and physicians whose job satisfaction, spirit, and effectiveness depend so much on the organization's service integrity. It is hoped that this book will spur you and your organization forward.

References

1. Von Oech, R. *A Kick in the Seat of the Pants.* New York City: Perennial Library, Harper & Row, 1986.

2. Senge, P. *The Fifth Discipline: The Art and Practice of the Learning Organization.* New York City: Doubleday, 1991.

Selected Bibliography:
Helpful Resources for Achieving
Service Excellence

Books

Albrecht, K. *At America's Service*. Homewood, IL: Dow Jones Irwin, 1988.

Albrecht, K. *The Only Thing That Matters*. New York City: Harper Business, 1992.

Albrecht, K., and Bradford, L. *The Service Advantage*. Homewood, IL: Dow Jones Irwin, 1990.

Bell, C., and Zemke, R. *Managing Knock Your Socks Off Service*. New York City: AMA-COM, 1992.

The Einstein Consulting Group. *Clip'n'Copy: 101 Camera-Ready Items for Your In-House Newsletter*. Philadelphia: The Einstein Consulting Group, 1989.

Garfield, C. *Second to None*. Homewood, IL: Business One Irwin, 1992.

Leebov, W., and Ersoz, C. J. *The Health Care Manager's Guide to Continuous Quality Improvement*. Chicago: American Hospital Publishing, 1991.

Leebov, W., and Scott, G. *Health Care Managers in Transition: Shifting Roles and Changing Organizations*. San Francisco, CA: Jossey-Bass, 1990.

Peterson, K. *The Strategic Approach to Quality Service in Health Care*. Rockville, MD: Aspen, 1988.

Sewell, C., and Brown, P. *Customers for Life*. New York City: Doubleday, 1990.

Steiber, S., and Krowinski, W. *Measuring and Managing Patient Satisfaction*. Chicago: American Hospital Publishing, 1990.

Whiteley, R. *The Customer-Driven Company*. Reading, MA: Addison-Wesley, 1991.

Zeithaml, V., Parasuraman, A., and Berry, L. *Delivering Quality Service.* London: Free Press, 1990.

Newsletters

The Service Edge, Lakewood Publications, Minneapolis.

Service/Quality Connection; National Society for Patient Representation and Consumer Affairs, American Hospital Association, Chicago.

ADDITIONAL BOOKS OF INTEREST

Measuring and Managing Patient Satisfaction

by Steven R. Steiber and William J. Krowinski

Directed to marketing, planning and quality assurance professionals, the text describes how patient satisfaction fits into the overall management and research strategies of the health care provider, and presents step-by-step strategies for the design and implementation of telephone and mail questionnaires that will provide practical and useful information. Readers will also learn of potential pitfalls in the survey processes, how to design research plans, interview, maximize the rate of return, and record and analyze data. Sampling techniques, how to estimate reliability and validity of the survey items, and how to manage the total survey process are also discussed.

1990. 191 pages, 63 figures, 11 tables, 1 appendix, bibliography, index.
Catalog No. E99-136106 $45.00 (AHA members, $35.00)

Measuring Outcomes in Ambulatory Care

by Dale S. Benson, M.D.

"This book is required reading for any physician executives involved in either the supervision or hands-on management of quality improvement in their organization." *Physician Executive*

Measuring Outcomes presents a practical approach to measuring effectiveness in the episodic environment of ambulatory care. Dr. Benson presents a detailed, step-by-step process for developing effective outcome indicators. Indicators are classified into four categories—disease specific, general health, patient performance, and patient satisfaction. This approach works for all types of ambulatory care in all kinds of settings. Emerging strategies are examined, health status index is defined and explored, and a summary of outcomes management strategies in the 1990s is presented.

1992. 192 pages, 6 appendixes, 31 figures and tables.
Catalog No. E99-169106 $49.95 (AHA members, $39.95)

Total Quality Management: The Health Care Pioneers

by Mara Minerva Melum and Marie Kuchuris Sinioris

"This book is definitely recommended. It deserves to be read cover to cover." *Leadership in Health Services*, the official journal of the Canadian Hospital Association

This book is an executive's guide to the principles of total quality management learned from the experiences and achievements of health care organizations and their pioneering leaders. Almost forty health care innovators contributed case studies or participated in personal interviews. Each case study presents real-world experiences—the successes, the experiments, the "things we'd do differently."

1992. 404 pages, 96 figures, 1 table
Catalog No. E99-169410 $69.00 (AHA members, $55.00)

To order, call TOLL FREE
1-800-AHA-2626